Advances in Proctology and Colorectal Surgery

Advances in Proctology and Colorectal Surgery

Editor

Shmuel Avital

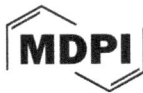

Basel • Beijing • Wuhan • Barcelona • Belgrade • Novi Sad • Cluj • Manchester

Editor
Shmuel Avital
Tel Aviv University
Tel Aviv
Israel

Editorial Office
MDPI
St. Alban-Anlage 66
4052 Basel, Switzerland

This is a reprint of articles from the Special Issue published online in the open access journal *Journal of Clinical Medicine* (ISSN 2077-0383) (available at: https://www.mdpi.com/journal/jcm/special_issues/Proctology_Colorectal_Surgery).

For citation purposes, cite each article independently as indicated on the article page online and as indicated below:

Lastname, A.A.; Lastname, B.B. Article Title. *Journal Name* **Year**, *Volume Number*, Page Range.

ISBN 978-3-0365-8840-7 (Hbk)
ISBN 978-3-0365-8841-4 (PDF)
doi.org/10.3390/books978-3-0365-8841-4

© 2023 by the authors. Articles in this book are Open Access and distributed under the Creative Commons Attribution (CC BY) license. The book as a whole is distributed by MDPI under the terms and conditions of the Creative Commons Attribution-NonCommercial-NoDerivs (CC BY-NC-ND) license.

Contents

Preface vii

Carlos Cerdan-Santacruz, Guilherme Pagin São Julião, Bruna Borba Vailati, Leonardo Corbi, Angelita Habr-Gama and Rodrigo Oliva Perez
Watch and Wait Approach for Rectal Cancer
Reprinted from: *J. Clin. Med.* **2023**, *12*, 2873, doi:10.3390/jcm12082873 1

Yaron Rudnicki, Nir Horesh, Assaf Harbi, Barak Lubianiker, Eraan Green, Guy Raveh, et al.
Rectal Cancer following Local Excision of Rectal Adenomas with Low-Grade Dysplasia—A Multicenter Study
Reprinted from: *J. Clin. Med.* **2023**, *12*, 1032, doi:10.3390/jcm12031032 19

Oscar Hernandez Dominguez, Sumeyye Yilmaz and Scott R. Steele
Stage IV Colorectal Cancer Management and Treatment
Reprinted from: *J. Clin. Med.* **2023**, *12*, 2072, doi:10.3390/jcm12052072 29

Ahmad Mahamid, Omar Abu-Zaydeh, Esther Kazlow, Dvir Froylich, Muneer Sawaied, Natalia Goldberg, et al.
The Effects of Primary Tumor Location on Survival after Liver Resection for Colorectal Liver Metastasis in the Mediterranean Population
Reprinted from: *J. Clin. Med.* **2023**, *12*, 5242, doi:10.3390/jcm12165242 55

Ilan Kent, Amandeep Ghuman, Luna Sadran, Adi Rov, Guy Lifschitz, et al.
Emergency Colectomies in the Elderly Population—Perioperative Mortality Risk-Factors and Long-Term Outcomes
Reprinted from: *J. Clin. Med.* **2023**, *12*, 2465, doi:10.3390/jcm12072465 65

Chun-Yen Hung, Chun-Yu Lin, Ming-Cheng Chen, Teng-Yi Chiu, Tzu-Wei Chiang and Feng-Fan Chiang
Developing a Robotic Surgical Platform Is Beneficial to the Implementation of the ERAS Program for Colorectal Surgery: An Outcome and Learning Curve Analysis
Reprinted from: *J. Clin. Med.* **2023**, *12*, 2661, doi:10.3390/jcm12072661 75

Yaron Rudnicki, Ron Pery, Sherief Shawki, Susanne Warner, Sean Patrick Cleary and Kevin T. Behm
A Synchronous Robotic Resection of Colorectal Cancer and Liver Metastases—Our Initial Experience
Reprinted from: *J. Clin. Med.* **2023**, *12*, 3255, doi:10.3390/jcm12093255 85

Zoe Garoufalia and Steven D. Wexner
Indocyanine Green Fluorescence Guided Surgery in Colorectal Surgery
Reprinted from: *J. Clin. Med.* **2023**, *12*, 494, doi:10.3390/jcm12020494 95

Martin Reichert, Lukas Eckerth, Moritz Fritzenwanker, Can Imirzalioglu, Anca-Laura Amati, Ingolf Askevold, et al.
New Perianal Sepsis Risk Score Predicts Outcome of Elderly Patients with Perianal Abscesses
Reprinted from: *J. Clin. Med.* **2023**, *12*, 5219, doi:10.3390/jcm12165219 111

Inese Fišere, Valērija Groma, Šimons Svirskis, Estere Strautmane and Andris Gardovskis
Evaluation of Clinical Manifestations of Hemorrhoidal Disease, Carried Out Surgeries and Prolapsed Anorectal Tissues: Associations with ABO Blood Groups of Patients
Reprinted from: *J. Clin. Med.* **2023**, *12*, 5119, doi:10.3390/jcm12155119 125

Paola Campennì, Angelo Alessandro Marra, Veronica De Simone, Francesco Litta, Angelo Parello and Carlo Ratto
Tunneling of Mesh during Ventral Rectopexy: Technical Aspects and Long-Term Functional Results
Reprinted from: *J. Clin. Med.* **2023**, *12*, 294, doi:10.3390/jcm12010294 . . . . **145**

Paola Campennì, Roberto Iezzi, Angelo Alessandro Marra, Alessandro Posa, Angelo Parello, Francesco Litta, et al.
The Emborrhoid Technique for Treatment of Bleeding Hemorrhoids in Patients with High Surgical Risk
Reprinted from: *J. Clin. Med.* **2022**, *11*, 5533, doi:10.3390/jcm11195533 . . . . **157**

Affifa Farrukh and John Francis Mayberry
Surgery for Ulcerative Colitis in the White British and South Asian Populations in Selected Trusts in England 2001–2020: An Absence of Disparate Care and a Need for Specialist Centres
Reprinted from: *J. Clin. Med.* **2022**, *11*, 4967, doi:10.3390/jcm11174967 . . . . **167**

Preface

Dear Readers,

I am very pleased with our recently published Special Issue entitled "Advances in Proctology and Colorectal Surgery".

In recent years, we have seen major changes in the treatment and surgical approach to colorectal pathologies. These changes were driven by technological developments, changes in concepts regarding treatment options, and the movement towards personalized treatment.

In this Special Issue, we tried to cover some of these ongoing changes in treatment concepts, the use of advanced technologies, as well as the specific outcomes for different patients.

Ten original articles were included in this Special Issue dealing with colorectal cancer patients' outcomes, the use of the robotic platform in colorectal surgery, and different aspects of treating and evaluation ano-rectal pathologies.

This Special Issue included, as well, three comprehensive review papers written by world-leading surgical groups. Dr Steven Wexner covered the use of Indocyanine Green Fluorescence in colorectal surgery, Dr Scott Steele's group reviewed different algorithms used to treat patients with metastatic colorectal disease, and Dr Rodrigo Oliva Perez together with Dr Angelita Habr-Gamaas and their group shared their experience with the "Watch and Wait" approach for rectal cancer.

I am sure that this Special Issue will aid surgeons focusing on treating colorectal pathologies.

Lastly, I want to thank Miss Shirley Chen from the JCM Editorial Office who assisted me along this journey. Last and not least, I want to thank Miss Elektra McDermott who helped me recruit some of the researchers that agreed to publish in our Special Issue.

Shmuel Avital
Editor

Review

Watch and Wait Approach for Rectal Cancer

Carlos Cerdan-Santacruz [1,2], Guilherme Pagin São Julião [3,4,5], Bruna Borba Vailati [3,4,5], Leonardo Corbi [3,4,5], Angelita Habr-Gama [3,4,5] and Rodrigo Oliva Perez [3,4,5,*]

1. Department of Coloproctology, Hospital Universitario de la Princesa, 28006 Madrid, Spain
2. Department of Coloproctology, Clínica Santa Elena, 28003 Madrid, Spain
3. Angelita and Joaquim Gama Institute, São Paulo 01329-020, Brazil; brunabvailati@gmail.com (B.B.V.); leonardo.corbi@hotmail.com (L.C.); gamange@uol.com.br (A.H.-G.)
4. Department of Coloproctology, Hospital Alemão Oswaldo Cruz, São Paulo 01323-020, Brazil
5. Department of Surgical Oncology, Hospital Beneficencia Portuguesa, São Paulo 01323-001, Brazil
* Correspondence: rodrigo.operez@gmail.com

Abstract: The administration of neoadjuvant chemoradiotherapy (nCRT) followed by total mesorrectal excision (TME) and selective use of adjuvant chemotherapy can still be considered the standard of care in locally advanced rectal cancer (LARC). However, avoiding sequelae of TME and entering a narrow follow-up program of watch and wait (W&W), in select cases that achieve a comparable clinical complete response (cCR) to nCRT, is now very attractive to both patients and clinicians. Many advances based on well-designed studies and long-term data coming from big multicenter cohorts have drawn some important conclusions and warnings regarding this strategy. In order to safely implement W&W, it is important consider proper selection of cases, best treatment options, surveillance strategy and the attitudes towards near complete responses or even tumor regrowth. The present review offers a comprehensive overview of W&W strategy from its origins to the most current literature, from a practical point of view focused on daily clinical practice, without losing sight of the most important future prospects in this area.

Keywords: rectal cancer; clinical complete response; watch and wait; organ preservation; total neoadjuvant therapy; immunotherapy; local recurrence; local tumor regrowth; near-complete response

1. Introduction

Management of rectal cancer has considerably changed over the last few decades [1]. While radical surgical resection with total mesorectal excision (TME) remains as one of the pillars of treatment, introduction of multimodality therapy with radiation and chemotherapy was fundamental for the development and proposal of organ-preservation strategies [2]. Initially used to improve local disease control, radiation alone or chemoradiation used in the preoperative (neoadjuvant) period was shown to be more effective than postoperative (adjuvant) treatment [3]. In addition to improvements in local disease control, preoperative treatment resulted in variable degrees of primary tumor response [4]. Observation of complete disappearance of the primary tumor (clinical complete response—cCR) led surgeons to consider avoiding immediate resection in select patients [5]. Since the initial reported outcomes of this non-operative treatment for patients who achieved a cCR, many changes have developed in terms of baseline assessment, neoadjuvant treatment regimens, assessment studies and timing of assessment. In addition, as long-term data become available, there is more information available regarding the risk of local regrowth of tumors which achieved a cCR and also regarding the risk of subsequent distant metastases development [6]. Finally, molecular markers have been able to distinguish a specific subtype of rectal cancer where a distinct treatment alternative may lead to an opportunity for organ-preservation in a significant proportion of cases [7].

2. Rationale

The reason why non-operative treatment of rectal cancer is attractive is related to the fact that TME surgery is associated with significant morbidity, mortality and functional consequences [8,9]. Significant disturbances associated with urinary and sexual function have been reported [10,11]. However, most relevant are the consequences associated with bowel function after surgery [12]. Depending on the level of the tumor in the rectum, level of the anastomosis and the requirement for partial or total intersphincteric resection, patients may experience variable levels of symptoms associated with Low Anterior Resection syndrome [13–15]. Finally, the requirement of a temporary or definitive stoma may be very critical to many of these patients and avoiding it remains an important, if not the most important, patients' expectation from rectal cancer treatment. Here, it should be considered that many patients who undergo primary anastomosis for rectal cancer with a temporary stoma may ultimately develop a failed anastomosis. Reasons for a failed anastomosis may include leaks, stenosis, recurrence and poor function. Therefore, a number of patients thought to have received a temporary stoma are ultimately faced with a definitive stoma. Over time, the rate of definitive stomas may be nearly triple initial estimates [16,17].

Non-operative treatment obviates many of these issues by avoidance of TME and therefore exposing patients to virtually no morbidity or mortality. However, caution should be taken as a proportion of patients entering a watch and wait (W&W) protocol will go on to develop a local regrowth of the primary tumor and therefore will require surgical resection [18,19]. This means not all patients with a cCR will avoid surgery. Second, even though functional outcomes among patients undergoing W&W are clearly and far better than TME or even local excision [20], function may ultimately not be as perfect as one would expect or hope [21]. Interesting data suggest that functional outcomes of patients undergoing W&W are not necessarily perfect, possibly due to the effects of radiation therapy to the rectum and anal sphincters [22]. The few studies that compared bowel function and quality of life between patients undergoing W&W and TME surgery were performed in at least 2 retrospective series. Both of them compared patients undergoing W&W to matched–controls among patients with incomplete clinical/pathological response followed by TME [20,21]. The results of these studies using different assessment tools were similar, suggesting superior functional and QoL outcomes for the W&W patients. However, one of the studies suggested that nearly one-third of patients within the W&W group reported severe LARS scores, suggesting potential long-term detrimental effects of RT to bowel function [20]. Altogether, these findings should be interpreted with caution. In addition to the limitations inherent to the studies' designs, one must consider that severe/poor LARS scores have also been reported by healthy individuals [23]. Finally, the comparison of W&W to TME patients may have compared apples to oranges. Ultimately, patients undergoing TME for residual disease would otherwise have never been candidates for W&W. This suggests that the control group may have been inappropriate for such comparison, with introduction of significant potential selection biases related to tumor response [24]. These issues should be taken into account when counseling patients for organ-preservation with W&W.

3. Baseline Features & Selection Criteria

3.1. Primary Reason for Neoadjuvant Therapy

Assessment of baseline features is critical for the selection of patients who are candidates for W&W. The initial experience of patients undergoing this strategy was accumulated before the availability of accurate staging tools [2,5]. Magnetic resonance imaging (MRI) was largely unavailable and not standardized. At that time, most patients with rectal cancer were considered for W&W based on response to therapy. This means that selection of patients was based on the final result rather than an intended outcome. Ultimately, patients were undergoing neoadjuvant chemoradiation for oncological purposes—to improve local disease control—and, by accident or chance, achieved a cCR. This was perhaps the only selection criterion at that time.

Progressively, staging modalities evolved over time and MRI interpretation became standardized, allowing for the stratification of patients and tumors based on risk factors for local and distant failure [25,26]. This led to a clearer distinction between patients with high-risk features—requiring nCRT for oncological purposes—and those with low-risk features—where perhaps the only benefit of nCRT would be the achievement of a cCR in an attempt to avoid TME surgery [27,28]. Even though these two scenarios have been referred to as an "accidental" versus an "intentional" organ-preservation approach, one could argue that W&W is never truly "intentional" as guaranteed achievement of cCR is not yet possible. Instead, the difference between the 2 scenarios is that the latter relates to the concept that the sole reason or sole benefit for the use of neoadjuvant therapy is achievement of cCR.

3.2. Baseline Features

In addition to the primary reason for the use of nCRT among these patients, assessment of baseline features is relevant for some additional reasons:

First, as findings consistent with cCR are largely subjective, it is highly recommended that comparable methods are used both at baseline and at the time of reassessment [29]. In this setting, detailed characterization of clinical, endoscopic and radiological features at baseline may be critical for the assessment of post-treatment response and identification of cCR or incomplete response [30].

Second, response to therapy seems to be a time-dependent phenomenon and not all patients achieve a cCR at the same time [31,32]. There are data to suggest that larger tumors take longer to respond. In this setting, it becomes relevant to understand the magnitude of response at each reassessment round. This is only possible when reassessment findings are comparable to baseline features. Ultimately, despite being largely subjective, quantification of response is an important piece of information. This is only possible when baseline assessment provides detailed information using the same tools expected to be used in reassessment rounds [33].

Finally, an important feature relates to the position of these tumors in the rectum. Since the beginning, the original description of W&W was restricted for tumors accessible to the finger during digital rectal examination (DRE), usually at an average of 7 cm from the anal verge, measured by rigid proctoscopy [5]. The reasons for these selection criteria relate to the risk-benefit balance. Tumors above/beyond the reach of the finger are probably best treated by TME surgery with far fewer functional consequences, less morbidity and lower risk of definitive stomas. Instead, distal tumors are at considerably higher risk for these negative functional outcomes and stoma requirements [34]. In the setting of risk of local regrowth and subsequent distant metastases, the authors believe that tumors located above this 7 cm distance are more likely to have risks that outweigh benefits of avoiding TME.

As MRI became widely available, in addition to being within the reach of DRE, tumors should be ideally located at the level of or below the insertion of the levator muscles in the pelvis. Tumors with the distal border located 1 cm above/beyond this anatomical landmark are in most cases best suited for TME with or without nCRT, indicated for oncological reasons [34] (Figure 1).

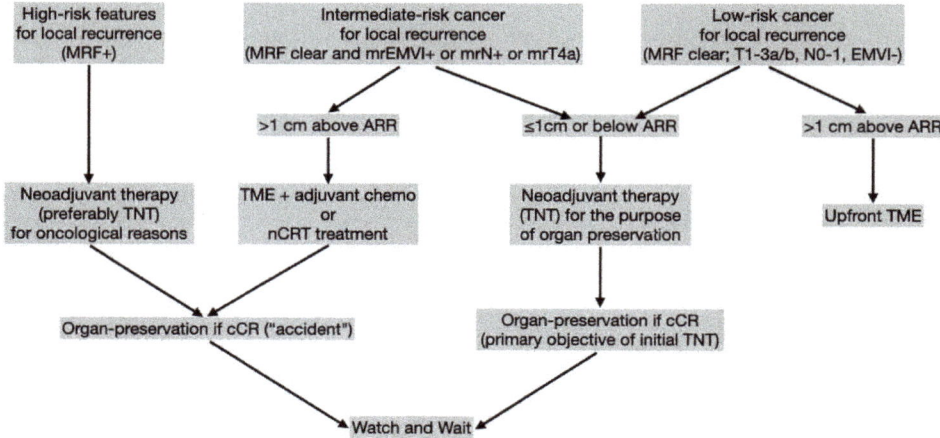

Figure 1. Algorithm for decision management based on risk factors for local recurrence and primary objective to achieve a cCR. ARR: anorectal ring; MRF: mesorectal fascia; mr: magnetic resonance; EMVI: extramural venous invasion; TNT: total neoadjuvant therapy; cCR: clinical complete response; TME: total mesorectal excision. While patients may undergo neoadjuvant therapy for different reasons, decision to W&W is based on the achievement of a cCR. Patients not achieving a cCR are usually recommended for surgical resection (most frequently TME).

3.3. Putting It All Together

Ultimately, baseline assessment is critical for the selection of patients that are being considered for W&W. The following necessary steps may be required before organ-preservation is even a consideration for these patients:

First, clinical (DRE) and endoscopic assessments should provide clear evidence of invasive cancer rather than benign polyps or lateral spreading tumors amenable to endoscopic/endoluminal resections [35]. The finding of mobile and soft lesions at DRE combined with clear endoscopic pit pattern classification may provide precise identification of patients that are candidates for endoscopic/endoluminal resection instead of neoadjuvant therapeutic approaches.

Second, once clinical and endoscopic findings of invasive cancer are present—beyond the scope of endoscopic/endoluminal resection—obtainment of endoscopic biopsies is mandatory. In addition to confirmation of adenocarcinoma histology, tumors are currently expected to be routinely tested for microsatellite instability, preferably through immunohistochemistry, for the presence/absence of the most frequently affected mismatch repair protein/genes [7,36].

Third, magnetic resonance is mandatory for proper staging of these patients and stratification into low-/high-risk categories. While several 2- and 3-tiered categories are available, our approach has been to clearly distinguish patients at high-risk for local recurrence based on mesorectal fascia (MRF) status (threatened when tumors are ≤1mm from the MRF) [28,37]. While tumors with extramural venous invasion (EMVI), lymph node metastases, tumor deposits and T4a may also be considered as high-risk; it is, as of yet, unclear whether these features are independently associated with the risk of local recurrence when there are unthreatened margins [28]. Therefore, MRF+ or positive circumferencial resection margin (CRM+) are patients where neoadjuvant therapy is clearly necessary and organ-preservation may be an additional benefit from this approach (in addition to improved local disease control in the event TME is required). The presence of any high-risk feature does not necessarily exclude the possibility of W&W once a cCR is achieved. This includes the presence of adverse pathological features such as high-grade adenocarcinoma or mucinous tumors (both in pathology and MRI imaging) frequently seen in baseline assessment. However, there is one exception to this rule: the presence of adverse features beyond the limits of the radiation field are clearly an exclusion criterion. The presence of nodal metastases, EMVI or tumor deposits above the cranial limit used for the radiation field should prompt post-treatment surgical resection in most patients, despite complete primary tumor response.

Finally, tumor location and distance from anal verge (by DRE and proctoscopy) and from the insertion of the levator ani (by MRI) are very relevant information to be taken into account to consider patients for W&W in the event of the achievement of a cCR [34] (Figure 1).

4. Preferred Treatment Strategy

Once patients have been properly assessed at baseline, one should be able to distinguish patients that are undergoing neoadjuvant therapy for sole purpose of achieving a cCR (distal and low-risk) from those that need therapy due to the high-risk of local recurrence (distal and threatened MRF) [28,37]. In both situations, maximal response is required to achieve a cCR and/or R0 resection (if surgery is ultimately required).

Maximal primary tumor response has been investigated in multiple studies, mostly by complete pathological response (pCR) as a surrogate for cCR [38,39].

Originally, the earliest experiences with cCR and W&W were derived from series using neoadjuvant chemoradiation (nCRT) with long-course radiation (RT) and concomitant 5FU-based chemotherapy [5]. While oxaliplatin has been associated with slightly higher pCR rates when used in combination with 5FU during RT, the significantly higher toxicity rates have limited its use in clinical practice [40,41]. As mentioned previously, response to treatment in rectal cancer after nCRT is a time-dependent phenomenon. In this setting, many systematic reviews and meta-analyses suggested that longer interval periods between the end of radiation and surgical resection were associated with higher rates of pCR [42,43]. This led to the consideration of the use of short-course RT followed by prolonged intervals (instead of the classic 1-week interval to TME) as an alternative to achieve similar rates of pCR as compared to standard nCRT using long-course RT [44]. While this did result in higher pCR rates, experience with cCR and W&W was largely unavailable using this particular regimen.

The concept of using longer intervals and additional chemotherapy during the resting period was investigated and did result in significantly higher rates of pCR and cCR rates in patients with rectal cancer [45]. The additional cycles of chemotherapy delivered between RT completion and assessment of tumor response were labelled as consolidation chemotherapy and were originally designed to improve primary tumor response [45]. Compared to standard nCRT regimens achieving pCR and cCR rates of nearly 15–30%, nCRT with consolidation chemotherapy initially reported pCR and cCR rates in the range of 30–50% [46–48].

Shortly thereafter, the concept of using systemic chemotherapy preoperatively was expanded to address the possibility of treating micrometastasic disease upfront (in addition to improving primary tumor response) and potentially improving survival of patients [49]. This concept, named as total neoadjuvant therapy, incorporated systemic chemotherapy being delivered immediately before (induction) or after (consolidation) chemoradiation in an attempt to improve survival and primary tumor response [50]. Elegantly-designed randomized clinical trials clearly demonstrated that TNT regimens resulted in higher chances of achieving a pCR when compared to patients undergoing standard nCRT regimens [51].

However, when TNT regimens were compared between them, consolidation chemotherapy regimens (in the setting of long-course RT) were more likely to result in pCR or even cCR when compared to induction regimens (also in the setting of long-course RT) [52,53].

There is still a question as to whether short-course or long-course RT TNT regimens are better in achieving a cCR and leading to organ-preservation. No RCT using short-course RT used cCR as a primary endpoint for that purpose and there are ongoing trials comparing these 2 regimens head-to-head in the setting of consolidation chemotherapy

(ACO/ARO/AIO-18.1 Trial; NCT04246684). Short-course RT would have the potential benefit of shorter treatment time (convenient for patients and allows more rational use of resources to deal with the considerable number of patients in need of treatment) [54]. However, little is known about the denominators of patients treated by short-course RT and consolidation chemotherapy that achieve a cCR and successfully undergo organ-preservation [55,56]. This contrasts with the recent estimates of nearly 50–60% of patients with locally advanced disease who avoid surgery in the setting of long-course RT and consolidation chemotherapy [53].

One important drawback of this treatment strategy using short-course RT has been recently reported in the setting of an RCT. Even though patients treated in the experimental arm had similar baseline staging features, underwent similar R0 resections and achieved a pCR 2× more frequently than the standard nCRT used in the control arm [55], local recurrence was significantly worse in the experimental arm [57]. One could argue that when using this approach to achieve a cCR, patients that eventually do not achieve a cCR may face higher chances of developing local recurrence even in the setting of an R0 resection.

All these studies have been performed for a population of patients with locally advanced rectal cancer—implying the oncological need for neoadjuvant therapy. However, studies have also reported on the outcomes of TNT regimens for cT2N0 disease. Apparently, patients with cT2N0 receiving TNT with long-course RT and consolidation chemotherapy have a significantly higher chance of achieving a cCR and avoiding TME [58].

More recently, nCRT regimens incorporating RT dose escalation techniques using contact radiation/brachytherapy (CxB) have been compared to standard nCRT in randomized trials using organ-preservation as their primary endpoint. Even though patients with cCR were grouped together with those achieving near-complete clinical response, organ-preservation rates were significantly higher in the experimental arm using CxB. While the ≥80% organ-preservation rate within the experimental arm in this study is quite remarkable, lack of widespread availability of the required CxB machine and expertise may considerably limit its implementation in clinical practice [59].

5. Assessment of Tumor Response

5.1. Assessment Tools

Assessment of tumor response to nCRT/TNT should be performed using the same assessment tools used at baseline assessment. Initial experiences with W&W were mainly derived from experience with clinical and endoscopic assessment tools, as radiological tools as we have available today were largely unavailable at that time [2,5].

5.2. Three-Pillar Assessment Criteria

Clinical assessment using DRE remains of critical relevance here. Findings consistent with a cCR include a smooth surface of the rectal wall at the area harboring the initial tumor and minimal induration of the rectal wall. There should be no ulceration, palpable mass or stenosis of the rectum [29]. It is the authors' experience that, sometimes, subtle irregularities are best felt by DRE than seen on endoscopy or radiological imaging modalities. We strongly advise surgeons who assessed the primary cancer at baseline to perform reassessment for tumor response to provide best possible comparison. Clearly, it should be stressed that tumors beyond the reach of the finger during DRE should perhaps be considered suboptimal candidates for W&W.

Endoscopic assessment is the second pillar in reassessment of response to nCRT/TNT. Usually, flexible endoscopy is currently preferred in order to (1) provide documentation of the endoscopic appearance of the residual scar/tumor; (2) to allow advanced imaging techniques such as narrow band imaging and (3) to allow retroflexive view of the anal canal (commonly performed using the gastroscope rather than the colonoscope) and fully appreciate tumors close to anal canal and dentate line. Endoscopic findings consistent with a cCR include a white scar, no ulceration of the rectal wall or no irregularities of the mucosa. There should be no stenosis of the rectum allowing for a smooth progression of the colonoscope through the area harboring the primary tumor. While teleangiectasias are often detected within the area of the original tumor, irregular redness of the mucosa should be perceived as suspicious and preferably disappear in subsequent reassessments if this is the only positive finding during endoscopic assessment [29] (Figure 2).

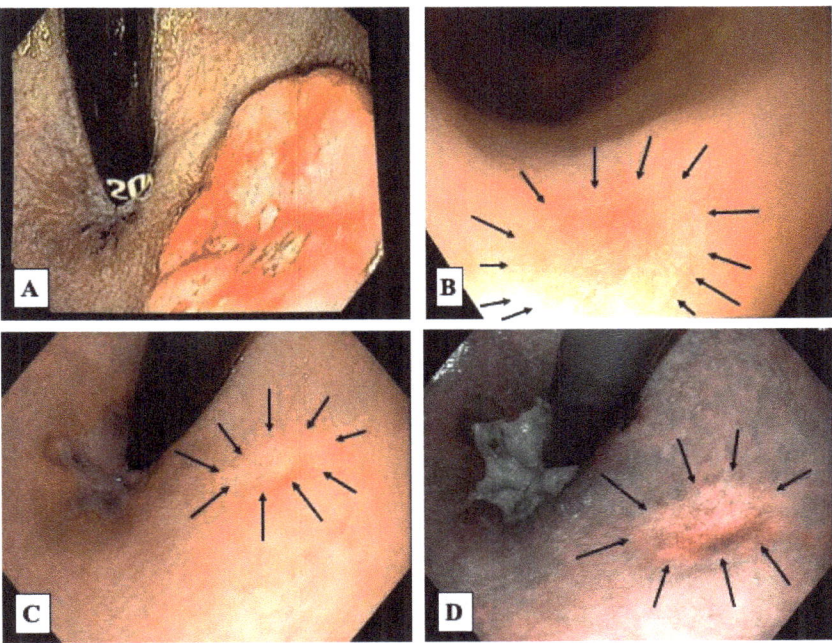

Figure 2. Endoscopic view of a baseline tumor (**A**) and post-treatment findings consistent with a cCR using direct view (**B**), retroflexive view (**C**) and narrow-band imaging (**D**). Throughout images (**B**–**D**), one can appreciate the presence of a white scar and significant telangiectasia (arrows). There are no ulcers or stenosis of the rectum.

The third pillar in reassessment is radiological imaging of the rectum, mesorectum and lateral pelvic compartment. Originally, imaging following neoadjuvant treatment was directed to assess almost exclusively the mesorectal and lateral pelvic compartment in the search for the presence of residual disease within lymph node, vascular structures (extramural vascular invasion—EMVI) and/or tumor deposits (replacement by tumor tissue within lymph nodes, blood and lymphatic vessels or nerves). However, as imaging techniques and interpretation have improved over the years, radiology can provide accurate information regarding the rectal wall itself. T2-weighted sequences often suffice for assessment of response without the need for intravenous contrast [60]. A proposed classification system has been commonly used to grade response (similarly to the pathological grading system; MRI Tumor regression grade - TRG) according to the presence of low-signal intensity areas. mrTRG1-2 are usually associated with complete or near-complete tumor response (suggesting a significant replacement by fibrotic tissue) in contrast with mrTRG3-5 [61]. Low-signal intensity areas may be regular or irregular and comparison with baseline imaging features may be helpful in assessment of response. While there is still controversy surrounding the usefulness of diffusion-weighted sequences [30,62–64], areas of restriction during this sequence may provide functional information and indicate the presence of residual cancer, adding to interpretation of T2-weighted sequences [65] (Figure 3).

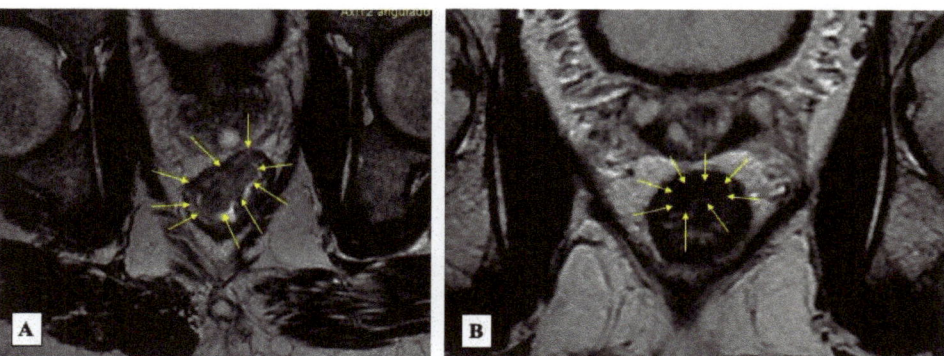

Figure 3. Radiological assessment using MR showing the baseline tumor (**A**—arrows) and an area of low-signal intensity areas consistent with a complete response in T2-weighted images (**B**—arrows).

PET–CT has been used for the purpose of tumor response assessment in several studies and may be useful for the identification of appropriate candidates for W&W in this setting [66–68]. However, as mentioned previously, reassessment by PET–CT preferably requires a baseline assessment using PET–CT. Considering the limitations in image resolution within this study (inferior to the high-resolution MRI images), considerable costs and the requirement of radiation associated with PET–CT (contrasting with MRI), the radiological study of choice has been high-resolution MRI in most cases.

Endoscopic biopsies are not included as one of the pillars for the diagnosis of a cCR. This means a negative endoscopic biopsy is not required to select patients for a W&W strategy if a cCR has otherwise been achieved [69]. This must be approached carefully, as surgeons often consider that an endoscopic biopsy is useless for the assessment of response. This is clearly not the case and often endoscopic biopsies may aid in the decision process in individual situations. In general, a negative endoscopic biopsy should not be considered as diagnostic for a complete response if there is INCOMPLETE clinical response. This is due to the low negative predictive value of this diagnostic tool in this setting (nearly only 20%). However, a positive endoscopic biopsy may be informative and useful in such patients with very significant yet incomplete responses ("near-complete" responses).

5.3. Timing

5.3.1. First Assessment

Tumor response is a time-dependent phenomenon. Still, it appears that response is not linear over time and majority of response is usually observed early on either during or immediately after completion of radiation [31]. This means that patients who achieve a cCR will exhibit the majority of tumor regression early on during or after treatment [32,70]. Tumors with poor response after completion or 6 weeks from RT completion are unlikely to present major further response after such period [31]. In this setting, we recommend a first assessment of response between 6–8 weeks to attest significant response taking place early on as a sign of promising outcomes in achieving a cCR and successful W&W [34]. Because local regrowth is a risk among these patients, an early initial assessment of response may be quite useful. Many of these patients may actually present with excellent response at this very first assessment round and subsequently develop a local regrowth (which remains very small on the 2nd reassessment round). The fact that a first reassessment has been performed may allow for the correct identification of a local regrowth [34]. Had a first early assessment of response not been performed, this small early regrowth could have been mistaken for a near-complete ongoing response leading to further delay in diagnosis and subsequent definitive treatment of the regrowth.

5.3.2. Reassessment Rounds

Even though the majority of response is observed within early time intervals from RT completion, it may actually take longer intervals for tumors to achieve all strict criteria for a cCR. One retrospective study indicated that the majority of cCR were only achieved after 16 weeks from RT completion in patients receiving CRT and consolidation chemotherapy [33]. Therefore, one has to consider that many of these patients will present with significant yet incomplete clinical responses in one or more of the reassessment rounds. It has been suggested that whenever patients achieved a near-complete clinical response, subsequent reassessment could lead to achievement of cCR in a rather high proportion of patients [33]. However, the "near-complete" response is a poorly-defined clinical entity with very little consensus in its definition [71]. Instead of labelling patients to harbor "near-complete" clinical response, the readership may perhaps consider the presence of the following features in deciding for subsequent reassessment of response rounds prior to definitive surgical resection of the primary:

First, tumors should have exhibited significant response in their very first assessment round. Comparison with baseline assessment information may be helpful in identifying patients who truly exhibit very significant responses (nearly 75–80% of the tumor volume is gone by endoscopic assessment and only a minor irregularity is detected) [32]. One should be careful, as small tumors that remain small may be less responsive when compared to large baseline tumors that nearly disappear. DRE should be questionable and only minor irregularities should be accepted. Radiology should be identifying patients with mrTRG1-2 only [61].

Second, there should be ongoing response in between rounds, meaning that there is no stable incomplete clinical response. Instead, clear subsequent regression needs to be clearly documented with any of the assessment studies [33].

Third, endoluminal response seems to be the driver of response. This means that endoscopy and DRE showing complete disappearance of the tumor should be considered more significant than radiological disappearance of the disease. In other words, if there is no evidence of cancer during DRE and endoscopy, even if there is suspicious residual cancer on MRI, we believe a subsequent reassessment may be harmless and offer the opportunity for achievement of all criteria of cCR (including radiological). However, patients with mrTRG1 and the presence of ulceration with elevated borders and highly suspicious areas palpable during DRE should probably undergo resection of the primary disease.

Finally, most cCR are usually achieved within 6 months from RT completion [33]. If incomplete response is still obvious after 24–26 weeks from RT completion, surgical resection of the primary is perhaps preferred [72].

6. Local Regrowth
6.1. Definition and Salvage

Local regrowth is, by definition, the reappearance of the primary tumors within the rectal wall, the mesorectum or within the lateral pelvic compartment after the achievement of a cCR [73]. It seems that nearly 25–30% of patients who achieve a cCR and are managed non-operatively will eventually develop a local regrowth [74]. This risk is highest within the 3 years immediately after the achievement of a cCR [6,18,19,74] (Figure 4).

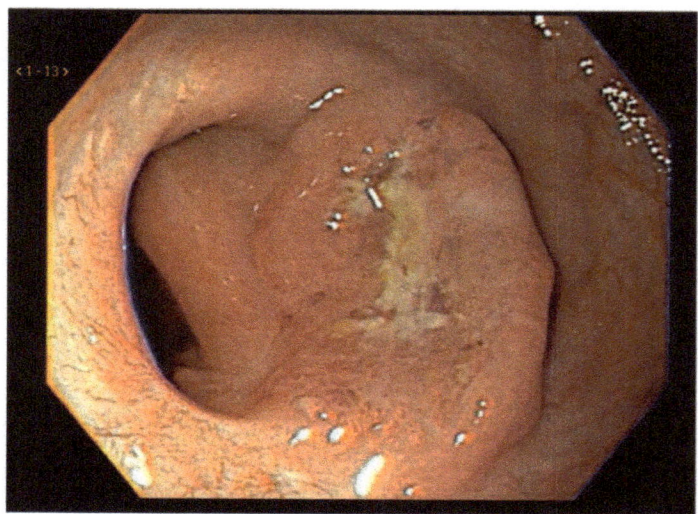

Figure 4. Endoscopic view of a local regrowth following the achievement of a cCR.

The term regrowth instead of recurrence was originally proposed to distinguish this clinical entity from local recurrences after TME surgery. The idea was to attempt to avoid the stigma associated with local recurrences following TME frequently associated with poor outcomes, often unresectable and frequently associated with debilitating condition [73]. Instead, local regrowth is, in the majority of the cases amenable to salvage resection, possible through an R0 resection in nearly 90% of the cases [75–78]. In fact, surgical salvage of local regrowth provides excellent local disease control with subsequent re-recurrence in ≤5% of the cases. A significant proportion of patients requiring salvage TME at the time of local regrowth ultimately require an abdominal perineal resection (APR) [79]. In fact, the rates of APR among regrowth seem to be higher than in patients proceeding straight to TME after treatment completion and incomplete clinical response [78]. These differences may be due to distinct features between patients being offered W&W versus those undergoing TME related to tumor location. Since ideal candidates for W&W are those with tumors located at the reach of the finger during DRE and located at the level of or below the insertion of the levator ani muscles, it is not surprising that local regrowth at this level would frequently require APR [80].

Still, a proportion of these patients may also be salvaged by a second opportunity for organ-preservation: transanal local excision of the regrowth. This has been recently reported in two independent series. Curiously, disease-free survival among local regrowth salvaged by local excision was better than patients undergoing TME for salvage. However, locally-excised regrowth was more likely to have early-stage disease at baseline. Therefore, such differences in survival may possibly be reflecting intrinsic differences in baseline stages rather than the actual type of salvage employed at the time of regrowth [81,82].

6.2. Risk Factors

Risk factors for development of local regrowth after the achievement of a cCR appear to be related exclusively to baseline T stage [83]. Apparently, there seems to be a 10% increase in the risk of local regrowth for every increase in T stage category: 20% for cT2, 30% for cT3 and 40% for cT4 [18]. Curiously, baseline N stage has not been associated with the risk of a local regrowth in these patients [84]. Interestingly, when patients sustain a cCR longer than 3 years, the risk of local recurrence becomes minimal. In addition, risk factors such as baseline T stage become irrelevant. This suggests that the main driver in the risk of local regrowth is primary response to treatment, overriding risk factors associated with baseline features or even treatment-related [85].

7. Distant Metastases

The risk of distant metastases among patients who achieve a cCR after treatment is considerably low [74]. In fact, an early report suggested that this risk was considerably higher among patients who developed local regrowth compared to those who did not [86]. In fact, subsequent studies examining larger datasets of patients with cCR looked for risk factors for development of distant metastases after entering a W&W program. Curiously, the only identifiable risk factor for development of distant metastases in this series was previous development of local regrowth [75,87]. However, one has to consider that these patients are biologically intrinsically different: cCR who never develop local regrowth are true complete responders; whereas local regrowth are necessarily incomplete responders that were mistaken for a cCR [88]. Therefore, it is not surprising that they have distinct risks for development of distant metastases.

However, the risk of distant metastases after cCR becomes very low after completion of 5 years of follow-up from the baseline cancer. Instead, local regrowth sustains a considerable risk for distant metastases until they complete 5 years, not from the baseline cancer but from the local regrowth [85,87]. This suggests that leaving the incomplete response in situ for variable periods of time may increase the risk of distant metastases already provided by the baseline cancer.

In order to address this question, patients with local regrowth managed by salvage resection at the time of local regrowth have been compared to incomplete responses managed by straight surgery after completion of treatment. There were no differences in survival both in retrospective and prospective series [53,79]. Still, such comparison may also not be fair since local regrowth had excellent initial response to treatment (it was even mistaken for a cCR). The control group (TME straight after treatment) did not necessarily have excellent response. Therefore, one could argue that local regrowth that was salvaged should have had better survival outcomes than all TMEs.

In this setting, an even more recent study compared the outcomes of salvage surgery for local regrowth to the outcomes of TME straight after treatment in the setting of excellent tumor response (to balance for response to treatment across groups). In this study, two independent risk factors were identified: local regrowth and ypT3-4 in the resected specimen. Combination of both features—local regrowth and ypT3-4—in the resected specimen led to significantly worse distant-metastases-free survival. This suggests that patients who have excellent (but incomplete) response managed by TME straight after treatment respond better than those undergoing salvage TME at the time of local regrowth. (Dis Colon & Rectum—accepted for publication—in press).

While this is restricted to a very small proportion of patients who achieve a cCR, patients need to be fully aware of the risks associated with W&W in this setting.

8. Surveillance Strategy

Considering the risk of local regrowth is most frequent within 3 years of follow-up after the achievement of a cCR, and the risk of subsequent distant metastases among this subgroup of patients, surveillance has been adapted to attempt to minimize these risks [85].

First, surveillance is more intensive during the first 3 years of follow-up. Usually, these patients are assessed for their primary tumors every 8 weeks. Second, surveillance is recommended for life even though the risk of regrowth becomes very low after 3 years being disease-free. Third, we want to avoid the risk of detecting a local regrowth harboring ypT3-4 disease within the resected specimen. Taking all this information into account, patients should preferably undergo a DRE, proctoscopy, CEA levels and MRI every 8–12 weeks during the first 3 years. After these 3 years, follow-up may perhaps be loosened to every 6 months and to include primary tumor response assessment [54]. Metastatic disease surveillance should follow the usual guidelines [89] and should only be intensified in the case of (1) a local regrowth and/or (2) clinical suspicion. After the 5th year, patients can follow-up yearly.

Ultimately, this surveillance program results in frequent visits required for clinical, endoscopic and radiological assessment particularly during the first 3 years of follow-up. Patients should be clearly and fully informed upfront of this recommended follow-up and understand the potential clinical and oncological consequences of local regrowth. Failure to comply with appropriate follow-up in a W&W program may constitute a relative contra-indication for any organ-preservation strategy. Still, surveillance strategies may differ across different institutions and have changed over time. Therefore, in line with any surveillance strategy for rectal cancer regardless of definitive surgical or non-surgical management, patients are not specifically asked to consent to a fixed surveillance program.

9. MSI Rectal Cancer and Watch and Wait

Patients with high-level microsatellite instability (MSI-high) adenocarcinomas were found to have worse rates of complete response to standard nCRT [36]. The development of PD1 checkpoint inhibitors led to the observation of significant tumor response in multiple tumors with MSI status. The idea is that activation of a specific immune response is capable of eliciting significant anti-tumoral effect of the host immune system, eventually leading to a significant proportion of complete response in multiple primary solid tumors. One recent single-arm clinical trial including primary MSI-high rectal adenocarcinoma offered PD-1 checkpoint inhibitors leading to a surprisingly 100% cCR rate among 14 patients, without the use of radiation or standard chemotherapy [7]. While these exciting and enthusiastic results await further longer follow-up and increase in the number of patients included, it creates a clear distinction based on molecular features of rectal cancers dependent on microsatellite instability and the possibility of treatment with immunotherapy potentially leading to avoidance of TME in the vast majority (if not all!) patients.

10. Conclusions

In conclusion, Watch & Wait is now considered as an attractive alternative to TME for patients with distal rectal cancer. Patients who achieve a cCR using strict clinical, endoscopic and radiological criteria may benefit from avoiding radical surgery when surgical alternatives are APR or intersphincteric resections. Functional outcomes after W&W appear to be superior to TME in this setting. Careful surveillance should be recommended for early detection of tumor regrowth, which appears to be observed in nearly 30% of patients entered in a W&W program within 3 years of completion of treatment. Salvage surgery seems to be safe for local regrowth and provides good long-term local disease control. The risk of distant metastases is overall low among patients undergoing W&W. However, the subset of patients who develop local regrowth may be at higher risk for developing subsequent metastatic disease.

Author Contributions: Conceptualization, C.C.-S., G.P.S.J., B.B.V., L.C., A.H.-G. and R.O.P.; Methodology, C.C.-S., G.P.S.J., B.B.V., L.C., A.H.-G. and R.O.P.; Validation, C.C.-S., G.P.S.J., B.B.V., L.C. and A.H.-G.; Formal analysis, C.C.-S., G.P.S.J., B.B.V., L.C., A.H.-G. and R.O.P.; Investigation, C.C.-S., G.P.S.J., B.B.V., L.C., A.H.-G. and R.O.P.; Data curation, C.C.-S., G.P.S.J., B.B.V., L.C., A.H.-G. and R.O.P.; Writing—original draft, C.C.-S., G.P.S.J., B.B.V., L.C., A.H.-G. and R.O.P.; Writing—review & editing, C.C.-S., G.P.S.J., B.B.V., L.C., A.H.-G. and R.O.P.; Supervision, R.O.P.; Project administration, A.H.-G. All authors have read and agreed to the published version of the manuscript.

Funding: This research received no external funding.

Institutional Review Board Statement: Not applicable.

Informed Consent Statement: Not applicable.

Data Availability Statement: Not applicable.

Conflicts of Interest: The authors declare no conflict of interest.

References

1. Srivastava, V.; Goswami, A.; Basu, S.; Shukla, V. Locally Advanced Rectal Cancer: What We Learned in the Last Two Decades and the Future Perspectives. *J. Gastrointest. Cancer* **2022**, 1–16. [CrossRef]
2. Habr-Gama, A.; de Souza, P.; Ribeiro, U., Jr.; Nadalin, W.; Gansl, R.; Sousa, A., Jr.; Campos, F.; Gama-Rodrigues, J. Low rectal cancer: Impact of radiation and chemotherapy on surgical treatment. *Dis. Colon Rectum* **1998**, *41*, 1087–1096. [CrossRef]
3. Sauer, R.; Becker, H.; Hohenberger, W.; Rödel, C.; Wittekind, C.; Fietkau, R.; Martus, P.; Tschmelitsch, J.; Hager, E.; Hess, C.; et al. Preoperative versus postoperative chemoradiotherapy for rectal cancer. *N. Engl. J. Med.* **2004**, *35*, 1731–1740. [CrossRef] [PubMed]
4. Quah, H.; Chou, J.; Gonen, M.; Shia, J.; Schrag, D.; Saltz, L.; Goodman, K.; Minsky, B.; Wong, W.; Weiser, M. Pathologic stage is most prognostic of disease-free survival in locally advanced rectal cancer patients after preoperative chemoradiation. *Cancer* **2008**, *113*, 57–64. [CrossRef] [PubMed]
5. Habr-Gama, A.; Perez, R.; Nadalin, W.; Sabbaga, J.; Ribeiro, U., Jr.; Sousa, A.S., Jr.; Campos, F.; Kiss, D.; Gama-Rodrigues, J. Operative versus nonoperative treatment for stage 0 distal rectal cancer following chemoradiation therapy: Long-term results. *Ann. Surg.* **2004**, *240*, 711–717; discussion 717–718. [CrossRef]
6. van der Valk, M.J.M.; E Hilling, D.; Bastiaannet, E.; Kranenbarg, E.M.-K.; Beets, G.L.; Figueiredo, N.L.; Habr-Gama, A.; O Perez, R.; Renehan, A.G.; van de Velde, C.J.H.; et al. Long-term outcomes of clinical complete responders after neoadjuvant treatment for rectal cancer in the International Watch & Wait Database (IWWD): An international multicentre registry study. *Lancet* **2018**, *391*, 2537–2545.
7. Cercek, A.; Lumish, M.; Sinopoli, J.; Weiss, J.; Shia, J.; Lamendola-Essel, M.; El Dika, I.; Segal, N.; Shcherba, M.; Sugarman, R.; et al. PD-1 Blockade in Mismatch Repair-Deficient, Locally Advanced Rectal Cancer. *N. Engl. J. Med.* **2022**, *386*, 2363–2376. [CrossRef] [PubMed]
8. Alimova, I.; Chernyshov, S.; Nagudov, M.; Rybakov, E. Comparison of oncological and functional outcomes and quality of life after transanal or laparoscopic total mesorectal excision for rectal cancer: A systematic review and meta-analysis. *Tech. Coloproctol.* **2021**, *25*, 901–913. [CrossRef]
9. Schnitzbauer, V.; Gerken, M.; Benz, S.; Volkel, V.; Draeger, T.; Furst, A.; Klinkhammer-Schalke, M. Laparoscopic and open surgery in rectal cancer patients in Germany: Short and long-term results of a large 10-year population-based cohort. *Surg. Endosc.* **2020**, *34*, 1132–1141. [CrossRef]
10. Celentano, V.; Cohen, R.; Warusavitarne, J.; Faiz, O.; Chand, M. Sexual dysfunction following rectal cancer surgery. *Int. J. Color. Dis.* **2017**, *32*, 1523–1530. [CrossRef]
11. Grass, J.; Persiani, R.; Tirelli, F.; Chen, C.; Caricato, M.; Pecorino, A.; Lang, I.; Kemper, M.; Izbicki, J.; Melling, N.; et al. Robotic versus transanal total mesorectal excision in sexual, anorectal, and urinary function: A multicenter, prospective, observational study. *Int. J. Color. Dis.* **2021**, *36*, 2749–2761. [CrossRef]
12. Al-Rashid, F.; Robitaille, S.; Liberman, A.; Charlebois, P.; Stein, B.; Feldman, L.; Fiore, J., Jr.; Lee, L. Trajectory of change of low anterior resection syndrome over time after restorative proctectomy for rectal adenocarcinoma. *Tech. Coloproctol.* **2022**, *26*, 195–203. [CrossRef]
13. Denost, Q.; Laurent, C.; Capdepont, M.; Zerbib, F.; Rullier, E. Risk factors for fecal incontinence after intersphincteric resection for rectal cancer. *Dis. Colon Rectum* **2011**, *54*, 963–968. [CrossRef]
14. Denost, Q.; Moreau, J.; Vendrely, V.; Celerier, B.; Rullier, A.; Assenat, V.; Rullier, E. Intersphincteric resection for low rectal cancer: The risk is functional rather than oncological. A 25-year experience from Bordeaux. *Color. Dis.* **2020**, *22*, 1603–1613. [CrossRef]
15. Trenti, L.; Galvez, A.; Biondo, S.; Solis, A.; Vallribera-Valls, F.; Espin-Basany, E.; Garcia-Granero, A.; Kreisler, E. Quality of life and anterior resection syndrome after surgery for mid to low rectal cancer: A cross-sectional study. *Eur. J. Surg. Oncol.* **2018**, *44*, 1031–1039. [CrossRef] [PubMed]
16. Back, E.; Haggstrom, J.; Holmgren, K.; Haapamaki, M.; Matthiessen, P.; Rutegard, J.; Rutegard, M. Permanent stoma rates after anterior resection for rectal cancer: Risk prediction scoring using preoperative variables. *Br. J. Surg.* **2021**, *108*, 1388–1395. [CrossRef]
17. Celerier, B.; Denost, Q.; Van Geluwe, B.; Pontallier, A.; Rullier, E. The risk of definitive stoma formation at 10 years after low and ultralow anterior resection for rectal cancer. *Color. Dis.* **2016**, *18*, 59–66. [CrossRef] [PubMed]
18. Chadi, S.; Malcomson, L.; Ensor, J.; Riley, R.D.; A Vaccaro, C.; Rossi, G.L.; Daniels, I.R.; Smart, N.J.; E Osborne, M.; Beets, G.L.; et al. Factors affecting local regrowth after watch and wait for patients with a clinical complete response following chemoradiotherapy in rectal cancer (InterCoRe consortium): An individual participant data meta-analysis. *Lancet Gastroenterol. Hepatol.* **2018**, *3*, 825–836. [CrossRef] [PubMed]
19. Renehan, A.G.; Malcomson, L.; Emsley, R.; Gollins, S.; Maw, A.; Myint, A.S.; Rooney, P.S.; Susnerwala, S.; Blower, A.; Saunders, M.P.; et al. Watch-and-wait approach versus surgical resection after chemoradiotherapy for patients with rectal cancer (the OnCoRe project): A propensity-score matched cohort analysis. *Lancet Oncol.* **2016**, *17*, 174–183. [CrossRef] [PubMed]
20. Hupkens, B.J.; Martens, M.H.; Stoot, J.H.; Berbee, M.; Melenhorst, J.; Beets-Tan, R.G.; Beets, G.L.; Breukink, S.O. Quality of Life in Rectal Cancer Patients After Chemoradiation: Watch-and-Wait Policy Versus Standard Resection—A Matched-Controlled Study. *Dis. Colon Rectum* **2017**, *60*, 1032–1040. [CrossRef]
21. Quezada-Diaz, F.F.; Smith, J.J.; Jimenez-Rodriguez, R.M.; Wasserman, I.; Pappou, E.P.; Patil, S.; Wei, I.H.; Nash, G.M.; Guillem, J.G.; Weiser, M.R.; et al. Patient-Reported Bowel Function in Patients With Rectal Cancer Managed by a Watch-and-Wait Strategy After Neoadjuvant Therapy: A Case-Control Study. *Dis. Colon Rectum* **2020**, *63*, 897–902. [CrossRef]

22. Pollack, J.; Holm, T.; Cedermark, B.; Holmstrom, B.; Mellgren, A. Long-term effect of preoperative radiation therapy on anorectal function. *Dis. Colon Rectum* **2006**, *49*, 345–352. [CrossRef] [PubMed]
23. Juul, T.; Elfeki, H.; Christensen, P.; Laurberg, S.; Emmertsen, K.; Bager, P. Normative Data for the Low Anterior Resection Syndrome Score (LARS Score). *Ann. Surg.* **2019**, *269*, 1124–1128. [CrossRef] [PubMed]
24. Vailati, B.; Habr-Gama, A.; Mattacheo, A.; Juliao, G.S.; Perez, R. Quality of Life in Patients With Rectal Cancer After Chemoradiation: Watch-and-Wait Policy Versus Standard Resection-Are We Comparing Apples to Oranges? *Dis. Colon Rectum* **2018**, *61*, e21. [CrossRef] [PubMed]
25. Taylor, F.; Swift, R.; Blomqvist, L.; Brown, G. A systematic approach to the interpretation of preoperative staging MRI for rectal cancer. *AJR Am. J. Roentgenol.* **2008**, *191*, 1827–1835. [CrossRef]
26. Brown, G.; Radcliffe, A.; Newcombe, R.; Dallimore, N.; Bourne, M.; Williams, G. Preoperative assessment of prognostic factors in rectal cancer using high-resolution magnetic resonance imaging. *Br. J. Surg.* **2003**, *90*, 355–364. [CrossRef]
27. Habr-Gama, A.; Juliao, G.S.; Gama-Rodrigues, J.; Vailati, B.; Ortega, C.; Fernandez, L.; Araujo, S.; Perez, R. Baseline T Classification Predicts Early Tumor Regrowth After Nonoperative Management in Distal Rectal Cancer After Extended Neoadjuvant Chemoradiation and Initial Complete Clinical Response. *Dis. Colon Rectum* **2017**, *60*, 586–594. [CrossRef]
28. Taylor, F.; Quirke, P.; Heald, R.; Moran, B.; Blomqvist, L.; Swift, I.; Sebag-Montefiore, D.; Tekkis, P.; Brown, G.; MERCURY Study group. Preoperative high-resolution magnetic resonance imaging can identify good prognosis stage I, II, and III rectal cancer best managed by surgery alone: A prospective, multicenter, European study. *Ann. Surg.* **2011**, *253*, 711–719. [CrossRef]
29. Habr-Gama, A.; Perez, R.; Wynn, G.; Marks, J.; Kessler, H.; Gama-Rodrigues, J. Complete clinical response after neoadjuvant chemoradiation therapy for distal rectal cancer: Characterization of clinical and endoscopic findings for standardization. *Dis. Colon Rectum* **2010**, *53*, 1692–1698. [CrossRef]
30. Maas, M.; Lambregts, D.M.J.; Nelemans, P.J.; Heijnen, L.A.; Martens, M.H.; Leijtens, J.W.A.; Sosef, M.; Hulsewé, K.W.E.; Hoff, C.; Breukink, S.O.; et al. Assessment of Clinical Complete Response After Chemoradiation for Rectal Cancer with Digital Rectal Examination, Endoscopy, and MRI: Selection for Organ-Saving Treatment. *Ann. Surg. Oncol.* **2015**, *22*, 3873–3880. [CrossRef] [PubMed]
31. Perez, R.O.; Habr-Gama, A.; Julião, G.P.S.; Gama-Rodrigues, J.; Sousa, A.H.; Campos, F.G.; Imperiale, A.R.; Lynn, P.B.; Proscurshim, I.; Nahas, S.C.; et al. Optimal timing for assessment of tumor response to neoadjuvant chemoradiation in patients with rectal cancer: Do all patients benefit from waiting longer than 6 weeks? *Int. J. Radiat. Oncol. Biol. Phys.* **2012**, *84*, 1159–1165. [CrossRef]
32. Perez, R.; Habr-Gama, A.; Juliao, G.S.; Lynn, P.; Sabbagh, C.; Proscurshim, I.; Campos, F.; Gama-Rodrigues, J.; Nahas, S.; Buchpiguel, C. Predicting complete response to neoadjuvant CRT for distal rectal cancer using sequential PET/CT imaging. *Tech. Coloproctol.* **2014**, *18*, 699–708. [CrossRef] [PubMed]
33. Habr-Gama, A.; Juliao, G.S.; Fernandez, L.; Vailati, B.; Andrade, A.; Araujo, S.; Gama-Rodrigues, J.; Perez, R. Achieving a Complete Clinical Response After Neoadjuvant Chemoradiation That Does Not Require Surgical Resection: It May Take Longer Than You Think! *Dis. Colon Rectum* **2019**, *62*, 802–808. [CrossRef] [PubMed]
34. Cerdan-Santacruz, C.; Vailati, B.; Juliao, G.S.; Habr-Gama, A.; Perez, R. Watch and wait: Why, to whom and how. *Surg. Oncol.* **2022**, *43*, 101774. [CrossRef]
35. Matsuda, T.; Fujii, T.; Saito, Y.; Nakajima, T.; Uraoka, T.; Kobayashi, N.; Ikehara, H.; Ikematsu, H.; Fu, K.; Emura, F.; et al. Efficacy of the invasive/non-invasive pattern by magnifying chromoendoscopy to estimate the depth of invasion of early colorectal neoplasms. *Am. J. Gastroenterol.* **2008**, *103*, 2700–2706. [CrossRef]
36. Cercek, A.; Fernandes, G.D.S.; Roxburgh, C.; Ganesh, K.; Ng, S.; Sanchez-Vega, F.; Yaeger, R.; Segal, N.; Reidy-Lagunes, D.; Varghese, A.; et al. Mismatch Repair-Deficient Rectal Cancer and Resistance to Neoadjuvant Chemotherapy. *Clin. Cancer Res.* **2020**, *26*, 3271–3279. [CrossRef] [PubMed]
37. Stelzner, S.; Ruppert, R.; Kube, R.; Strassburg, J.; Lewin, A.; Baral, J.; Maurer, C.; Sauer, J.; Lauscher, J.; Winde, G.; et al. Selection of patients with rectal cancer for neoadjuvant therapy using pre-therapeutic MRI-Results from OCUM trial. *Eur. J. Radiol.* **2022**, *147*, 110113. [CrossRef] [PubMed]
38. Wan, L.; Peng, W.; Zou, S.; Ye, F.; Geng, Y.; Ouyang, H.; Zhao, X.; Zhang, H. MRI-based delta-radiomics are predictive of pathological complete response after neoadjuvant chemoradiotherapy in locally advanced rectal cancer. *Acad. Radiol.* **2021**, *28* (Suppl. 1), S95–S104. [CrossRef] [PubMed]
39. Yuan, Y.; Zheng, K.; Zhou, L.; Chen, F.; Zhang, S.; Lu, H.; Lu, J.; Shao, C.; Meng, R.; Zhang, W.; et al. Predictive value of modified MRI-based split scar sign (mrSSS) score for pathological complete response after neoadjuvant chemoradiotherapy for patients with rectal cancer. *Int. J. Colorectal. Dis.* **2023**, *38*, 40. [CrossRef]
40. Grabenbauer, A.; Aigner, T.; Gobel, H.; Leibl, B.; Lamberti, C.; Grabenbauer, G.; Distel, L. Preoperative Radiochemotherapy in Rectal Cancer: Is There an Impact of Oxaliplatin on Pathologic Complete Response and Survival Rates under "Real World" Conditions? *Cells* **2023**, *12*, 399. [CrossRef]
41. Diefenhardt, M.; Ludmir, E.; Hofheinz, R.; Ghadimi, M.; Minsky, B.; Rodel, C.; Fokas, E. Association of Treatment Adherence With Oncologic Outcomes for Patients With Rectal Cancer: A Post Hoc Analysis of the CAO/ARO/AIO-04 Phase 3 Randomized Clinical Trial. *JAMA Oncol.* **2020**, *6*, 1416–1421. [CrossRef] [PubMed]
42. Yu, M.; Wang, D.; Li, S.; Huang, L.; Wei, J. Does a long interval between neoadjuvant chemoradiotherapy and surgery benefit the clinical outcomes of locally advanced rectal cancer? A systematic review and meta analyses. *Int. J. Colorectal. Dis.* **2022**, *37*, 855–868. [CrossRef]

43. Foster, J.; Jones, E.; Falk, S.; Cooper, E.; Francis, N. Timing of surgery after long-course neoadjuvant chemoradiotherapy for rectal cancer: A systematic review of the literature. *Dis. Colon Rectum* **2013**, *57*, 921–930. [CrossRef] [PubMed]
44. Erlandsson, J.; Holm, T.; Pettersson, D.; Berglund, A.; Cedermark, B.; Radu, C.; Johansson, H.; Machado, M.; Hjern, F.; Hallbook, O.; et al. Optimal fractionation of preoperative radiotherapy and timing to surgery for rectal cancer (Stockholm III): A multicentre, randomised, non-blinded, phase 3, non-inferiority trial. *Lancet Oncol.* **2017**, *18*, 336–346. [CrossRef] [PubMed]
45. Habr-Gama, A.; Perez, R.; Sabbaga, J.; Nadalin, W.; Juliao, G.S.; Gama-Rodrigues, J. Increasing the rates of complete response to neoadjuvant chemoradiotherapy for distal rectal cancer: Results of a prospective study using additional chemotherapy during the resting period. *Dis. Colon Rectum* **2009**, *52*, 1927–1934. [CrossRef]
46. Gao, Y.; Zhang, X.; An, X.; Cai, M.; Zeng, Z.; Chen, G.; Kong, L.; Lin, J.; Wan, D.; Pan, Z.; et al. Oxaliplatin and capecitabine concomitant with neoadjuvant radiotherapy and extended to the resting period in high risk locally advanced rectal cancer. *Strahlenther Onkol* **2014**, *190*, 158–164. [CrossRef]
47. Habr-Gama, A.; Perez, R.; Juliao, G.S.; Proscurshim, I.; Fernandez, L.; Figueiredo, M.; Gama-Rodrigues, J.; Buchpiguel, C.A. Consolidation chemotherapy during neoadjuvant chemoradiation (CRT) for distal rectal cancer leads to sustained decrease in tumor metabolism when compared to standard CRT regimen. *Radiat. Oncol.* **2016**, *11*, 24. [CrossRef]
48. Asoglu, O.; Tokmak, H.; Bakir, B.; Demir, G.; Ozyar, E.; Atalar, B.; Goksel, S.; Koza, B.; Mert, A.G.; Demir, A.; et al. The impact of total neo-adjuvant treatment on nonoperative management in patients with locally advanced rectal cancer: The evaluation of 66 cases. *Eur. J. Surg. Oncol.* **2020**, *46*, 402–409. [CrossRef]
49. Juliao, G.S.; Habr-Gama, A.; Vailati, B.; Aguilar, P.; Sabbaga, J.; Araujo, S.; Mattacheo, A.; Alexandre, F.; Fernandez, L.; Gomes, D.; et al. Is neoadjuvant chemoradiation with dose-escalation and consolidation chemotherapy sufficient to increase surgery-free and distant metastases-free survival in baseline cT3 rectal cancer? *Eur. J. Surg. Oncol.* **2018**, *44*, 93–99. [CrossRef]
50. Fernandez-Martos, C.; Garcia-Albeniz, X.; Pericay, C.; Maurel, J.; Aparicio, J.; Montagut, C.; Safont, M.; Salud, A.; Vera, R.; Massuti, B.; et al. Chemoradiation, surgery and adjuvant chemotherapy versus induction chemotherapy followed by chemoradiation and surgery: Long-term results of the Spanish GCR-3 phase II randomized trialdagger. *Ann. Oncol.* **2015**, *26*, 1722–1728. [CrossRef]
51. Fokas, E.; Allgauer, M.; Polat, B.; Klautke, G.; Grabenbauer, G.; Fietkau, R.; Kuhnt, T.; Staib, L.; Brunner, T.; Grosu, A.; et al. German Rectal Cancer Study, Randomized Phase II Trial of Chemoradiotherapy Plus Induction or Consolidation Chemotherapy as Total Neoadjuvant Therapy for Locally Advanced Rectal Cancer: CAO/ARO/AIO-12. *J. Clin. Oncol.* **2019**, *37*, 3212–3222. [CrossRef] [PubMed]
52. Fokas, E.; Schlenska-Lange, A.; Polat, B.; Klautke, G.; Grabenbauer, G.; Fietkau, R.; Kuhnt, T.; Staib, L.; Brunner, T.; Grosu, A.; et al. German Rectal Cancer Study, Chemoradiotherapy Plus Induction or Consolidation Chemotherapy as Total Neoadjuvant Therapy for Patients With Locally Advanced Rectal Cancer: Long-term Results of the CAO/ARO/AIO-12 Randomized Clinical Trial. *JAMA Oncol.* **2022**, *8*, e215445. [CrossRef] [PubMed]
53. Garcia-Aguilar, J.; Patil, S.; Gollub, M.; Kim, J.; Yuval, J.; Thompson, H.; Verheij, F.; Omer, D.; Lee, M.; Dunne, R.; et al. Organ Preservation in Patients With Rectal Adenocarcinoma Treated With Total Neoadjuvant Therapy. *J. Clin. Oncol.* **2022**, *40*, 2546–2556. [CrossRef]
54. Chakrabarti, D.; Rajan, S.; Akhtar, N.; Qayoom, S.; Gupta, S.; Verma, M.; Srivastava, K.; Kumar, V.; Bhatt, M.; Gupta, R. Short-course radiotherapy with consolidation chemotherapy versus conventionally fractionated long-course chemoradiotherapy for locally advanced rectal cancer: Randomized clinical trial. *Br. J. Surg.* **2021**, *108*, 511–520. [CrossRef]
55. Bahadoer, R.R.; A Dijkstra, E.; van Etten, B.; Marijnen, C.A.M.; Putter, H.; Kranenbarg, E.M.-K.; Roodvoets, A.G.H.; Nagtegaal, I.D.; Beets-Tan, R.G.H.; Blomqvist, L.K.; et al. Short-course radiotherapy followed by chemotherapy before total mesorectal excision (TME) versus preoperative chemoradiotherapy, TME, and optional adjuvant chemotherapy in locally advanced rectal cancer (RAPIDO): A randomised, open-label, phase 3 trial. *Lancet Oncol.* **2021**, *22*, 29–42. [CrossRef] [PubMed]
56. Chin, R.-I.; Roy, A.; Pedersen, K.S.; Huang, Y.; Hunt, S.R.; Glasgow, S.C.; Tan, B.R.; Wise, P.E.; Silviera, M.L.; Smith, R.K.; et al. Clinical Complete Response in Patients With Rectal Adenocarcinoma Treated With Short-Course Radiation Therapy and Nonoperative Management. *Int. J. Radiat. Oncol. Biol. Phys.* **2022**, *112*, 715–725. [CrossRef]
57. Dijkstra, E.A.; Nilsson, P.J.; Hospers, G.A.; Bahadoer, R.R.; Kranenbarg, E.M.-K.; Roodvoets, A.G.; Putter, H.; Berglund, Å.M.; Cervantes, A.; Crolla, R.M.; et al. Locoregional Failure During and After Short-course Radiotherapy followed by Chemotherapy and Surgery Compared to Long-course Chemoradiotherapy and Surgery—A Five-year Follow-up of the RAPIDO Trial. *Ann. Surg.* **2023**. [CrossRef]
58. Habr-Gama, A.; Juliao, G.S.; Vailati, B.; Sabbaga, J.; Aguilar, P.; Fernandez, L.; Araujo, S.; Perez, R.O. Organ Preservation in cT2N0 Rectal Cancer After Neoadjuvant Chemoradiation Therapy: The Impact of Radiation Therapy Dose-escalation and Consolidation Chemotherapy. *Ann. Surg.* **2019**, *269*, 102–107. [CrossRef]
59. Gerard, J.; Barbet, N.; Schiappa, R.; Magne, N.; Martel, I.; Mineur, L.; Deberne, M.; Zilli, T.; Dhadda, A.; Myint, A.; et al. Neoadjuvant chemoradiotherapy with radiation dose escalation with contact x-ray brachytherapy boost or external beam radiotherapy boost for organ preservation in early cT2-cT3 rectal adenocarcinoma (OPERA): A phase 3, randomised controlled trial. *Lancet Gastroenterol Hepatol* **2023**, *8*, 356–367. [CrossRef]
60. Patel, U.; Brown, G.; Rutten, H.; West, N.; Sebag-Montefiore, D.; Glynne-Jones, R.; Rullier, E.; Peeters, M.; Van Cutsem, E.; Ricci, S.; et al. Comparison of magnetic resonance imaging and histopathological response to chemoradiotherapy in locally advanced rectal cancer. *Ann. Surg. Oncol.* **2012**, *19*, 2842–2852. [CrossRef]

61. Patel, U.; Blomqvist, L.; Taylor, F.; George, C.; Guthrie, A.; Bees, N.; Brown, G. MRI after treatment of locally advanced rectal cancer: How to report tumor response–the MERCURY experience. *AJR Am. J. Roentgenol.* **2012**, *199*, W486–W495. [CrossRef] [PubMed]
62. Lambregts, D.; Lahaye, M.; Heijnen, L.; Martens, M.; Maas, M.; Beets, G.; Beets-Tan, R.G. MRI and diffusion-weighted MRI to diagnose a local tumour regrowth during long-term follow-up of rectal cancer patients treated with organ preservation after chemoradiotherapy. *Eur. Radiol.* **2016**, *26*, 2118–2125. [CrossRef] [PubMed]
63. Lambregts, D.; Maas, M.; Bakers, F.; Cappendijk, V.; Lammering, G.; Beets, G.; Beets-Tan, R. Long-term follow-up features on rectal MRI during a wait-and-see approach after a clinical complete response in patients with rectal cancer treated with chemoradiotherapy. *Dis. Colon Rectum* **2011**, *54*, 1521–1528. [CrossRef] [PubMed]
64. Lambregts, D.; Rao, S.; Sassen, S.; Martens, M.; Heijnen, L.; Buijsen, J.; Sosef, M.; Beets, G.; Vliegen, R.; Beets-Tan, R.G. MRI and Diffusion-weighted MRI Volumetry for Identification of Complete Tumor Responders After Preoperative Chemoradiotherapy in Patients With Rectal Cancer: A Bi-institutional Validation Study. *Ann. Surg.* **2015**, *262*, 1034–1039. [CrossRef]
65. Lambregts, D.M.J.; Van Heeswijk, M.M.; Pizzi, A.D.; Van Elderen, S.G.C.; Andrade, L.; Peters, N.H.G.M.; Kint, P.A.M.; Jong, M.O.-D.; Bipat, S.; Ooms, R.; et al. Diffusion-weighted MRI to assess response to chemoradiotherapy in rectal cancer: Main interpretation pitfalls and their use for teaching. *Eur. Radiol.* **2017**, *27*, 4445–4454. [CrossRef]
66. dos Anjos, D.A.; Perez, R.O.; Habr-Gama, A.; Julião, G.P.S.; Vailati, B.B.; Fernandez, L.M.; de Sousa, J.B.; Buchpiguel, C.A. Semi-quantitative Volumetry by Sequential PET/CT May Improve Prediction of Complete Response to Neoadjuvant Chemoradiation in Patients With Distal Rectal Cancer. *Dis. Colon Rectum* **2016**, *59*, 805–812. [CrossRef]
67. Perez, R.; Habr-Gama, A.; Gama-Rodrigues, J.; Proscurshim, I.; Juliao, G.; Lynn, P.; Ono, C.; Campos, F.; Sousa, A.S., Jr.; Imperiale, A.; et al. Accuracy of positron emission tomography/computed tomography and clinical assessment in the detection of complete rectal tumor regression after neoadjuvant chemoradiation: Long-term results of a prospective trial (National Clinical Trial 00254683). *Cancer* **2012**, *118*, 3501–3511. [CrossRef]
68. Rymer, B.; Curtis, N.; Siddiqui, M.; Chand, M. FDG PET/CT Can Assess the Response of Locally Advanced Rectal Cancer to Neoadjuvant Chemoradiotherapy: Evidence From Meta-analysis and Systematic Review. *Clin. Nucl. Med.* **2016**, *41*, 371–375. [CrossRef]
69. Perez, R.O.; Habr-Gama, A.; Pereira, G.V.; Lynn, P.B.; Alves, P.A.; Proscurshim, I.; Rawet, V.; Gama-Rodrigues, J. Role of biopsies in patients with residual rectal cancer following neoadjuvant chemoradiation after downsizing: Can they rule out persisting cancer? *Color. Dis.* **2012**, *14*, 714–720. [CrossRef]
70. Van Den Begin, R.; Kleijnen, J.-P.; Engels, B.; Philippens, M.; Van Asselen, B.; Raaymakers, B.; Reerink, O.; De Ridder, M.; Intven, M. Tumor volume regression during preoperative chemoradiotherapy for rectal cancer: A prospective observational study with weekly MRI. *Acta Oncol.* **2018**, *57*, 723–727. [CrossRef]
71. Custers, P.A.; Geubels, B.M.; Beets, G.L.; Lambregts, D.M.J.; E van Leerdam, M.; van Triest, B.; Maas, M. Defining near-complete response following (chemo)radiotherapy for rectal cancer: Systematic review. *Br. J. Surg.* **2022**, *110*, 43–49. [CrossRef]
72. Deidda, S.; Elmore, U.; Rosati, R.; De Nardi, P.; Vignali, A.; Puccetti, F.; Spolverato, G.; Capelli, G.; Zuin, M.; Muratore, A.; et al. Association of Delayed Surgery With Oncologic Long-term Outcomes in Patients With Locally Advanced Rectal Cancer Not Responding to Preoperative Chemoradiation. *JAMA Surg.* **2021**, *156*, 1141–1149. [CrossRef] [PubMed]
73. Heald, R.; Beets, G.; Carvalho, C. Report from a consensus meeting: Response to chemoradiotherapy in rectal cancer-predictor of cure and a crucial new choice for the patient: On behalf of the Champalimaud 2014 Faculty for 'Rectal cancer: When NOT to operate'. *Color. Dis.* **2014**, *16*, 334–337. [CrossRef]
74. Dattani, M.; Heald, R.; Goussous, G.; Broadhurst, J.; Julião, G.S.; Habr-Gama, A.; Perez, R.; Moran, B.J. Oncological and Survival Outcomes in Watch and Wait Patients With a Clinical Complete Response After Neoadjuvant Chemoradiotherapy for Rectal Cancer: A Systematic Review and Pooled Analysis. *Ann. Surg.* **2018**, *268*, 955–967. [CrossRef]
75. Fernandez, L.M.M.; Figueiredo, N.L.M.; Habr-Gama, A.M.; Julião, G.P.M.S.; Vieira, P.M.; Vailati, B.B.M.; Nasir, I.M.; Parés, O.M.; Santiago, I.M.; Castillo-Martin, M.M.; et al. Salvage Surgery With Organ Preservation for Patients With Local Regrowth After Watch and Wait: Is It Still Possible? *Dis. Colon Rectum* **2020**, *63*, 1053–1062. [CrossRef]
76. Habr-Gama, A.; Gama-Rodrigues, J.; Juliao, G.S.; Proscurshim, I.; Sabbagh, C.; Lynn, P.; Perez, R.O. Local recurrence after complete clinical response and watch and wait in rectal cancer after neoadjuvant chemoradiation: Impact of salvage therapy on local disease control. *Int. J. Radiat. Oncol. Biol. Phys.* **2014**, *88*, 822–828. [CrossRef]
77. Kong, J.C.; Guerra, G.R.; Warrier, S.K.; Ramsay, R.G.; Heriot, A.G. Outcome and Salvage Surgery Following "Watch and Wait" for Rectal Cancer after Neoadjuvant Therapy: A Systematic Review. *Dis. Colon Rectum* **2017**, *60*, 335–345. [CrossRef] [PubMed]
78. Nasir, I.; Fernandez, L.; Vieira, P.; Parés, O.; Santiago, I.; Castillo-Martin, M.; Domingos, H.; Cunha, J.F.; Carvalho, C.; Heald, R.J.; et al. Salvage surgery for local regrowths in Watch & Wait-Are we harming our patients by deferring the surgery? *Eur. J. Surg. Oncol.* **2019**, *45*, 1559–1566. [PubMed]
79. Habr-Gama, A.; Perez, R.O.; Proscurshim, I.; dos Santos, R.M.N.; Kiss, D.; Gama-Rodrigues, J.; Cecconello, I. Interval between surgery and neoadjuvant chemoradiation therapy for distal rectal cancer: Does delayed surgery have an impact on outcome? *Int. J. Radiat. Oncol.* **2008**, *71*, 1181–1188. [CrossRef]
80. Smith, F.M.; Ahad, A.; Perez, R.O.; Marks, J.; Bujko, K.; Heald, R.J. Local Excision Techniques for Rectal Cancer After Neoadjuvant Chemoradiotherapy: What Are We Doing? *Dis. Colon Rectum* **2017**, *60*, 228–239. [CrossRef]

81. Garcia-Aguilar, J.; Chow, O.S.; Smith, D.D.; Marcet, J.E.; Cataldo, P.A.; Varma, M.G.; Kumar, A.S.; Oommen, S.; Coutsoftides, T.; Hunt, S.R.; et al. Timing of Rectal Cancer Response to Chemoradiation, Effect of adding mFOLFOX6 after neoadjuvant chemoradiation in locally advanced rectal cancer: A multicentre, phase 2 trial. *Lancet Oncol.* **2015**, *16*, 957–966. [CrossRef] [PubMed]
82. Lefevre, J.H.; Mineur, L.; Kotti, S.; Rullier, E.; Rouanet, P.; de Chaisemartin, C.; Meunier, B.; Mehrdad, J.; Cotte, E.; Desrame, J.; et al. Effect of Interval (7 or 11 weeks) Between Neoadjuvant Radiochemotherapy and Surgery on Complete Pathologic Response in Rectal Cancer: A Multicenter, Randomized, Controlled Trial (GRECCAR-6). *J. Clin. Oncol.* **2016**, *34*, 3773–3780. [CrossRef]
83. Juliao, G.S.; Karagkounis, G.; Fernandez, L.; Habr-Gama, A.; Vailati, B.; Dattani, M.; Kalady, M.; Perez, R.O. Conditional Survival in Patients With Rectal Cancer and Complete Clinical Response Managed by Watch and Wait After Chemoradiation: Recurrence Risk Over Time. *Ann. Surg.* **2020**, *272*, 138–144. [CrossRef]
84. Habr-Gama, A.; Julião, G.P.S.; Vailati, B.B.; Fernandez, L.M.; Ortega, C.D.; Figueiredo, N.; Gama-Rodrigues, J.; Perez, R.O. Organ Preservation Among Patients With Clinically Node-Positive Rectal Cancer: Is It Really More Dangerous? *Dis. Colon Rectum* **2019**, *62*, 675–683. [CrossRef]
85. Fernandez, L.M.; Julião, G.P.S.; Figueiredo, N.L.; Beets, G.L.; van der Valk, M.J.M.; Bahadoer, R.R.; E Hilling, D.; Kranenbarg, E.M.-K.; Roodvoets, A.G.H.; Renehan, A.G.; et al. Conditional recurrence-free survival of clinical complete responders managed by watch and wait after neoadjuvant chemoradiotherapy for rectal cancer in the International Watch & Wait Database: A retrospective, international, multicentre registry study. *Lancet Oncol.* **2021**, *22*, 43–50.
86. Smith, J.J.; Strombom, P.; Chow, O.S.; Roxburgh, C.S.; Lynn, P.; Eaton, A.; Widmar, M.; Ganesh, K.; Yaeger, R.; Cercek, A.; et al. Assessment of a Watch-and-Wait Strategy for Rectal Cancer in Patients With a Complete Response After Neoadjuvant Therapy. *JAMA Oncol.* **2019**, *5*, e185896. [CrossRef] [PubMed]
87. Fernandez, L.M.; Julião, G.P.S.; Renehan, A.G.; Beets, G.L.; Papoila, A.L.; Vailati, B.B.; Bahadoer, R R.; Kranenbarg, E.M.-K.; Roodvoets, A.G.H.; Figueiredo, N.L.; et al. The Risk of Distant Metastases in Patients With Clinical Complete Response Managed by Watch and Wait After Neoadjuvant Therapy for Rectal Cancer: The Influence of Local Regrowth in the International Watch and Wait Database. *Dis. Colon Rectum* **2023**, *66*, 41–49. [CrossRef]
88. Cerdán-Santacruz, C.; Vailati, B.B.; Julião, G.P.S.; Habr-Gama, A.; Perez, R.O. Local tumor regrowth after clinical complete response following neoadjuvant therapy for rectal cancer: What happens when organ preservation fails short. *Tech. Coloproctol.* **2023**, *27*, 1–9. [CrossRef] [PubMed]
89. Kennedy, E.; Zwaal, C.; Asmis, T.; Cho, C.; Galica, J.; Ginty, A.; Govindarajan, A. An Evidence-Based Guideline for Surveillance of Patients after Curative Treatment for Colon and Rectal Cancer. *Curr. Oncol.* **2022**, *29*, 724–740. [CrossRef]

Disclaimer/Publisher's Note: The statements, opinions and data contained in all publications are solely those of the individual author(s) and contributor(s) and not of MDPI and/or the editor(s). MDPI and/or the editor(s) disclaim responsibility for any injury to people or property resulting from any ideas, methods, instructions or products referred to in the content.

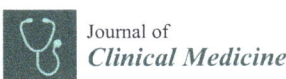

Article

Rectal Cancer following Local Excision of Rectal Adenomas with Low-Grade Dysplasia—A Multicenter Study

Yaron Rudnicki [1,*], Nir Horesh [2], Assaf Harbi [3], Barak Lubianiker [4], Eraan Green [5], Guy Raveh [6], Moran Slavin [1], Lior Segev [2], Haim Gilshtein [3], Muhammad Khalifa [4], Alexander Barenboim [5], Nir Wasserberg [6], Marat Khaikin [2], Hagit Tulchinsky [5], Nidal Issa [4], Daniel Duek [3], Shmuel Avital [1] and Ian White [6]

1. Meir Medical Center, Department of Surgery, Faculty of Medicine, Tel Aviv University, Kfar Saba 4428164, Israel
2. Sheba Medical Center, Department of General Surgery B and Organ Transplantation, Faculty of Medicine, Tel Aviv University, Ramat Gan 5265601, Israel
3. Rambam Health Care Campus, Department of General Surgery, Rappaport Faculty of Medicine, Technion-Israel Institute of Technology, Haifa 3109601, Israel
4. Rabin Medical Center-Hasharon Hospital, Department of Surgery, Faculty of Medicine, Tel Aviv University, Petach Tikva 49100, Israel
5. Tel Aviv Sourasky Medical Center, Department of Surgery, Faculty of Medicine, Tel Aviv University, Tel Aviv 69978, Israel
6. Rabin Medical Center-Beilinson Hospital, Department of Surgery, Faculty of Medicine, Tel Aviv University, Petach Tikva 4941492, Israel
* Correspondence: yaron217@gmail.com

Abstract: Purpose: Rectal polyps with low-grade dysplasia (LGD) can be removed by local excision surgery (LE). It is unclear whether these lesions pose a higher risk for recurrence and cancer development and might warrant an early repeat rectal endoscopy. This study aims to assess the rectal cancer rate following local excision of LGD rectal lesions. **Methods**: A retrospective multicenter study including all patients that underwent LE for rectal polyps over a period of 11 years was conducted. Demographic, clinical, and surgical data of patients with LGD were collected and analyzed. **Results**: Out of 274 patients that underwent LE of rectal lesions, 81 (30%) had a pathology of LGD. The mean patient age was 65 ± 11 years, and 52 (64%) were male. The mean distance from the anal verge was 7.2 ± 4.3 cm, and the average lesion was 3.2 ± 1.8 cm. Full thickness resection was achieved in 68 patients (84%), and four (5%) had involved margins for LGD. Nine patients (11%) had local recurrence and developed rectal cancer in an average time interval of 19.3 ± 14.5 months, with seven of them (78%) diagnosed less than two years after the initial LE. Seven of the nine patients were treated with another local excision, whilst one had a low anterior resection, and one was treated with radiation. The mean follow-up time was 25.3 ± 22.4 months. **Conclusions**: Locally resected rectal polyps with LGD may carry a significant risk of recurring and developing cancer within two years. This data suggests patients should have a closer surveillance protocol in place.

Keywords: low-grade dysplasia; rectal cancer; rectal polyps; local excision; recurrence

1. Introduction

A rectal polyp is considered a precursor for rectal cancer according to the adenoma-adenocarcinoma sequence. The timely removal of these lesions is considered essential for preventing advancement to malignancy in up to 90% of cases [1,2]. After successfully removing a polyp, it is recommended to continue surveillance at certain time intervals due to the increased risk for recurrence and advancement to malignancy [3]. The time interval for endoscopic surveillance is extrapolated from multiple studies trying to define the level of risk by features such as the number of polyps, the size, personal and family history of colorectal cancer (CRC), and the grade of dysplasia [4–7]. Guidelines for post-polypectomy surveillance after removing a dysplastic lesion are often ambiguous regarding the distinction between rectal and colonic polyps, the implications of resection margins with dysplasia, depth of resection, and whether the resection was performed endoscopically or surgically. Some post-polypectomy surveillance guidelines recommend an interval of three years for repeat colonoscopy after removal of a dysplastic lesion to detect early recurrence of adenomas or even CRC [8].

To date, most rectal lesions are removed endoscopically. However, distal rectal lesions; large or suspicious rectal lesions, including polyps larger than 1 cm; sessile adenomas; and early-stage rectal cancerous masses are better served by surgical removal. LE surgery can be performed with a standard transanal excision (TAE) or minimally invasive surgery (MIS). Local excision surgery allows for a full-thickness resection, negative resection margins, and the ability to close the defect in the rectal wall following resection [9]. The reported rate of LGD histology in LE rectal lesions varies from 7% to 51% [10,11]. As transanal MIS platforms became more and more common, the ability to remove larger masses transanally grew, which in turn led to a much higher number of LGD lesions being excised. It is unknown whether these LGD rectal lesions pose a higher risk of recurrence and development of rectal cancer.

This study aimed to assess the rate of rectal malignancy following LE of LGD lesions in the rectum.

2. Materials and Methods

A multicenter retrospective study following all patients with rectal lesions resected with a transanal local excision approach was conducted from October 2010 to March 2020 (11 years) in six academic medical centers in Israel. A subsequent analysis of patients with a final pathology of low-grade dysplasia was conducted. The data collected included the operative platforms used (a standard transanal excision (TAE), a transanal minimally invasive surgery (TAMIS), and a transanal endoscopic microsurgery (TEM)); demographics characteristics (age, gender, body mass index (BMI); co-morbidities; American Society of Anesthesiology (ASA) score); preoperative studies performed, including endoscopy with rectal lesion biopsy (rigid proctoscopy, Flexible Sigmoidoscopy, Colonoscopy); abdominal and pelvic CT; and endorectal ultrasound (ERUS) or pelvic magnetic resonance imaging (MRI), or both.

Operative and postoperative data were collected, including operative approach, surgical findings, length of hospital stay, postoperative complications, morbidity, and mortality. The Clavien-Dindo classification of surgical complications score was used to classify postoperative complications [12]. Pathology reports were reviewed for histological characteristics such as size and resection margins. Out-patient visits and follow-up charts were reviewed for malignant recurrence and treatment after diagnosis of rectal malignancy. There was no standardized follow-up protocol, and various surveillance protocols were noted among the various centers. Polyps with any other pathology except low-grade dysplasia were excluded from the cohort.

Approval of the institutional review boards of all six participating centers was attained for the study (IRB 0179-20-MMC). All respective institutional review boards waived the need for individual informed consent by each patient for this retrospective study.

Statistical analyses were performed using EZR (Version 1.55) and R software (version 4.1.2) (Chugai Igakusha: Tokyo, Japan). Continuous data were expressed as mean and standard deviation when normally distributed or otherwise as the median and interquartile range (IQR). Student-t test or Mann–Whitney U test was used to analyze continuous variables. Categorical data were expressed as numbers and proportions and analyzed using Fisher exact or Chi-Square test. A p-value < 0.05 was considered significant.

3. Results

During the study, 274 patients underwent transanal local excision of rectal tumors. The histological findings in the pathology reports of 81 patients (30%) were polyps with low-grade dysplasia and are the focus of this study. The other 193 patients had lesions with malignancy or high-grade dysplasia (Figure 1). The mean patient age at diagnosis was 65 ± 11 years, 52 patients (64%) were male, and the mean body mass index (BMI) was 26.6 ± 4.8 kg/m². Patient demographics and preoperative data are detailed in Table 1. The mean and SD follow-up time was 25.3 ± 22.4 months.

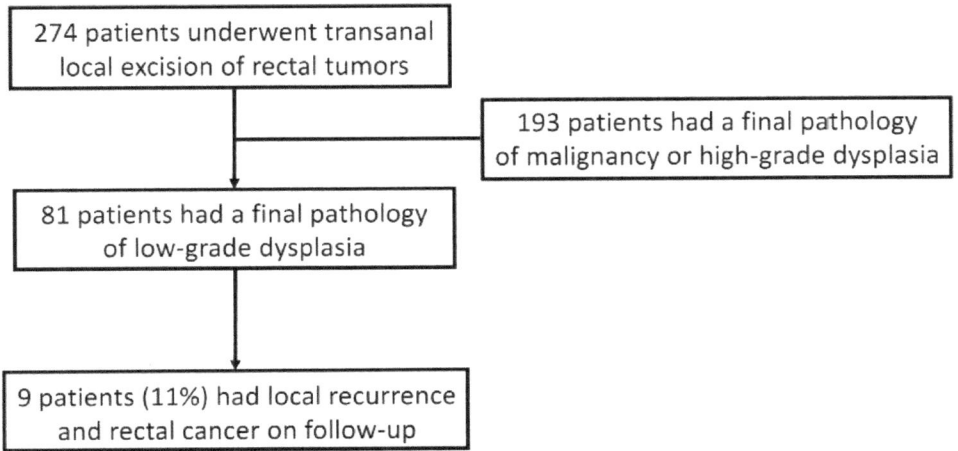

Figure 1. Flow chart of participation in the study, recurrence with rectal cancer.

Table 1. Baseline demographic and clinical and imaging characteristics of patients.

Characteristic	(n = 81)
Number of patients	81
Age at operation (years)—mean ± SD	65 ± 11
Male sex—n (%)	52 (64%)
Body mass index (BMI)—mean ± SD	26.6 ± 4.8
Co-morbidities ≥ 1 — n (%)	54 (67%)
ASA class I—n (%)	6
ASA class II—n (%)	47
ASA class III—n (%)	8
ASA class IV—n (%)	3
Missing data on ASA	17
Preoperative assessment (Endoscopy)	
Distance from anal verge (cm)—mean ± SD	7 ± 3.5
Largest diameter of lesion (cm)—mean ± SD	3.3 ± 3.1
Type of polyp	
Sessile polyp—n (%)	40 (49%)
Pedunculated polyp—n (%)	13 (16%)
Missing data—n (%)	28 (35%)
Preoperative biopsy report	
Low-grade dysplasia (LGD)	49 (60%)
High-grade dysplasia (HGD)	12 (15%)
Well-differentiated adenocarcinoma	3 (4%)
Moderately differentiated adenocarcinoma	2 (2%)
Poorly differentiated adenocarcinoma	0
Missing data	15 (19%)
Preoperative imaging	
ERUS was performed—n (%)	37 (46%)
MRI Pelvis was performed—n (%)	8 (10%)

ASA—American Society of Anesthesiology score; ERUS—Endorectal ultrasound; MRI—Magnetic resonance imaging.

3.1. Preoperative Workup

All 81 patients with final pathology of LGD underwent a colonoscopy for surveillance or colorectal symptoms that showed a rectal polyp with a mean size of 3.3 ± 3.1 cm, at an average distance of 7 ± 3.5 cm from the anal verge. Endoscopy reports of the type of polyps seen were 40 (49%) sessile polyps and 13 (16%) pedunculated polyps, and 28 (35%) had missing endoscopic data. Although the final pathology was low-grade dysplasia for all cases, the initial preoperative biopsy reports were low-grade dysplasia for 49 patients (60%), 12 (15%) high-grade dysplasia, 3 (4%) well-differentiated adenocarcinoma, 2 (2%) moderately differentiated adenocarcinomas, and 15 (19%) had missing biopsy data. Thirty-seven of the 81 patients (46%) had imaging with endorectal ultrasound (ERUS), and eight of 81 (10%) had pelvic magnetic resonance imaging (MRI), seven of whom had also undergone a ERUS (Table 1).

3.2. Surgical Techniques and Operational Findings

The rectal lesions were resected using three main platforms. Twenty of eighty-one patients (25%) underwent a standard "open" transanal excision, 36 (44%) were operated on using the TAMIS platform, and 25 (31%) via the TEM platform. The mean distance of the lesions from the anal verge was 7.2 ± 4.3 cm, with a mean lesion size of 2.8 ± 1.6 cm. The depth of resection was a full thickness resection in 68 (84%) patients, partial thickness resection in 6 (7%), mucosal resection in 4 (5%), and a piecemeal resection in 3 (4%) patients. The rectal wall defect after resection was closed with a running suture in 49 (61%) cases, with interrupted sutures in 27 (33%), and was left open in 5 (6%). There were no intraoperative complications, and only one case (1%) had an added laparoscopy that ruled out intraabdominal penetration.

3.3. Complication and Pathology Reports

The average length of hospital stay was 3.6 ± 1.8 days, and there were 12 (15%) cases with postoperative complications. Two cases of bleeding, six of wound infection or abscesses, two of cardiac or respiratory complications, and two of transient fecal incontinence. Only four (5%) cases were regarded as a Clavien-Dindo complication score of 3b or more. From the pathology reports, the mean diameter of the lesions was 3.2 ± 1.8 cm. Forty-seven lesions (58%) had a clear margin of over 3 mm; 18 (22%) had clear margins, but were under 3 mm; four (5%) had involved margins; and margin data was missing in 12 patients (15%). One patient (1%) with an involved margin underwent a repeat local excision attempt (Table 2).

3.4. Follow-Up, Recurrence, and Rectal Cancer Rate

Nine (11%) patients with LGD were found to have local intraluminal rectal cancer on follow-up. The mean follow-up was 25.3 ± 22.4 months. The average time interval from the first local excision to the diagnosis of the cancerous recurrence was 19.3 ± 14.5 months (range 5.2–54 months), with seven of nine (78%) of them diagnosed within less than two years from the initial LE. Reviewing the original reports of these nine cases showed that they all had an original low-grade dysplasia on the preoperative endoscopic biopsy and on final postoperative pathology. The average size of the original lesions was 3.5 cm (range 1.4–7 cm). Six patients had a clear margin of over 3 mm, and three had involved margins with low-grade dysplasia. The original resection depth was full-thickness resection in four patients, one had a partial thickness resection, one had a mucosal resection, and three had a piecemeal resection in more than one piece. The treatment modality chosen following rectal cancer diagnosis was a redo local excision in seven patients, one underwent a low anterior resection, and one got radiotherapy alone (Table 3).

Table 2. Surgical techniques, operational findings, complications, and pathology reports.

Characteristic	(n = 81)
Operative technique	
TAE—n (%)	20 (25%)
TAMIS—n (%)	36 (44%)
TEM—n (%)	25 (31%)
Distance from anal verge (cm)—mean ± SD	7.2 ± 4.3
Largest diameter of lesion (cm)—mean ± SD	2.8 ± 1.6
Predominant rectal wall location	
Posterior wall	19 (23%)
Anterior wall	18 (22%)
Lt lateral wall	21 (26%)
Rt lateral wall	13 (16%)
Unknown	10 (13%)
Depth of resection	
Full-thickness resection	68 (84%)
Partial-thickness resection	6 (7%)
Mucosal resection	4 (5%)
Piecemeal (in >1 piece)	3 (4%)
Defect closure approach	
Running suture	49 (61%)
Interrupted sutures	27 (33%)
Defect left open	5 (6%)
Intra-operative complications	0
Laparoscopy added—no complication found	1 (1%)
LOS—Length of stay (days)—mean ± SD	3.6 ± 1.8
Postoperative complications	12 (15%)
Bleeding	2 (2%)
Wound infection/Abscess	6 (7%)
Cardiac/Respiratory complication	2 (2%)
Transient fecal incontinence	2 (2%)
Clavien-Dindo ≥ 3B	4 (5%)
Final pathology	
Largest diameter of lesion (cm)—mean ± SD	3.2 ± 1.8
Margins	
Clear margins >3 mm	47 (58%)
Clear margins <3 mm	18 (22%)
Involved margins	4 (5%)
Missing data	12 (15%)
Added treatment after pathology—Redo LE	1 (1%)

TEA—Transanal excision; TAMIS—Transanal minimally invasive surgery; TEM—Transanal endoscopic microsurgery; Clavien-Dindo—The Clavien-Dindo classification of surgical complications; LE—Local excision.

Table 3. Characteristics of recurrence cases.

Characteristic	(n = 9)
Local recurrence	9
Systemic recurrence	0
Time interval from LE to cancerous recurrence (months)—mean ± SD (range)	19.3 ± 14.5 (5.2–54)
Number of patients that recurred under 24 months	7 (78%)
Original largest diameter of lesion (cm)—mean (range)	3.5 (1.5–7)
Original margins	
Clear margins >3 mm	6/9
Clear margins <3 mm	0
Involved margins	3/9
Original depth of resection	
Full-thickness resection	4/9
Partial-thickness resection	1/9
Mucosal resection	1/9

Table 3. *Cont.*

Characteristic	(n = 9)
Piecemeal (in >1 piece)	3/9
Original operative platform used	
TAE—p/n	6/9
TAMIS—p/n	1/9
TEM—p/n	2/9
Treatment after recurrence	
Re-do local excision	7
LAR	1
Radiotherapy	1
Follow-up time (months)—mean ± SD	25.3 ± 22.4

LE—Local excision; SD—Standard deviation; p—Positive; n—Number; TEA—Transanal excision; TAMIS—Transanal minimally invasive surgery; TEM—Transanal endoscopic microsurgery; LAR—Low anterior resection.

4. Discussion

This study demonstrates a high risk (11%) for local recurrence and the development of rectal cancer in patients with low-grade dysplastic adenoma resected transanally from the rectum. Seven of the nine patients that developed cancer were diagnosed within two years of the original local excision of the pre-cancerous rectal lesion. Unlike high grade dysplastic rectal lesions that are suspected of cancer until proven otherwise and those with an involved dysplastic margin prompting re-excision, low-grade dysplastic lesions are not considered cancerous and might lead to a less stern approach and follow up. There is little data in the literature on the risk of these LGD patients and therefore at what intervals they should be endoscopically or clinically followed up with. Studies focusing on the risk of developing a possible malignant tumor seen on surveillance colonoscopies after three years showed that patients that had mild or mild/moderate dysplasia at the index polypectomy had a 3.5–5.5% risk of developing an advanced adenoma, not necessarily cancer, throughout the colon and rectum, mainly in the proximal colon [13,14]. It is important to state that these studies relate to endoscopic polypectomies and not specifically to surgically removed lesions, which are usually not endoscopically resectable.

A meta-analysis by Saini et al. tried to quantify the risk factors for an advanced adenoma to be found during a three-year surveillance colonoscopy. He found that patients with ≥3 adenomas, a large adenoma (≥1 cm), or a high-grade dysplasia at the index polypectomy are at an increased risk for recurrence of advanced adenomas and therefore might benefit from close surveillance colonoscopies [15]. Most colonoscopy surveillance guidelines for patients with a history of resected adenomas stratify patients into low or high risk for recurrent advanced adenomas and cancer. The allocation to low or high risk is based mainly on the size, the number of adenomas, and having an advanced adenoma at the index colonoscopy. However, they do not draw any distinction between colonic and rectal polyps [5,7].

The definition of an advanced adenoma in the gastroenterology literature is usually an adenoma that is ≥1 cm, has villous histology, has a high-grade dysplasia feature, or even colorectal cancer in it [16–18]. Adenomas with low-grade dysplasia are not considered advanced adenomas and, presumably, do not place the patient in the high-risk group. Often, LGD adenomas are larger than 1 cm and then are considered high risk. Most guidelines do not take colonic vs. rectal origin of the polyp, or even positive dysplastic margins, into account for risk stratification. All patients that developed rectal cancer in this cohort had original adenomas that were larger than one centimeter and would have been classified as high risk for recurrence and, according to local recommendations, would have been advised to return for a repeat colonoscopy in three years. Having said that, the data in this study showed that almost all patients who developed rectal cancer after resection of the LGD lesion had done so in under two years from the index LE.

Unlike rectal polyps, large unresectable colonic polyps are usually referred to surgery for segmental colonic resection. By doing so, we not only gain a proper histological diagnosis of the polyp but also employ a preventive measure for recurrence in that segment of large bowel (as surgical resection also includes lymph node clearance). As transanal local excision surgeries found their place in treating rectal lesions, especially MIS platforms such as TEM and TAMIS, it brought about a plethora of new challenges in how to regard pre-cancerous rectal polyps. Unlike endoscopic polypectomy from the rectum, LE surgery allows for larger polyps, full-thickness resection, and a higher regard for margins [10,19]. LE of these "unresectable" polyps replaced anterior resection, which would have been a more oncologically complete surgical treatment. Therefore, as these large rectal polyps can be removed entirely with the rectum left in place, is the patient at a higher risk, which leads to the question: should these patients adhere to a different surveillance time interval?

The US Multi-Society Task Force of Colorectal Cancer (MSTF), the American Society of Colon and Rectal Surgeons (ASCRS), and the National Comprehensive Cancer Network (NCCN) guidelines all recommend a repeat surveillance colonoscopy after removing a dysplastic lesion after three years, to detect and prevent CRC with no distinction between colon and rectum or modus of resection [20–22].

Our data suggest that large rectal polyps (≥ 1 cm) with LGD should be viewed in a different light, and it would be prudent to address them as highly suspicious lesions with a high risk for rectal cancer. Most of the polyps in the cohort were sessile polyps, some had a high suspicion of adenocarcinoma from the endoscopic biopsy, and most did not undergo specific pelvic imaging such as ERUS or pelvic MRI. From a technical point of view, not all lesions had a full-thickness resection, as five out of the nine patients that developed cancer had a partial thickness or piecemeal resection of the lesions, and six out of the nine patients that developed cancer had a transanal excision (TEA), a non-MIS technique, which is less common today. There were some postoperative complications, and not all lesions had clear dysplastic margins. These factors might account for seeding of free dysplastic cells or involved margins in the rectum that may explain the development of rectal cancer later in life.

From a pathology point of view, a lenient approach to non-cancerous lesions is prevalent, as they are not regarded as dangerous and, as such, lead to a more cursory pathological report [23]. The International Collaboration on Cancer Reporting (ICCR) recently published recommendations on pathology reporting of colorectal local excision specimens. There is little emphasis on grading dysplastic lesions and no specific recommendation for low-grade dysplasia [24]. In contrast to these findings, it is important to state that most of the diagnosed rectal cancer lesions were found to be early rectal cancer and were treated with another local excision. One patient underwent a low anterior resection, and one had radiotherapy. There was no distant disease found and no disease-related deaths.

The study's limitations revolve around its retrospective nature and its prolonged eleven-year period, during which time MIS LE has evolved and might have changed the approach to different lesions, as seen by the fact that more than half of recurrences occurred after TAE, with a non-full thickness resection and positive dysplastic margins but representing real-life practices. Although the multicentricity nature of the study is considered an advantage, it might allow for differences in patient selection and treatment choice that might have influenced the results. The relatively small sample size did not allow for a risk factors analysis. Adding to that, there was no active search for patients that recurred with only an adenoma (LGD or HGD) with no cancer, which might have augmented our findings' strengths.

5. Conclusions

Locally resected rectal polyps with low-grade dysplasia may carry a significant risk of recurring and developing cancer within two years. A more meticulous approach to the preoperative assessment, a full-thickness resection, the resection margins, and the didactic pathological report might aid in reducing this occurrence. These data suggest that these patients should adhere to a closer surveillance protocol Future studies should focus on assessing the optimal surveillance protocols and adherence for early detection of recurrence.

Author Contributions: Conceptualization, Y.R.; methodology, Y.R. and I.W.; data curation, N.H., A.H., B.L., E.G., G.R., M.S., L.S., H.G., M.K. (Muhammad Khalifa), A.B., N.W., M.K. (Marat Khaikin), H.T., N.I., D.D., S.A.; writing—original draft preparation, Y.R.; writing—review and editing, Y.R., N.H., A.H., B.L., E.G., G.R., M.S., L.S., H.G., M.K. (Muhammad Khalifa), A.B., N.W., M.K. (Marat Khaikin), H.T., N.I., D.D., S.A. and I.W.; All authors have read and agreed to the published version of the manuscript.

Funding: This research received no external funding.

Institutional Review Board Statement: The study was conducted in accordance with the Declaration of Helsinki and approved by the Institutional Review Board of Meir Medical Center (MMC-0179-20, 18/6/2020). This study was conducted in accordance with the ethical principles of the Declaration of Helsinki (Edinburgh 2000) and the approval of the Institutional Review Boards.

Informed Consent Statement: Patient consent was waived due to the retrospective nature of the study and the analysis used anonymous clinical data.

Data Availability Statement: Data will be available upon request from authors.

Conflicts of Interest: The authors have no related conflicts of interest to declare. The authors declare they do not have any financial or non-financial interests that are directly or indirectly related to this work.

References

1. Vogelstein, B.; Fearon, E.R.; Hamilton, S.R.; Kern, S.E.; Preisinger, A.C.; Leppert, M.; Smits, A.M.; Bos, J.L. Genetic alterations during colorectal-tumor development. *N. Engl. J. Med.* **1988**, *319*, 525–532. [CrossRef] [PubMed]
2. Winawer, S.J.; Zauber, A.G.; O'Brien, M.J.; Ho, M.N.; Gottlieb, L.; Sternberg, S.S.; Waye, J.D.; Bond, J.; Schapiro, M.; Stewart, E.T.; et al. Randomized Comparison of Surveillance Intervals after Colonoscopic Removal of Newly Diagnosed Adenomatous Polyps. *N. Engl. J. Med.* **1993**, *328*, 901–906. [CrossRef] [PubMed]
3. Robertson, D.J.; Greenberg, E.R.; Beach, M.; Sandler, R.S.; Ahnen, D.; Haile, R.W.; Burke, C.A.; Snover, D.C.; Bresalier, R.S.; McKeown-Eyssen, G.; et al. Colorectal cancer in patients under close colonoscopic surveillance. *Gastroenterology* **2005**, *129*, 34–41. [CrossRef] [PubMed]
4. Arditi, C.; Gonvers, J.-J.; Burnand, B.; Minoli, G.; Oertli, D.; Lacaine, F.; Dubois, R.; Vader, J.-P.; Filliettaz, S.S.; Peytremann-Bridevaux, I.; et al. Appropriateness of colonoscopy in Europe (EPAGE II) – Surveillance after polypectomy and after resection of colorectal cancer. *Endoscopy* **2009**, *41*, 209–217. [CrossRef]
5. Lieberman, D.A.; Rex, D.K.; Winawer, S.J.; Giardiello, F.M.; Johnson, D.A.; Levin, T.R. Guidelines for Colonoscopy Surveillance After Screening and Polypectomy: A Consensus Update by the US Multi-Society Task Force on Colorectal Cancer. *Gastroenterology* **2012**, *143*, 844–857. [CrossRef]
6. Waye, J.D.; Braunfeld, S. Surveillance Intervals after Colonoscopic Polypectomy. *Endoscopy* **1982**, *14*, 79–81. [CrossRef]
7. Winawer, S.J.; Zauber, A.G.; Fletcher, R.H.; Stillman, J.S.; O'Brien, M.J.; Levin, B.; Smith, R.A.; Lieberman, D.A.; Burt, R.W.; Levin, T.R.; et al. Guidelines for Colonoscopy Surveillance after Polypectomy: A Consensus Update by the US Multi-Society Task Force on Colorectal Cancer and the American Cancer Society. *CA: A Cancer J. Clin.* **2006**, *56*, 143–159.
8. Affi Koprowski, M.; Lu, K.C. Colorectal Cancer Screening and Postpolypectomy Surveillance. *Dis. Colon Rectum* **2021**, *64*, 932–935. [CrossRef]
9. Atallah, S.; Keller, D. Why the conventional parks transanal excision for early stage rectal cancer should be abandoned. *Dis. Colon Rectum* **2015**, *58*, 1211–1214. [CrossRef]
10. Leonard, D.; Colin, J.-F.; Remue, C.; Jamart, J.; Kartheuser, A. Transanal endoscopic microsurgery: Long-term experience, indication expansion, and technical improvements. *Surg. Endosc.* **2012**, *26*, 312–322. [CrossRef]
11. Khoury, W.; Igov, I.; Issa, N.; Gimelfarb, Y.; Duek, S.D. Transanal endoscopic microsurgery for upper rectal tumors. *Surg. Endosc.* **2014**, *28*, 2066–2071. [CrossRef]
12. Clavien, P.A.; Barkun, J.; De Oliveira, M.L.; Vauthey, J.N.; Dindo, D.; Schulick, R.D.; De Santibañes, E.; Pekolj, J.; Slankamenac, K.; Bassi, C.; et al. The Clavien-Dindo classification of surgical complications: Five-year experience. *Ann. Surg.* **2009**, *250*, 187–196. [CrossRef]
13. Bonithon-Kopp, C.; Piard, F.; Fenger, C.; Cabeza, E.; O'Morain, C.; Kronborg, O.; Faivre, J. Colorectal adenoma characteristics as predictors of recurrence. *Dis. Colon Rectum* **2004**, *47*, 323–333. [CrossRef] [PubMed]
14. van Stolk, R.U.; Beck, G.J.; Baron, J.A.; Haile, R.; Summers, R.; Group, P.P.S. Adenoma characteristics at first colonoscopy as predictors of adenoma recurrence and characteristics at follow-up. *Gastroenterology* **1998**, *115*, 13–18. [CrossRef] [PubMed]
15. Saini, S.D.; Kim, H.M.; Schoenfeld, P. Incidence of advanced adenomas at surveillance colonoscopy in patients with a personal history of colon adenomas: A meta-analysis and systematic review. *Gastrointest. Endosc.* **2006**, *64*, 614–626. [CrossRef] [PubMed]

16. Cordero, C.; Leo, E.; Cayuela, A.; Bozada, J.M.; Garcia, E.; Pizarro, M.A. Validity of early colonoscopy for the treatment of adenomas missed by initial endoscopic examination. *Rev. Esp. De Enferm. Dig.* **2001**, *93*, 519–528.
17. Nusko, G.; Mansmann, U.; Kirchner, T.; Hahn, E.G. Risk related surveillance following colorectal polypectomy. *Gut* **2002**, *51*, 424–428. [CrossRef]
18. Schatzkin, A.; Lanza, E.; Corle, D.; Lance, P.; Iber, F.; Caan, B.; Shike, M.; Weissfeld, J.; Burt, R.; Cooper, M.R.; et al. Lack of Effect of a Low-Fat, High-Fiber Diet on the Recurrence of Colorectal Adenomas. *N. Engl. J. Med.* **2000**, *342*, 1149–1155. [CrossRef]
19. Martin-Perez, B.; Andrade-Ribeiro, G.D.; Hunter, L.; Atallah, S. A systematic review of transanal minimally invasive surgery (TAMIS) from 2010 to 2013. *Tech. Coloproctol.* **2014**, *18*, 775–788. [CrossRef]
20. Rex, D.K.; Boland, C.R.; Dominitz, J.A.; Giardiello, F.M.; Johnson, D.A.; Kaltenbach, T.; Levin, T.R.; Lieberman, D.; Robertson, D.J. Colorectal Cancer Screening: Recommendations for Physicians and Patients from the U.S. Multi-Society Task Force on Colorectal Cancer. *Gastroenterology* **2017**, *153*, 307–323. [CrossRef]
21. Steele, S.R.; Hull, T.L.; Hyman, N.; Maykel, J.A.; Read, T.E.; Whitlow, C.B. *The ASCRS Manual of Colon and Rectal Surgery*; Springer: Berlin/Heidelberg, Germany, 2019.
22. Provenzale, D.; Ness, R.M.; Llor, X.; Weiss, J.M.; Abbadessa, B.; Cooper, G.; Early, D.S.; Friedman, M.; Giardiello, F.M.; Glaser, K.; et al. NCCN Guidelines Insights: Colorectal Cancer Screening, Version 2.2020. *J. Natl. Compr. Cancer Netw.* **2020**, *18*, 1312–1320. [CrossRef] [PubMed]
23. Khoury, R.; Duek, S.D.; Issa, N.; Khoury, W. Transanal endoscopic microsurgery for large benign rectal tumors; where are the limits? *Int. J. Surg.* **2016**, *29*, 128–131. [CrossRef] [PubMed]
24. Rosty, C.; Webster, F.; Nagtegaal, I.D.; Dataset Authoring Committee for the development of the IDfPRoCEB. Pathology Reporting of Colorectal Local Excision Specimens: Recommendations from the International Collaboration on Cancer Reporting (ICCR). *Gastroenterology* **2021**, *161*, 382–387. [CrossRef] [PubMed]

Disclaimer/Publisher's Note: The statements, opinions and data contained in all publications are solely those of the individual author(s) and contributor(s) and not of MDPI and/or the editor(s). MDPI and/or the editor(s) disclaim responsibility for any injury to people or property resulting from any ideas, methods, instructions or products referred to in the content.

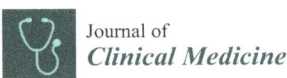 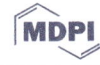

Review

Stage IV Colorectal Cancer Management and Treatment

Oscar Hernandez Dominguez [†], Sumeyye Yilmaz [†] and Scott R. Steele *

Department of Colorectal Surgery, Digestive Disease and Surgery Institute, Cleveland Clinic, Cleveland, OH 44195, USA
* Correspondence: steeles3@ccf.org; Tel.: +1-216-444-4715
† These authors contributed equally to this work.

Abstract: (1) Background: Colorectal cancer (CRC) is the third most common cancer and the second leading cause of cancer-related mortality worldwide. Up to 50% of patients with CRC develop metastatic CRC (mCRC). Surgical and systemic therapy advances can now offer significant survival advantages. Understanding the evolving treatment options is essential for decreasing mCRC mortality. We aim to summarize current evidence and guidelines regarding the management of mCRC to provide utility when making a treatment plan for the heterogenous spectrum of mCRC. (2) Methods: A comprehensive literature search of PubMed and current guidelines written by major cancer and surgical societies were reviewed. The references of the included studies were screened to identify additional studies that were incorporated as appropriate. (3) Results: The standard of care for mCRC primarily consists of surgical resection and systemic therapy. Complete resection of liver, lung, and peritoneal metastases is associated with better disease control and survival. Systemic therapy now includes chemotherapy, targeted therapy, and immunotherapy options that can be tailored by molecular profiling. Differences between colon and rectal metastasis management exist between major guidelines. (4) Conclusions: With the advances in surgical and systemic therapy, as well as a better understanding of tumor biology and the importance of molecular profiling, more patients can anticipate prolonged survival. We provide a summary of available evidence for the management of mCRC, highlighting the similarities and presenting the difference in available literature. Ultimately, a multidisciplinary evaluation of patients with mCRC is crucial to selecting the appropriate pathway.

Keywords: metastatic colorectal cancer; stage IV colon cancer; stage IV rectal cancer; treatment of stage IV colorectal cancer

Citation: Hernandez Dominguez, O.; Yilmaz, S.; Steele, S.R. Stage IV Colorectal Cancer Management and Treatment. *J. Clin. Med.* **2023**, *12*, 2072. https://doi.org/10.3390/jcm12052072

Academic Editor: Shmuel Avital

Received: 8 February 2023
Revised: 2 March 2023
Accepted: 4 March 2023
Published: 6 March 2023

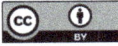

Copyright: © 2023 by the authors. Licensee MDPI, Basel, Switzerland. This article is an open access article distributed under the terms and conditions of the Creative Commons Attribution (CC BY) license (https://creativecommons.org/licenses/by/4.0/).

1. Introduction

Colorectal cancer (CRC) is the third most common cancer and the second leading cause of cancer-related mortality worldwide, with an estimated 1.9 million cases and 935,000 deaths annually [1,2]. In the United States, close to 1.37 million people were living with CRC and it is estimated that there were 52,580 deaths in 2022, making CRC the second most common cause of cancer-related deaths [3,4]. The average 5-year relative survival rate for all stages of CRC is 65.1% [3]. However, the cancer stage has a strong influence on survival. In stage IV CRC (metastatic CRC (mCRC)), defined as cancer spread to distant sites or organs or peritoneal metastasis, the 5-year survival rate significantly drops to 15.1% [3].

Approximately 22% of CRC cases have metastasis at presentation, and 19% will develop metachronous metastasis [3–6]. The most common sites of metastasis listed in order are the liver, lung, and peritoneum [5,7]. The site of metastasis has an impact on survival. To reflect this, stage IV mCRC is further classified based on metastasis to one site or organ (IVa), multiple sites or organs (IVb), or whether peritoneal metastasis is present (IVc). In addition to the site of metastasis, studies have also shown that the timing, number, and originating location of metastasis may also impact survival [6–8]. The heterogeneity of mCRC has demanded continued development in diagnosis and pretreatment testing as this is crucial in facilitating a multi-disciplinary approach to treatment.

The standard of care for mCRC primarily consists of surgical resection and systemic therapy. Unlike other stage IV cancers, surgical resection of mCRC can significantly prolong survival. In some cases, resection of liver and lung mCRC can even be curative [9–11]. A survival advantage has even been shown in peritoneal metastasis versus palliative care [12,13]. Additionally, the evolution of systemic therapy has improved mCRC survival or allowed the conversion of unresectable mCRC to resectable [14]. More recent additions of treatments targeted therapy of specific genetic tumor mutations (e.g., EGFR, VEGF, KRAS) and immunotherapy agents have also provided survival benefits in certain mCRC [9,11,15–18]. As the spectrum of treatment options for mCRC has grown, the cost of treating mCRC has also widened. Studies report the average costs of treatment can range from $12,000 to almost $300,000 due to the heterogeneity of treatment plans [19].

As research continues to uncover tumor-specific treatment options in mCRC, understanding the variety of treatment options is essential for increasing patient survival and decreasing the healthcare burden. This review summarizes current evidence regarding the management of mCRC to provide critical aid when making a treatment plan for the heterogenous spectrum of mCRC.

2. Materials and Methods

A comprehensive literature search of the Cochrane Database of Collected Research, PubMed, and EMBASE was performed. Our search strategy included different combinations of terms related to 'stage IV CRC', 'colorectal metastases', 'diagnosis of stage IV CRC', 'surgery for mCRC', 'systemic treatment for mCRC' in "All fields", and the related Mesh terms to identify English-language publications. Current guidelines written by major cancer societies, including the National Comprehensive Cancer Network (NCCN) [20,21], the European Society of Medical Oncology (ESMO) [22], the Japanese Society for Cancer of the Colon and Rectum (JSCCR) [23], the American Society of Colon and Rectal Surgeons (ASCRS) [24] are also reviewed. The references of the included studies were screened to identify additional studies that were incorporated as appropriate.

We did not seek Institutional Review Board approval as this type of study, a literature review does not require approval since no patient data are accessed or analyzed.

3. Diagnosis of Stage IV Colorectal Cancer

Staging has critical implications for the treatment plan and survivability of patients with mCRC. Diagnostic staging of mCRC mainly consists of laboratory tests and imaging, with a similar foundation as CRC staging. Adjunct imaging is mostly required to determine if a patient with mCRC can undergo curative resection.

For suspected or proven synchronous mCRC, guidelines suggest a total colonoscopy with biopsy be completed. Laboratory tests should include a complete blood count (CBC), a chemistry panel, and baseline carcinoembryonic antigen (CEA). In recent studies, elevated carbohydrate antigen (CA) 19-9 levels have been reported to be a predictor of poor survival [25,26]. Nevertheless, obtaining a CA 19-9 is optional per ESMO guidelines and not required by NCCN guidelines [20–22]. A computed tomography (CT) with intravenous (IV) and oral contrast of the chest, abdomen, and pelvis has long been the staple imaging modality for CRC [27]. Magnetic resonance imaging (MRI) with IV contrast of the abdomen can be helpful in cases where CT is insufficient in evaluating a metastatic lesion, particularly for the operative evaluation of metastatic liver lesions [28]. A positron emission tomography (PET)/CT scan is not recommended in routine diagnosis, staging, or surveillance. PET/CT should mainly be reserved for select cases of potentially resectable mCRC lesions. For example, during the preoperative evaluation of patients with high suspicion of previously unrecognized, or high extent mCRC that would exclude surgery [20,22]. The same laboratory testing and imaging recommendations apply to metachronous mCRC.

Subtle, but essential differences are present between colon and rectal cancer diagnostic staging. For the evaluation of rectal cancer, a pelvic MRI with contrast is a crucial addition for diagnosis, treatment, and surveillance due to its superior capability of evaluating tumor depth and prediction of circumferential resection margin (CRM) [21,29–31]. Furthermore, MRI detection of involved CRM has been reported to have a significant association with distant metastatic disease [30]. Endoscopic ultrasound (EUS) can also be used to evaluate rectal cancer. However, due to its decreased accuracy in staging and operator dependence, recent guidelines recommend EUS be reserved mainly when MRI is contraindicated [32,33]. A proctoscopy can be considered for the evaluation of rectal cancer. Proctoscopy can help determine an accurate distance between the anal verge and the primary tumor, which is important when determining if it is a low colon versus rectal cancer [34].

4. Treatment Strategies for Stage IV Colorectal Cancer

Treatment of mCRC is challenging and involves different modalities such as chemotherapy, radiotherapy (RT), and surgery. Multidisciplinary evaluation of patients is crucial, as there is no absolute treatment strategy [24]. Treatment strategies and goals are determined according to:

Tumor- and disease-related factors (e.g., synchronous or metachronous metastases, location and resectability of metastases and the primary tumor, presence of primary tumor-related symptoms, pathology, and molecular profiling).

Patient-related factors (e.g., Eastern Cooperative Oncology Group (ECOG) performance status [35], co-morbidities, patient expectations).

Treatment-related factors (e.g., toxicity) [20–23].

4.1. Treatment of Synchronous Metastases

Treatment of synchronous mCRC largely depends on the location and resectability of metastases. As a general rule, surgical resection combined with systemic treatment achieves the best cure in patients with resectable metastases. Whereas in the setting of unresectable disease, management depends on the degree of primary tumor-related symptoms. The treatment algorithm based on NCCN [20,21] and ASCRS [24] guidelines is summarized in Figure 1.

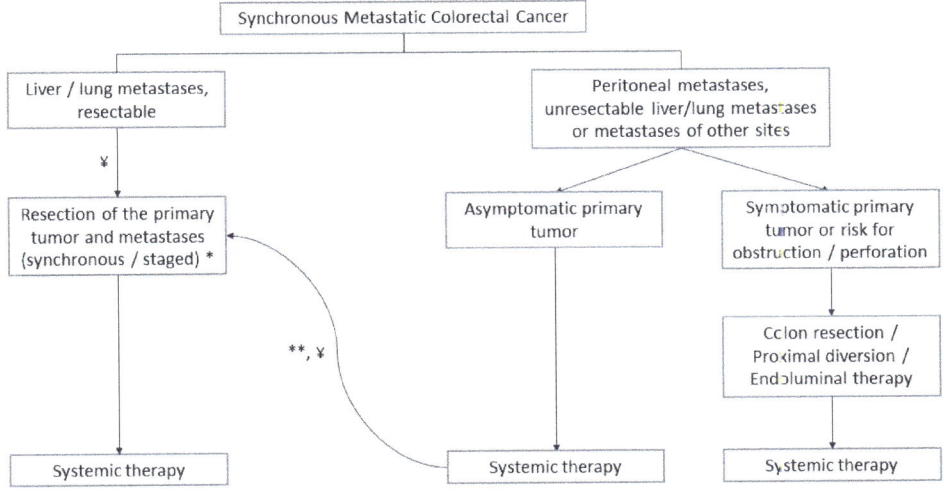

*Perioperative chemotherapy (neoadjuvant or between colectomy and metastasectomy) can be considered.
**Patients with unresectable liver/lung metastases should be re-evaluated every 2 months and surgery should be considered if conversion to resectable disease occurs.
¥If the primary tumor is in rectum, short course radiotherapy (preceded by chemotherapy if no previous systemic treatment) is given before resection of the primary tumor.

Figure 1. Treatment Algorithm for Metastatic Synchronous Adenocarcinoma of the Colon and Rectum.

4.1.1. Management of the Primary Tumor in the Setting of Unresectable Disease

The most common symptoms associated with CRC are bleeding, obstruction, and perforation. Chronic bleeding oftentimes presents itself with anemia, which can be managed non-operatively. However, acute significant blood loss requires intervention. For proximal cancers, resection is preferred [24]. Other treatments such as endovascular procedures (e.g., embolization, coiling, stents) [36,37] and radiation [38] can provide quick and effective palliation, with the latter being particularly effective in the rectum.

About 8–30% of patients with CRC present with partial or complete obstruction [24]. Further, up to 6% of patients with unresectable mCRC eventually require urgent surgical treatment due to obstruction or perforation [39], which is associated with reduced overall survival (OS) [24,40]. Compared to surgery, treating malignant obstruction with a colonic stent is associated with faster recovery, fewer complications, and a shorter time to chemotherapy onset, which is an important predictor of OS [41–43]. However, distal rectal tumors may not be amenable to stenting. Primary tumors that cause bowel perforation are associated with a poor prognosis [44], and resection is the preferred treatment.

Resection of the primary asymptomatic tumor in the presence of unresectable mCRC is not recommended [20,21]. In their review, Cirocchi et al. [39] failed to show an association between primary tumor resection with OS. Kanemitsu et al. [45] published a randomized controlled trial (RCT) showing no survival benefit of primary tumor resection in the setting of unresectable mCRC. It seems like these patients die as a result of their systemic disease rather than primary tumor-related complications [39].

4.1.2. Liver Metastases

The liver is the most common metastatic site for mCRC. Around 11.8–14.4% of patients with colon and 9.5–12.5% with rectum cancer has liver metastases at the time of diagnosis [23,46]. The most common route of dissemination is hematogenous via the portal system [47].

According to European Colorectal Metastases Treatment Group (ECMTG), colorectal liver metastases (CRLMs) are classified into four groups: M0 (no metastases), M1a (resectable metastases), M1b (potentially resectable liver metastases), and M1c (liver metastases that are unlikely to ever become resectable) [48]. At the time of diagnosis, 20–25% of patients with CRLMs have resectable or potentially resectable lesions [24,49]. Surgery represents the only curative option for resectable CRLM. Current guidelines recommend performing a CRLM resection when curative resection (R0—resection with microscopically negative margins) is possible [20–24], there are no uncontrollable extrahepatic metastases, the function of the remaining liver is adequate, and the patient is capable of tolerating surgery [20,23]. Alternative to upfront resection, perioperative chemotherapy can be administered, which may increase progression-free survival (PFS) and OS [50,51]. Five-year OS rates following surgery are above 30% [52,53], approaching 58% in selected patients [23,54,55].

In the setting of unresectable synchronous liver metastases, systemic chemotherapy is recommended, with surgery being reserved for patients with primary tumor-related symptoms [20,22,24]. Re-evaluation should be performed every two months [20,22], as conversion from unresectable to resectable disease can be observed in 15–50% of patients [47]. Following conversion chemotherapy, R0 resection of hepatic metastases is associated with better survival than if resection was not performed [22,56]. Therefore, synchronous or staged resection of the primary tumor and metastases is recommended if conversion to resectable disease occurs [20,24]. The treatment algorithm and goals for colorectal liver or lung metastases are summarized in Figure 1 and Table 1.

Table 1. Treatment of Colorectal Cancer with Liver/Lung Metastases.

Resectability of Metastases	Treatment Goal	Treatment Strategy
R0-resectable liver or lung metastases	Cure/No evidence of disease	R0 resection of the primary tumor and all metastases *Possible better long-term outcomes with perioperative ChT* Adjuvant therapy/Observation
Potentially resectable metastatic disease	Cure/No evidence of disease	Doublet/Triplet ChT ± targeted therapy R0 resection after conversion to resectable disease Adjuvant therapy/Observation
Unlikely to ever become resectable disease	Symptom control Prolonged survival Better QoL	Doublet/Triplet ChT ± targeted therapy *Surgery in the presence of (or high-risk for) primary tumor-related symptoms*

ChT: Chemotherapy, QoL: Quality of Life. R0 resection: Resection with histologically proven negative margins, in which no gross or microscopic tumor remains in the primary tumor bed. Conversion: Downstaging from unresectable to resectable disease.

Ideally, R0 resection of CRLMs should be performed while maintaining adequate hepatic function. To maintain adequate liver function and prevent post-hepatectomy liver failure, future liver remnant (FLR) should be more than 20% of the total liver volume in a healthy, chemotherapy-naïve patient, 30% in a chemotherapy-treated patient, and 40% in patients with any evidence of cirrhosis or fibrosis [9,57]. Increasing emphasis on preserving the volume of FLR has led to several treatment strategies. Parenchymal-sparing hepatectomy (PSH), one of these strategies, is a widely-practiced surgical approach aiming to achieve R0 resection of the tumor while maintaining as much liver parenchyma as possible. Deng et al. [58] conducted a meta-analysis comparing the outcomes of PSH vs. non-PSH and reported comparable 3-year and 5-year OS and recurrence-free survival (RFS) rates. Furthermore, non-PSH was associated with higher postoperative complications and 90-day mortality rates. In their systematic review, Moris et al. [59] also reported comparable OS rates for PSH vs. anatomic resection. Nevertheless, the decision to proceed with PSH or non-PSH is made based on multiple factors such as tumor number, size, location [60,61], and the presence of specific mutations [62]. There is no clear consensus regarding the resection margin during PSH [20,24,63].

Regarding the timing of the surgery, simultaneous or staged (metachronous) resection of the primary tumor and metastases can be performed. Traditionally, resection of the primary tumor followed by systemic chemotherapy and resection of metastases (bowel-first) has been preferred. The liver-first strategy was proposed to address metastatic disease first, as it is the primary determinant of OS [64]. Depending on the difficulty of the colectomy or hepatectomy, the medical condition of the patient, and the surgeon's expertise, simultaneous colon and liver resection can safely be performed without compromising long-term oncological outcomes [65–67]. However, simultaneous resection is avoided when there is a primary tumor-related complication such as bleeding, obstruction, and perforation [52].

Dealing with a higher volume of total liver tumors or multiple bilobar liver disease requires more advanced strategies, as extended hepatectomy might result in post-hepatectomy liver failure [9]. When hepatic metastases are considered unresectable due to inadequate FLR, two-stage hepatectomy with or without portal vein embolization (PVE) can be considered [68]. This technique involves complete resection of metastases from the FLR (first stage hepatectomy), followed by PVE 2–5 weeks after the first stage hepatectomy, and second stage hepatectomy [69,70]. Dropout after the first stage is the major drawback of this operation, which can be seen in up to 35% of the patients [71], majorly due to tumor progression and sometimes insufficient FLR volume. Nevertheless, a 5-year survival rate of up to 64% for patients who complete the second stage reinforces the benefit of this procedure [72].

Associating liver partition and portal vein ligation for staged hepatectomy (ALPPS) involves portal vein ligation with tumoral clearance of the FLR and in situ splitting of the liver parenchyma, followed by a second operation 1–2 weeks later [70]. Compared to other techniques, ALPPS is associated with the highest growth rate for the FLR [73,74]. With ALPPS, more patients complete the second stage of hepatectomy, and the waiting interval between the two stages is shorter [74–78]. Although some RCTs and meta-analyses reported similar outcomes [75,76], the major concern about ALPPS remains to be the high postoperative morbidity and mortality rates [74,78]. Nevertheless, OS and RFS rates seem to be similar for two-stage hepatectomy and ALPPS [77,78].

Local ablative treatments (e.g., radiofrequency ablation (RFA), microwave ablation (MWA)) are commonly used in the treatment of CRLMs to increase resectability and achieve curative treatment in poor surgical candidates and patients with unresectable disease due to unfavorable tumor location or multilobar metastases. When combined with systemic therapy, RFA and MWA offer better disease-free survival and OS compared to chemotherapy alone [79–81]. These techniques may also be safely used as an adjunct to surgery in the presence of CRLMs, providing RFS and OS rates similar to surgery alone [82]. Transarterial chemoembolization (TACE) and radioembolization (TARE) are considered salvage therapies for patients with CRLMs not amenable to surgery or ablation who fail systemic chemotherapy [24]. Stereotactic body radiation therapy (SBRT) delivers high-dose radiation to tumoral tissues. It may be considered for the treatment of unresectable CRLMs and in the setting of oligometastatic disease (OMD), however, limited data exists on the outcomes of SBRT for CRLMs [83,84].

Liver transplantation has previously been proposed as a treatment option for unresectable CRLMs [85]. However, due to the high recurrence rate and poor OS, liver transplantation for CRLMs was abandoned. Groundbreaking research from Oslo [86] reintroduced liver transplantation for CRLMs, with 5-year OS rates reaching 60%. Predictors of survival in the first study led authors to define the Oslo Score (Table 2) and design the second study (SECA-II), which showed that with more strict selection criteria, 5-year OS rates of 83% can be achieved [87]. Although limited by organ availability, liver transplantation may offer a promising treatment option for patients with unresectable CRLMs.

Table 2. Oslo Score.

Maximum tumor diameter > 5.5 cm
CEA levels > 80 µg/L
Time from primary cancer surgery to liver transplantation < 2 years
Progression under chemotherapy

Each risk factor is equal to 1 point. An Oslo Score of 0–2 is associated with better overall survival.

4.1.3. Lung Metastases

Lungs are the second most common site for mCRC after the liver. Approximately 10–22% of patients with CRC have lung metastases at the time of diagnosis [24,52,88]. While cancers of the colon and upper rectum drain into the liver via the portal system, cancers of the middle and lower rectum can metastasize directly to the lungs via the inferior hemorrhoidal vein and inferior vena cava [89]. Due to this anatomical difference, pulmonary metastases are seen more frequently in rectal cancer than in colon cancer [52,89]. Pulmonary metastases have slower growth and better survival than other metastases [90]. Following pulmonary metastasectomy, 5-year OS is usually above 50%, reaching up to 68% in patients with isolated lung metastases [24,52,89–91].

Management of lung metastases is similar to CRLMs (Figure 1 and Table 1) with surgical resection being the preferred practice in the setting of resectable disease [20,24,92]. However, unlike CRLMs, the literature on the outcomes of pulmonary metastasectomy is limited to retrospective case series, without a single prospective RCT [24,92]. The goal is to achieve R0 resection with the preservation of adequate pulmonary function. Usually, the tumor is amenable to wedge resection or segmental resection. A resection margin of 10 mm is recommended by several studies [93]. Studies reported no difference in RFS and OS after video-assisted thoracoscopic surgery (VATS) vs. open thoracotomy. However, lack of intraoperative palpation during VATS may preclude the detection of small metastases [94]. Pulmonary lobectomy in the setting of metastatic disease may be associated with poor prognosis [90]; therefore, is not recommended [93].

Mediastinal and hilar lymph node positivity can be seen in up to 44% of patients with pulmonary metastases, and it is associated with poor prognosis [89,90,95]. Dissection of the mediastinal and hilar lymph nodes can be considered; however, this has not improved survival [90].

Local ablative treatments can be used either alone or in conjunction with surgery for resectable pulmonary metastases. They can also be considered for OMD, unresectable metastases, or patients with high operative risk [20,24]. When surgical resection is not feasible, RFA and MWA are associated with improved survival [96]. For tumors larger than 3 cm, MWA and SBRT seem to be more effective in achieving local tumor control [97]. Data comparing SBRT to other techniques is scarce, nevertheless, it can be considered in highly selected cases such as centrally located lesions in the setting of OMD [97].

4.1.4. Peritoneal Metastases

Peritoneal metastases are seen in 5–17% of mCRC patients [9,52,98,99]. Underlying mechanisms include spontaneous seeding of tumor cells from a T4 CRC, extravasation of tumor cells as a result of either spontaneous or iatrogenic perforation, and transection of lymphatics during colon resection [100]. The most frequent signs and symptoms are ascites and intestinal obstruction [99]. Peritoneal metastasis is a well-known predictor of poor prognosis in CRC patients [101]. In fact, until recent advances in therapy, the presence of peritoneal metastases was thought to be representing a terminal disease [9].

According to NCCN guidelines, the primary treatment of peritoneal metastases is systemic chemotherapy. Surgical resection of the primary tumor should be considered in the presence of primary tumor-related symptoms, or imminent risk for obstruction (Figure 1) [20].

More recently, cytoreductive surgery (CRS) with or without hyperthermic intraperitoneal chemotherapy (HIPEC) has been performed for the treatment of CRC peritoneal metastases. CRS involves the removal of all macroscopic tumor tissue, involving peritonectomy, resection of involved organs, and omentectomy. HIPEC comprises intraperitoneal circulation of chemotherapeutics (most commonly oxaliplatin or mitomycin-C (MMC) based) to eradicate microscopically remnant tumor cells [52,99]. In their RCT, Verwaal et al. [102] reported increased OS for patients undergoing CRS + HIPEC (MMC-based) + adjuvant therapy vs. systemic therapy alone. Their study was limited by the inclusion of appendiceal carcinomas and patients discontinuing treatment due to toxicity or disease progression. Cashin et al. [103] designed an RCT comparing outcomes for patients undergoing CRS + HIPEC vs. systemic chemotherapy. Although terminated prematurely, their study managed to prove increased OS for patients undergoing CRS + HIPEC. However, it seems the completeness of cytoreduction is the predictor of OS [102–104]. PRODIGE 7 RCT [105] evaluated the role of HIPEC by comparing CRS + HIPEC vs. CRS alone. Their results showed no difference in OS. Additionally, Grade 3+ adverse events at 60 days were higher in the CRS + HIPEC group. Today, several guidelines recommend CRS plus chemotherapy for selected patients (Table 3) with peritoneal metastases [9,99,106]. However, HIPEC is not routinely recommended as an addition to CRS [22,83].

Synchronous colorectal liver and peritoneal metastases (CLPM) can be seen in 8% of stage IV CRC patients [98]. Studies report OS ranging from 13 to 45.7 months with a combination of CRS + HIPEC with liver resection (or ablation) for synchronous CLPM [107,108]. Nevertheless, the best strategy for the treatment of CLPM remains unclear [107].

Table 3. Selection Criteria for CRS ± HIPEC for CRC with Peritoneal Metastases.

ECOG performance status < 2
No major comorbidities (medically fit for surgery)
None-mild symptoms
Stable disease (no tumor progression) under chemotherapy
No extra-abdominal metastases *
Completeness of cytoreduction (CC score 0–1) possible
Peritoneal cancer index < 20
Patient's motivation and informed consent

CRC: Colorectal Cancer, CRS: Cytoreductive Surgery, ECOG: Eastern Cooperative Oncology Group, HIPEC: Hyperthermic Intraperitoneal Chemotherapy. * Presence of resectable hepatic metastases is not a contraindication to CRS and HIPEC.

4.1.5. Other Metastases

Approximately 5–10% of women with CRC develop ovarian metastasis, which is associated with a median OS of 19–27 months [109]. Ovarian metastasis can reach significant sizes without becoming symptomatic. Compared to other sites, ovarian metastasis is disproportionately unresponsive to chemotherapy. Several studies report better survival outcomes with surgical oophorectomy and cytoreduction, especially when R0 resection is achieved [109,110]. Routine prophylactic oophorectomy can be offered to postmenopausal women with mCRC, however, is not recommended for premenopausal women [24]. Recently, a Dutch trial has been proposed, aiming to evaluate the role of prophylactic oophorectomy in postmenopausal women, but no results have been published yet [111].

In addition to ovarian metastasis, CRC can metastasize to several other organs, including bone, brain, adrenal glands, and retroperitoneal lymph nodes. Bone metastasis is seen in 6–10.4% of the cases and is associated with poor OS [112]. Palliation of pain is an important part of treatment in patients with bone metastasis. Brain metastasis is rare (1–4%). Surgical resection of solitary metastasis is associated with OS of 30–40 weeks [23], and a local recurrence rate of 50–60% [24]. Stereotactic radiation therapy can achieve an 80–90% local control rate in patients with no more than 3–4 metastases that are <3 cm in diameter [23,24]. Whole brain radiation therapy (WBRT) can be an option for patients with multiple brain metastases, however, it is associated with increased side effects, and no improvement in OS [113]. Although there are controversies regarding the treatment of retroperitoneal and para-aortic lymph node metastases, a meta-analysis recently has shown improved OS following the resection of para-aortic lymph nodes, with no increase in postoperative complication rates [114].

4.1.6. Rectal Cancer

Management of stage IV rectal cancer with synchronous lung and/or liver metastases is different from colon cancer by the addition of RT to the treatment algorithm [21] (Figure 2). RT can be given either as short-course RT (25 Gy in five daily treatment fractions) or long-course chemoradiotherapy (CRT) (45–50.4 Gy in 25–28 fractions over 5–6 weeks with concurrent 5-FU infusion or capecitabine). Perioperative RT combined with surgery results in better OS [45,115]. Furthermore, preoperative RT is preferred over postoperative RT, because it is associated with reduced local recurrence risk [116–118]. In some patients, a complete response of the primary tumor to RT can be seen. In these patients, the watch-and-wait (W&W) approach can be considered. However, this approach can be associated with a high local regrowth rate [119]. Moreover, literature regarding the use of the W&W approach in stage IV rectal cancer is very limited.

Surgery can be performed immediately (within 1 week) or delayed (4–6 weeks) after RT. The ideal timing of surgery in relation to RT remains controversial. In the Stockholm III trial [120], patients with stage IV rectal cancer were divided into three groups (short-course RT (SCRT) with immediate surgery, SCRT with delayed surgery, and long-course RT with delayed surgery) to address this question. The results of this trial showed no difference between the three groups in cumulative incidences of local recurrence, distant metastases, and OS. In two-arm randomization, postoperative complications were more common in SCRT with delayed surgery group compared to SCRT with immediate surgery.

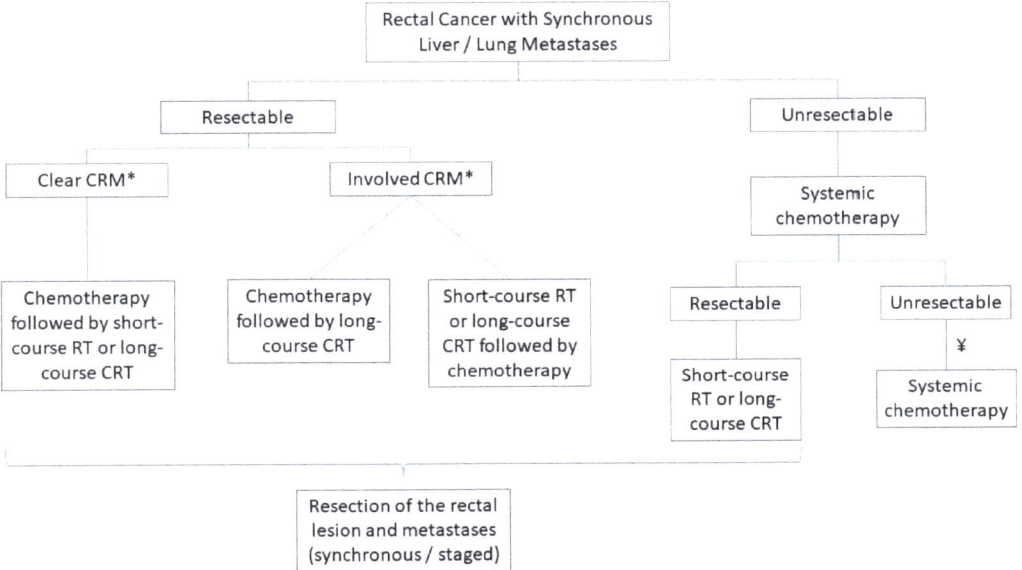

Figure 2. Treatment Algorithm for Stage IV Rectal Cancer with Synchronous Liver/Lung Metastases.

Although the timing of surgery is not important according to the Stockholm III trial [120], delaying hepatic resection until completion of systemic chemotherapy is concerning due to chemotherapy-induced liver changes, which may increase the risk for post-hepatectomy liver failure. Therefore, the current ASCRS guideline's recommendation is to perform immediate surgery following chemotherapy and SCRT if RT is planned after chemotherapy [24]. Another possible option can be to perform hepatic resection after 2–3 months of neoadjuvant chemotherapy, with an additional 3 months of chemotherapy followed by RT and then resection of the primary tumor.

4.2. Treatment of Metachronous Metastases

Up to 14–34% of patients with non-metastatic CRC will ultimately develop metachronous metastases [121]. Like synchronous metastases, the liver and lung are the most common site for metachronous metastases. The prognosis of CRC with metachronous metastases is better than CRC with synchronous metastases, with a recent study reporting 49.9% vs. 41.8% 1-year OS, and 13.2% vs. 6.2% 5-year OS in favor of metachronous CRLMs [122].

The treatment algorithm for CRC with metachronous metastases is summarized in Figure 3. When possible, resection of metastases is preferred. Whereas if the disease is unresectable, systemic therapy is the main treatment. Patients with an unresectable disease should be followed every 2 months for conversion to resectable disease. If conversion to resectable disease occurs, resection followed by observation or systemic therapy is recommended [20,21].

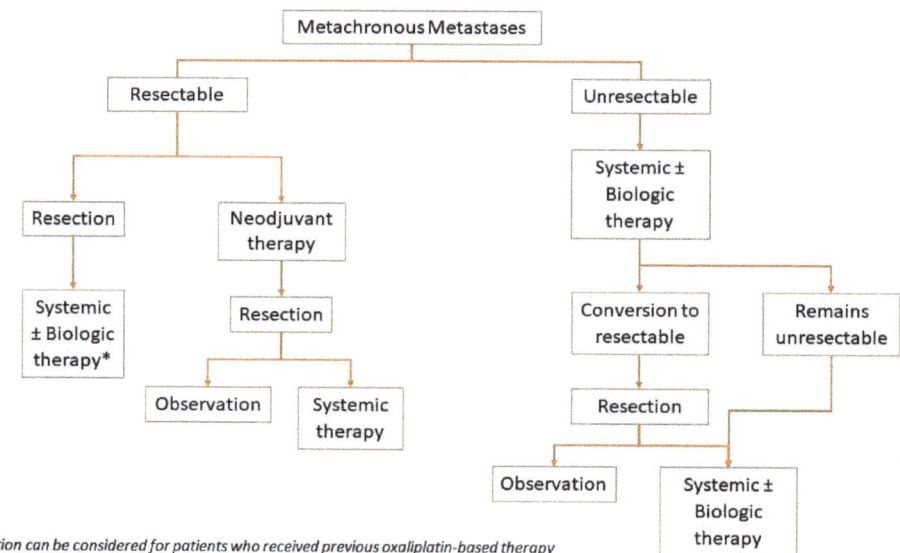

Figure 3. Treatment Algorithm for Metastatic Metachronous Adenocarcinoma of the Colon and Rectum.

4.3. Systemic Therapy

Along with surgery, systemic therapy is one of the primary components of mCRC treatments (Figures 4 and 5). Systemic therapy can offer a curative option or a palliative treatment. Advances in systemic therapy options and efficacy improved survival from 6 to 12 months to 2 to 3 years [16]. More recently, systemic therapy has played a growing role in unresectable mCRC, where it is increasingly being used to convert patients with an unresectable disease into suitable candidates for resection. Even among patients who initially undergo resection, systemic therapy is used to target occult nodal infiltration and micro-metastasis. Given the constant evolution and high complexity of systemic therapy, all patients with mCRC should be evaluated in a center with multidisciplinary specialists to help them determine the best combination of chemotherapy, targeted therapy, radiation, and available clinical trials.

Chemotherapy is the mainstay of systemic treatment for mCRC. Chemotherapy regimens will typically consist of a fluoropyrimidine (5-FU or capecitabine) paired in a two-drug regimen (doublet) with irinotecan or oxaliplatin. Treatment regimens can be 5-FU- or capecitabine-based and can be either oxaliplatin-based (FOLFOX or CAPEOX) or irinotecan-based (FOLFIRI or CAPIRI) with no difference in survival [123–126]. With similar efficacy between combinations, toxicity profiles can distinguish the optimal treatment regimen for individual patients. It is not uncommon for patients to transition between chemotherapy combinations due to intolerance of side effects or disease progression.

Bevacizumab, a monoclonal antibody that targets vascular endothelial growth factor (VEGF), has become a part of mCRC treatment starting in 2004 after an RCT showed OS advantages when bevacizumab was paired with 5-FU-based chemotherapy [127,128]. Treatment with fluoropyrimidine and bevacizumab has been shown to provide longer PFS in elderly patients unable to tolerate more aggressive doublet first-line treatments [129,130]. Bevacizumab can also be added to doublet chemotherapy in first-line therapy for select patients [131–133]. However, bevacizumab is not recommended in the perioperative period due to the risk of wound healing complications [128]. NCCN guidelines recommend holding bevacizumab 6 weeks before surgery and 6 to 8 weeks post-surgery after several studies found no difference in perioperative complications when bevacizumab was held during this period [20,21,134,135].

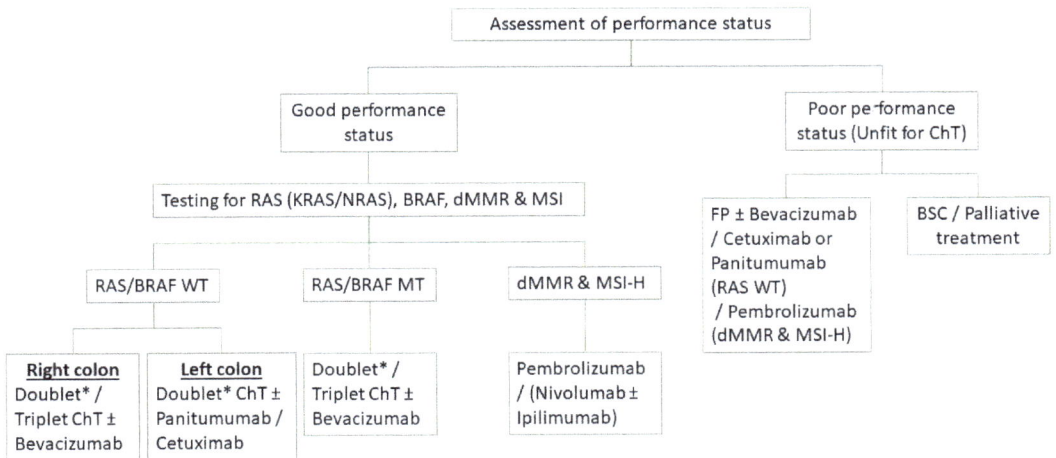

Figure 4. First-line Systemic Treatment for Stage IV CRC with Unresectable Metastases.

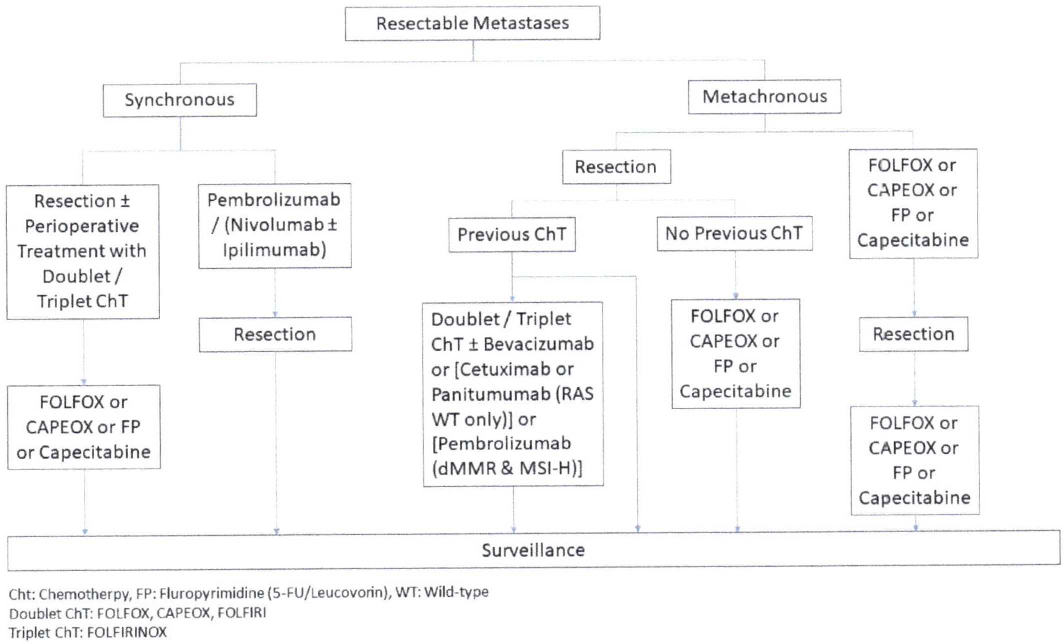

Figure 5. First-line Systemic Treatment for Stage IV CRC with Resectable Metastases.

Regimens with a three-drug (triplet) combination, FOLFIRINOX or FOLFOXIRI, are also available as first-line therapy and are commonly paired with bevacizumab. Major clinical guidelines recommend triplet therapy in patients that are optimally fit and without significant comorbidities [20–23]. NCCN recently updated their guidelines to replace the higher 5-FU dose in FOLFOXIRI with a lower 5-FU-dosed FOLFIRINOX due to patients in the USA having greater toxicity with 5-FU [20,21]. A meta-analysis by Cremolini et al. [136] evaluated unresectable mCRC European-based patients randomly assigned to either FOLFOXIRI plus bevacizumab or doublet regimen plus bevacizumab and found a significant benefit in OS and R0 resection rate in the FOLFOXIRI group. Of note, higher rates of neutropenia, mucositis, nausea, and diarrhea were observed and 99% of the patients in this analysis had an ECOG performance status from 0 to 1. However, the randomized phase III TRIPLETE study recently showed that modified FOLFOXIRI failed to provide benefits in overall response rate or R0 resection rates when compared to modified FOLFOX, but significantly increased GI toxicity side effects were seen with triplet therapy [137].

4.3.1. Molecular Profiling

The ability to analyze individual tumors for biomarkers (genes, proteins, or other molecules) has driven the growth of targeted therapy for mCRC. Currently, aberrations in microsatellite instability (MSI), mismatch repair (MMR), KRAS, NRAS, BRAF, and HER2 genes have been identified as significant biomarkers impacting therapy response. As a result, all major guidelines uniformly recommend that mCRC cases undergo molecular profiling at initial diagnosis to help personalize the most favorable systemic therapy regimen [20–23].

All major guidelines recommend patients with mCRC undergo testing for MMR deficiency (dMMR) or high MSI (MSI-H) [20–23], a mutation found in up to 5% of mCRC [138]. Universal testing of dMMR/MSI-H can help identify and counsel patients with Lynch syndrome, the most common cause of hereditary CRC, and it can also be a predictive marker for immunotherapy susceptible tumors. Tumors with dMMR/MSI-H evade immune-system destruction by blocking the PD-1 receptors on host T cells. PD-1 inhibitors (e.g., Nivolumab, Pembrolizumab) and cytotoxic T-lymphocyte associated protein 4 (CTLA-4) inhibitors (e.g., Ipilimumab) are immunotherapy treatments aimed at preventing dMMR/MSI-H tumors from escaping destruction. Clinical trials have shown that targeting dMMR/MSI-H mCRC with PD-1 inhibitors and CTLA-4 inhibitors results in a beneficial clinical response and improved survival [139,140]. Based on a recent analysis of the KEYNOTE-177 trial [141], most guidelines now recommend that pembrolizumab alone can be used as first-line therapy in dMMR/MSI-H mCRC.

Molecular profiling can also identify mutations that predict ineffective therapies. For example, mCRC tumors with mutations in the RAS gene (KRAS or NRAS), seen in approximately 40% of mCRC [142], have shown no treatment benefit from epidermal growth factor receptor (EGFR) inhibitors (e.g., panitumumab, cetuximab) [143,144]. Therefore, EGFR inhibitors are not recommended in patients with RAS-mutated mCRC. Moreover, determining RAS status with primary tumor location has been shown to affect treatment response. Wild-type RAS mCRC whose primary tumor originated in the right colon (cecum to hepatic flexure) has shown little benefit when treated with EGFR inhibitors but did show a favorable response with Bevacizumab [145–147]. Therefore, current guidelines suggest EGFR inhibitor treatment should only be first-line for wild-type RAS mCRC whose primary tumor originated from the left colon (splenic flexure to rectum) and bevacizumab for right-side originating mCRC [20–23,148].

BRAF V600E-variant tumors, found in approximately 6–9% of patients with mCRC [138], also do not benefit from treatment with EGFR inhibitors [149,150]. As a result, EGFR inhibitors are no longer included in the first-line treatment of the BRAF variant mCRC. However, longer survival and improved treatment response rates have been observed when the BRAF variant mCRC is treated simultaneously with EGFR inhibitors and BRAF inhibitors (e.g., encorafenib) [151,152]. EGFR inhibitors paired with BRAF inhibitors can be used as second-line treatment for wild-type RAS and BRAF V600E-variant mCRC. Additionally, BRAF mutations are a marker of a more aggressive phenotype and poor prognosis [153]. Multidisciplinary boards should consider the poor prognosis of this variant when determining therapy or inclusion in clinical trials.

Most recent ESMO and NCCN guidelines recommend testing wild-type RAS and wild-type BRAF mCRC patients for human epidermal growth factor receptor 2 (HER2) amplification, which is found in less than 5% of mCRC [20–22,154,155]. This recommendation comes as several studies have shown that mCRC tumors without mutations in RAS or BRAF, but exhibiting HER2 amplification, have favorable responses when treated with HER2 antagonists (e.g., trastuzumab, pertuzumab) [156,157]. When feasible, guidelines also recommend testing for NTRK fusions, which are found in less than 1% of CRC [158]. This is supported by multiple studies showing mCRC solid tumors with NTRK fusions had a favorable response rate when treated with NTRK inhibitors (e.g., larotrectinib and entrectinib) [159,160].

4.3.2. Maintenance Therapy

Continuation of induction therapy becomes difficult after achieving maximum response due to neuropathy and fatigue associated with oxaliplatin-based chemotherapy and FOLFIRI, respectively [161]. The concept of maintenance therapy includes reducing treatment intensity without compromising disease control [22]. It is used after first-line therapy for patients with unresectable mCRC until disease progression. Additionally, compared to a chemotherapy-free interval, maintenance therapy is associated with better PFS [162–167]. Several trials [162–173] including different maintenance strategies have been published (Table 4). Major guidelines recommend discussing maintenance therapy with patients and explaining side effect profiles of common options 5-FU/Leucovorin ± bevacizumab, cetuximab, or panitumumab [20–22].

4.3.3. Second-Line and Subsequent Therapy

Failure of systemic therapy is defined by the progression of metastatic disease. Second-line therapy describes systemic therapy options available after the failure of the first-line chemotherapy. Second-line therapy is tailored according to previous therapies (Figure 6). In general, patients who receive oxaliplatin-based chemotherapy upfront should be treated with irinotecan-based chemotherapy and vice versa [20–22]. The addition of biologics based on molecular profiling should be considered, given their association with increased OS [174–176]. Aflibercept and ramucirumab (in combination with FOLFIRI) can be considered as alternatives to bevacizumab for patients treated with oxaliplatin previously [175,176].

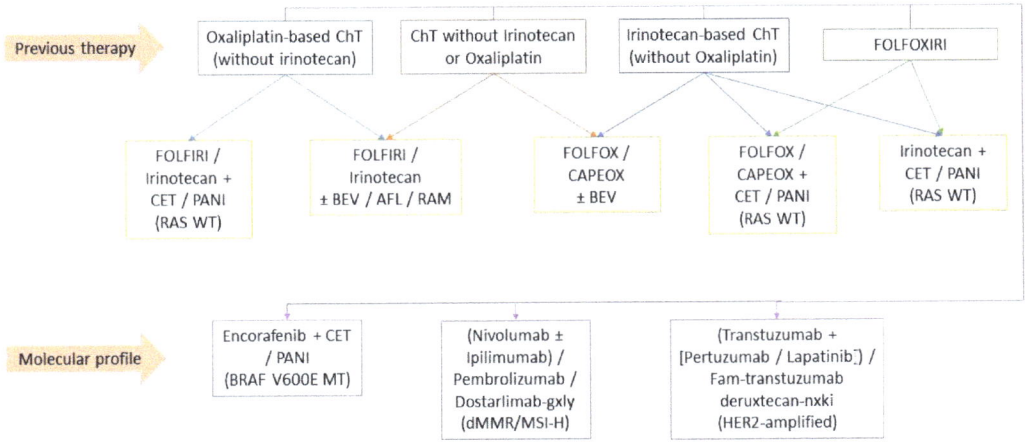

ChT: Chemotherapy, MT: Mutated, WT: Wild type

Figure 6. Second-line Systemic Treatment for Stage IV CRC.

Table 4. Trials on Different Regimens for Maintenance Therapy.

Study (Trial Name)	Induction Chemotherapy	Maintenance Therapy	Outcomes	Results	Significance
Chibaudel 2009 [162] (GERCOR OPTIMOX2)	mFOLFOX7	FP vs. No treatment	PFS OS	8.6 vs. 6.6 months, HR 0.61 23.8 vs. 19.5 months, HR 0.88	$p = 0.0017$ $p = NS$
Hegewisch-Becker 2015 [163] (AIO 0207 #)	CAPOX/FOLFOX + BEVA	FP + BEVA vs. BEVA vs. No treatment	PFS OS Grade 3–4 AEs	6.3 vs. 4.6 vs. 3.5 months 20.2 vs. 21.9 vs. 23.1 30.4% vs. 24.3% vs. 13.3%	$p < 0.0001$ $p = NS$ N/A *
Koeberle 2015 [164] (SAKK 41/06)	FP/FOLFOX/FOLFIRI + BEVA	BEVA vs. No treatment	PFS OS Grade 3–4 AEs	9.5 vs. 8.5 months, HR 0.75 25.4 vs. 23.8 months, HR 0.83 6.1% vs. 0.8%	$p = 0.025$ $p = NS$ N/A *
Simkens 2015 [165] (CAIRO3)	CAPOX + BEVA	CAP/BEVA vs. No treatment	PFS OS Grade 3–4 AEs	8.5 vs. 4.1 months, HR 0.4 25.9 vs. 22.4 months, HR 0.83 60% vs. 34%	$p < 0.0001$ $p = 0.06$ $p < 0.0001$
Luo 2016 [166]	CAPOX/FOLFOX	CAP vs. No treatment	PFS OS Grade 3–4 AEs	6.4 vs. 3.4 months, HR 0.54 25.6 vs. 23.3 months, HR 0.85 41.9% vs. 22.4%	$p < 0.001$ $p = NS$ N/A *
Aparicio 2018 [167] (PRODIGE 9)	FOLFIRI + BEVA	BEVA vs. No treatment	PFS PFS rate (12 months) OS	9.2 vs. 8.9 months, HR 0.91 30.2% vs. 21% 21.7 vs. 22 months, HR 1.11	$p = NS$ $p = NS$ $p = NS$
Diaz-Rubio 2012 [168] (MACRO TTD)	CAPOX + BEVA	BEVA vs. Continuation of ChT	PFS OS Grade 3–4 AEs	9.7 vs. 10.4 months, HR 1.10 20 vs. 23.2 months, HR 1.05 55% vs. 47%	$p = NS$ $p = NS$ N/A *
Yalcin 2013 [169] (Stop and Go)	CAPOX + BEVA	CAP + BEVA vs. Continuation of ChT	PFS OS Grade 3–4 AEs	11.0 vs. 8.3 months, HR 0.6 23.8 vs. 20.2 months 34.4% vs. 48.4%	$p = 0.002$ $p = NS$ $p = NS$
Hagman 2016 [170] (Nordic ACT2)	CAPOX/FOLFOX or CAPIRI/FOLFIRI ± BEVA	BEVA vs. BEVA + ERLO (KRAS WT)	PFS PFS rate (3 months) OS Grade 3–4 AEs	3.6 vs. 5.7 months, HR 0.93 64.7% vs. 63.6% 30.7 vs. 20.6 months, HR 0.58 25.7% vs. 58.2%	$p = NS$ $p = NS$ $p = 0.051$ N/A *
		BEVA vs. CAP (KRAS MT)	PFS PFS rate (3 months) OS Grade 3–4 AEs	3.9 vs. 3.7 months, HR 1.19 75% vs. 66.7% 26.4 vs. 28.0 months, HR 1.57 20.6% vs. 15.2%	$p = NS$ $p = NS$ $p = NS$ N/A *

Table 4. *Cont.*

Study (Trial Name)	Induction Chemotherapy	Maintenance Therapy	Outcomes	Results	Significance
Cremolini 2018 [171]	mFOLFOXIRI + CET	CET vs. BEVA (KRAS WT)	PFS OS Grade 3–4 AEs	13.3 vs. 10.8 months, HR 0.73 37.5 vs. 37 months, HR 0.98 25% vs. 8%	p = NS p = NS N/A *
Pietrantonio 2019 [172]	FOLFOX + PANI	FP + PANI vs. PANI	PFS rate (10 months) OS rate (18 months) Grade 3–4 AEs	59.9% vs. 49% 66.4% vs. 62.4% 42.4% vs. 20.3%	***p* = 0.01** p = NS N/A *
Modest 2021 [173] (PANAMA)	FOLFOX + PANI	FP + PANI vs. FP	PFS OS	8.8 vs. 5.7 months, HR 0.72 28.7 vs. 25.7 months, HR 0.84	***p* = 0.014** p = NS

BEVA: Bevacizumab, CAP: Capecitabine, CET: Cetuximab, ChT: Chemotherapy, ERLO: Erlotinib, FP: Fluoropyrimidine, PANI: Panitumumab, AE: Adverse events, HR: Hazard ratio, MT: Mutated, NS: Non-significant, OS: Overall survival, PFS: Progression-free survival, WT: Wild-type. * No information regarding significance level. # BEVA alone was non-inferior to FP + BEVA, whereas no treatment was not. Bold indicates that the difference between the results are statistically significant.

After progression on second-line therapy, patients with RAS/BRAF wild-type disease should receive an EGFR inhibitor combined with irinotecan. Alternatively, if they have HER2 mutation, transtuzumab can be preferred. If patients have BRAF V600E mutation, the encorafenib-cetuximab regimen should be considered [20,22]. Patients with RAS mutation who progressed under second-line therapy are considered to have the refractory disease [16]. Treatment with regorafenib or trifluridine and tipiracil is recommended for patients with refractory disease [16,20,22] as they may provide survival benefits compared to placebo [177,178].

5. Surveillance

The goal of surveillance in mCRC is to identify potentially resectable mCRC recurrences or new metachronous mCRC lesions. Surveillance protocols generally include follow-up visits with a clinical exam, tumor markers, imaging, and endoscopy. Generally, these follow-up visits occur up to 5 years after treatment, with more frequent surveillance in the first 2–3 years. This surveillance period is supported by evidence showing that 80–85% of CRC recurrence happens in the first 3 years, and less than 5% recur after 5 years [23,179,180]. Surveillance of mCRC is further justified by evidence showing surgical resection of recurrent mCRC can provide survival benefits. Butte et al. reported that up to 25% of patients that had resection of their mCRC recurrence were disease free at 36 months [181]. Therefore, surveillance can also help identify patients that are potentially curable of recurrent mCRC. It is important to note that evidence-based surveillance recommendations for mCRC are limited in the literature and the available recommendations are many times extrapolated from stage III CRC recommendations [182].

NCCN and ESMO have similar surveillance recommendations for history and physical (H&P) examination and CEA. Per NCCN, an H&P and CEA are recommended every 3 to 6 months (every 3 months per ESMO) for the first 2 years and then every 6 months for a total of 5 years. The ASCRS released guidelines in 2021, recommending an H&P and CEA every 3 to 12 months for the first 2 years and then every 6 to 12 months for the next 3 years. CEA surveillance routines are supported by the RCT, CEAwatch, which showed a significantly higher proportion of recurrence detected by CEA [183].

Most mCRC surveillance protocols recommend CT as the imaging modality of choice due to its ability to detect liver metastasis and resectable lung lesions [184]. For both colon and rectal cancer, NCCN and ESMO recommend a contrast-enhanced CT chest, abdomen, and pelvis every 3 to 6 months (3 months per ESMO) in the first 2 years and then every 6 to 12 months (6 months per ESMO) for up to a total of 5 years [20–22]. ASCRS has a less intense interval, recommending twice in 5 years or up to annually for 5 years in those with previously resected mCRC [185]. The variability in imaging frequency can likely be explained by a study from 2013, which showed that a higher frequency of imaging within 5 years did not result in increased survival in previously resected liver mCRC [186].

NCCN and ASCRS guidelines recommend colonoscopy 1 year after treatment, repeated in 3 years, and then every 5 years thereafter. For patients that did not have a preoperative colonoscopy due to an obstructing lesion, NCCN recommends a colonoscopy 3 to 6 months after surgery (1–6 months per ASCRS). Rectal cancer patients have additional surveillance depending on their treatment choice. For patients with transanal excision, NCCN recommends a rectal MRI or EUS every 3 to 6 months for 2 years, then every 6 months for a total of 5 years. ASCRS recommends a proctoscopy, possible rectal EUS, every 6 to 12 months for a total of 3 to 5 years in patients who underwent resection with anastomosis.

Other adjunct surveillance methods are being explored; however, no current evidence supports the addition of these to recent guidelines. PET/CT scans for routine surveillance are not recommended as they have not been shown to decrease mortality or detect resectable recurrence to justify the increased cost [187]. Additionally, there is insufficient evidence at the moment to recommend circulating DNA (ctDNA) as a surveillance method.

6. Future Direction of Stage IV Management

Although ctDNA does not have a role in the management of mCRC according to current guidelines, a recent large, prospective observational study including stage IV CRC patients demonstrated that postsurgical ctDNA at 4 weeks was a significant prognostic biomarker of recurrence. Kotani et al. [188] believe that ctDNA may be incorporated into staging criteria and predict adjuvant chemotherapy benefits in the future; however, randomized trials are lacking. Cancer stem cells are also being explored as a target of mCRC treatment due to their role in tumor growth, therapy resistance, metastasis, and relapse. However, no current clinical trials targeting CRC stem cells have been able to show relevant clinical activity in CRC treatment. Several trials were discontinued due to high toxicity and lack of anticancer activity [189]. Additionally, cancer stem cell biomarkers, like STAT3, are being explored for prognosis and patient-specific surveillance markers [190]. Tumor-driven changes have been observed in metabolic pathways such as glycolysis, lipid metabolism, and gut microbiota are also being explored as novel CRC treatment targets, but like cancer stem cells, pre-clinical research has not translated to promising clinical utility just yet [191].

7. Conclusions

CRC is the third most common cancer and the second cause of cancer-related mortality worldwide. Approximately 22% of patients with CRC have metastases at initial diagnosis. Management of mCRC is challenging, due to variable tumor extent and molecular characteristics. Unlike other stage IV cancers, surgical resection of metastases with curative intent is strongly recommended. Complete resection of liver, lung, and peritoneal metastases is associated with better disease control and survival. With the advances in systemic therapy, as well as a better understanding of tumor biology and the importance of molecular profiling, more patients can anticipate prolonged survival. Ultimately, a multidisciplinary evaluation of patients with mCRC is crucial to selecting the appropriate pathway.

Author Contributions: Conceptualization, O.H.D., S.Y. and S.R.S.; design/methodology, O.H.D., S.Y. and S.R.S.; investigation, O.H.D. and S.Y.; resources, O.H.D. and S.Y.; data curation, O.H.D. and S.Y.; writing—original draft preparation, O.H.D. and S.Y.; writing—review and editing, O.H.D., S.Y. and S.R.S.; visualization, O.H.D., S.Y. and S.R.S.; supervision, S.R.S.; project administration, S.R.S. All authors have read and agreed to the published version of the manuscript.

Funding: This research received no external funding.

Institutional Review Board Statement: Ethical review and approval were waived for this study due to this article being a literature review, hence requiring no Institutional Review Board approval since no patient data are accessed or analyzed.

Informed Consent Statement: Not applicable.

Data Availability Statement: No new data was created as this article was a literature review.

Conflicts of Interest: The authors declare no conflict of interest.

References

1. Morgan, E.; Arnold, M.; Gini, A.; Lorenzoni, V.; Cabasag, C.J.; Laversanne, M.; Vignat, J.; Ferlay, J.; Murphy, N.; Bray, F. Global burden of colorectal cancer in 2020 and 2040: Incidence and mortality estimates from GLOBOCAN. *Gut* **2022**, *72*, 338–344. [CrossRef]
2. Sung, H.; Ferlay, J.; Siegel, R.L.; Laversanne, M.; Soerjomataram, I.; Jemal, A.; Bray, F. Global Cancer Statistics 2020: GLOBOCAN Estimates of Incidence and Mortality Worldwide for 36 Cancers in 185 Countries. *CA Cancer J. Clin.* **2021**, *71*, 209–249. [CrossRef] [PubMed]
3. National Cancer Institute—SEER Program. Colorectal Cancer—Cancer Stat Facts. Available online: https://seer.cancer.gov/statfacts/html/colorect.html (accessed on 7 January 2023).
4. Siegel, R.L.; Miller, K.D.; Fuchs, H.E.; Jemal, A. Cancer statistics. *CA Cancer J. Clin.* **2022**, *72*, 7–33. [CrossRef] [PubMed]
5. Väyrynen, V.; Wirta, E.; Seppälä, T.; Sihvo, E.; Mecklin, J.; Vasala, K.; Kellokumpu, I. Incidence and management of patients with colorectal cancer and synchronous and metachronous colorectal metastases: A population-based study. *BJS Open* **2020**, *4*, 685–692. [CrossRef] [PubMed]

6. Elferink, M.A.G.; de Jong, K.P.; Klaase, J.M.; Siemerink, E.J.; de Wilt, J.H.W. Metachronous metastases from colorectal cancer: A population-based study in North-East Netherlands. *Int. J. Color. Dis.* **2014**, *30*, 205–212. [CrossRef]
7. Riihimäki, M.; Hemminki, A.; Sundquist, J.; Hemminki, K. Patterns of metastasis in colon and rectal cancer. *Sci. Rep.* **2016**, *6*, 29765. [CrossRef] [PubMed]
8. Brouwer, N.P.M.; Van Der Kruijssen, D.E.W.; Hugen, N.; De Hingh, I.H.J.T.; Nagtegaal, I.; Verhoeven, R.; Koopman, M.; De Wilt, J.H.W. The Impact of Primary Tumor Location in Synchronous Metastatic Colorectal Cancer: Differences in Metastatic Sites and Survival. *Ann. Surg. Oncol.* **2019**, *27*, 1580–1588. [CrossRef] [PubMed]
9. Chakedis, J.; Schmidt, C.R. Surgical Treatment of Metastatic Colorectal Cancer. *Surg. Oncol. Clin. N. Am.* **2018**, *27*, 377–399. [CrossRef]
10. Van Der Geest, L.G.M.; Lam-Boer, J.; Koopman, M.; Verhoef, C.; Elferink, M.A.G.; De Wilt, J.H.W. Nationwide trends in incidence, treatment and survival of colorectal cancer patients with synchronous metastases. *Clin. Exp. Metastasis* **2015**, *32*, 457–465. [CrossRef]
11. Lee, R.M.; Cardona, K.; Russell, M.C. Historical perspective: Two decades of progress in treating metastatic colorectal cancer. *J. Surg. Oncol.* **2019**, *119*, 549–563. [CrossRef]
12. Razenberg, L.; van Gestel, Y.; Creemers, G.-J.; Verwaal, V.; Lemmens, V.; de Hingh, I. Trends in cytoreductive surgery and hyperthermic intraperitoneal chemotherapy for the treatment of synchronous peritoneal carcinomatosis of colorectal origin in the Netherlands. *Eur. J. Surg. Oncol. (EJSO)* **2015**, *41*, 466–471. [CrossRef] [PubMed]
13. Simkens, G.A.; Van Oudheusden, T.R.; Nieboer, D.; Steyerberg, E.W.; Rutten, H.J.; Luyer, M.D.; Nienhuijs, S.W.; De Hingh, I.H. Development of a Prognostic Nomogram for Patients with Peritoneally Metastasized Colorectal Cancer Treated with Cytoreductive Surgery and HIPEC. *Ann. Surg. Oncol.* **2016**, *23*, 4214–4221. [CrossRef]
14. Jawed, I.; Wilkerson, J.; Prasad, V.; Duffy, A.G.; Fojo, T. Colorectal Cancer Survival Gains and Novel Treatment Regimens: A Systematic Review and Analysis. *JAMA Oncol.* **2015**, *1*, 787–795. [CrossRef]
15. Zhang, G.Q.; Taylor, J.P.; Stem, M.; Almaazmi, H.; Efron, J.E.; Atallah, C.; Safar, B. Aggressive Multimodal Treatment and Metastatic Colorectal Cancer Survival. *J. Am. Coll. Surg.* **2020**, *230*, 689–698. [CrossRef] [PubMed]
16. Biller, L.H.; Schrag, D. Diagnosis and Treatment of Metastatic Colorectal Cancer: A review. *JAMA* **2021**, *325*, 669–685. [CrossRef]
17. Breugom, A.; Bastiaannet, E.; Guren, M.; Kørner, H.; Boelens, P.; Dekker, F.; Kapiteijn, E.; Gelderblom, H.; Larsen, I.; Liefers, G.; et al. Treatment strategies and overall survival for incurable metastatic colorectal cancer—A EURECCA international comparison including 21,196 patients from the Netherlands and Norway. *Eur. J. Surg. Oncol. (EJSO)* **2020**, *46*, 1167–1173. [CrossRef] [PubMed]
18. Eisterer, W.; Prager, G. Chemotherapy, Still an Option in the Twenty-First Century in Metastatic Colorectal Cancer? *Cardiovasc. Interv. Radiol.* **2019**, *42*, 1213–1220. [CrossRef]
19. Bhimani, N.; Wong, G.; Molloy, C.; Pavlakis, N.; Diakos, C.; Clarke, S.; Dieng, M.; Hugh, T. Cost of treating metastatic colorectal cancer: A systematic review. *Public Health* **2022**, *211*, 97–104. [CrossRef]
20. Benson, A.B.; Al-Hawary, M.M.; Azad, N.; Chen, Y.-J.; Ciombor, K.K.; Cohen, S.; Cooper, H.S.; Deming, D.; Farkas, L.; Garrido-Laguna, I.; et al. NCCN Guidelines Version 2.2022 Colon Cancer Continue NCCN Guidelines Panel Disclosures. 2022. Available online: https://www.nccn.org/home/member- (accessed on 7 January 2023).
21. Benson, A.B.; Al-Hawary, M.M.; Azad, N.; Chen, Y.-J.; Ciombor, K.K.; Cohen, S.; Cooper, H.S.; Deming, D.; Farkas, L.; Garrido-Laguna, I.; et al. NCCN Guidelines Version 3.2022 Rectal Cancer Continue NCCN Guidelines Panel Disclosures; 2022. Available online: https://www.nccn.org/home/member- (accessed on 7 January 2023).
22. Cervantes, A.; Adam, R.; Roselló, S.; Arnold, D.; Normanno, N.; Taïeb, J.; Seligmann, J.; De Baere, T.; Osterlund, P.; Yoshino, T.; et al. Metastatic colorectal cancer: ESMO Clinical Practice Guideline for diagnosis, treatment and follow-up. *Ann. Oncol.* **2022**, *34*, 10–32. [CrossRef]
23. Hashiguchi, Y.; Muro, K.; Saito, Y.; Ito, Y.; Ajioka, Y.; Hamaguchi, T.; Hasegawa, K.; Hotta, K.; Ishida, H.; Ishiguro, M.; et al. Japanese Society for Cancer of the Colon and Rectum (JSCCR) guidelines 2019 for the treatment of colorectal cancer. *Int. J. Clin. Oncol.* **2020**, *25*, 1. [CrossRef]
24. Hedrick, T.L. *The ASCRS Manual of Colon and Rectal Surgery*, 4th ed.; Steele, S.R., Hull, T.L., Hyman, N., Maykel, J.A., Read, T.E., Whitlow, C.B., Eds.; Springer: Cham, Switzerland, 2022; p. 547.
25. Lakemeyer, L.; Sander, S.; Wittau, M.; Henne-Bruns, D.; Kornmann, M.; Lemke, J. Diagnostic and Prognostic Value of CEA and CA19-9 in Colorectal Cancer. *Diseases* **2021**, *9*, 21. [CrossRef]
26. Yu, Z.; Chen, Z.; Wu, J.; Li, Z.; Wu, Y. Prognostic value of pretreatment serum carbohydrate antigen 19-9 level in patients with colorectal cancer: A meta-analysis. *PLoS ONE* **2017**, *12*, e0188139. [CrossRef] [PubMed]
27. Balthazar, E.; Megibow, A.; Hulnick, D.; Naidich, D. Carcinoma of the colon: Detection and preoperative staging by CT. *Am. J. Roentgenol.* **1988**, *150*, 301–306. [CrossRef] [PubMed]
28. Niekel, M.C.; Bipat, S.; Stoker, J. Diagnostic Imaging of Colorectal Liver Metastases with CT, MR Imaging, FDG PET, and/or FDG PET/CT: A Meta-Analysis of Prospective Studies Including Patients Who Have Not Previously Undergone Treatment 1. *Radiology* **2010**, *257*, 674–684. [CrossRef] [PubMed]
29. Zhang, G.; Cai, Y.-Z.; Xu, G.-H. Diagnostic Accuracy of MRI for Assessment of T Category and Circumferential Resection Margin Involvement in Patients with Rectal Cancer. *Dis. Colon Rectum* **2016**, *59*, 789–799. [CrossRef]

30. Taylor, F.G.; Quirke, P.; Heald, R.J.; Moran, B.J.; Blomqvist, L.; Swift, I.R.; Sebag-Montefiore, D.; Tekkis, P.; Brown, G. Preoperative Magnetic Resonance Imaging Assessment of Circumferential Resection Margin Predicts Disease-Free Survival and Local Recurrence: 5-Year Follow-Up Results of the MERCURY Study. *J. Clin. Oncol.* **2014**, *32*, 34–43. [CrossRef]
31. Faletti, R.; Gatti, M.; Arezzo, A.; Stola, S.; Benedini, M.C.; Bergamasco, L.; Morino, M.; Fonio, P. Preoperative staging of rectal cancer using magnetic resonance imaging: Comparison with pathological staging. *Int. J. Clin. Rev.* **2018**, *73*, 13–19. [CrossRef]
32. Ashraf, S.; Hompes, R.; Slater, A.; Lindsey, I.; Bach, S.; Mortensen, N.J.; Cunningham, C.; on behalf of the Association of Coloproctology of Great Britain and Ireland Transanal Endoscopic Microsurgery (TEM) Collaboration. A critical appraisal of endorectal ultrasound and transanal endoscopic microsurgery and decision-making in early rectal cancer. *Color. Dis.* **2011**, *14*, 821–826. [CrossRef]
33. Bipat, S.; Glas, A.S.; Slors, F.J.M.; Zwinderman, A.H.; Bossuyt, P.M.M.; Stoker, J. Rectal Cancer: Local Staging and Assessment of Lymph Node Involvement with Endoluminal US, CT, and MR Imaging—A Meta-Analysis. *Radiology* **2004**, *232*, 773–783. [CrossRef] [PubMed]
34. Tanaka, A.; Sadahiro, S.; Suzuki, T.; Okada, K.; Saito, G. Comparisons of Rigid Proctoscopy, Flexible Colonoscopy, and Digital Rectal Examination for Determining the Localization of Rectal Cancers. *Dis. Colon Rectum* **2018**, *61*, 202–206. [CrossRef] [PubMed]
35. Mischel, A.-M.; Rosielle, D.A. Eastern Cooperative Oncology Group Performance Status #434. *J. Palliat. Med.* **2022**, *25*, 508–510. [CrossRef] [PubMed]
36. Corvino, F.; Giurazza, F.; Cangiano, G.; Silvestre, M.; Cavaglià, E.; de Magistris, G.; Amodio, F.; Corvino, A.; Niola, R. Endovascular Treatment of Peripheral Vascular Blowout Syndrome in End-Stage Malignancies. *Ann. Vasc. Surg.* **2019**, *58*, 382.e1–382.e5. [CrossRef] [PubMed]
37. Huntress, L.A.; Kogan, S.; Nagarsheth, K.; Nassiri, N. Palliative Endovascular Techniques for Management of Peripheral Vascular Blowout Syndrome in End-Stage Malignancies. *Vasc. Endovasc. Surg.* **2017**, *51*, 394–399. [CrossRef]
38. Cameron, M.G.; Kersten, C.; Vistad, I.; Fosså, S.; Guren, M.G. Palliative pelvic radiotherapy of symptomatic incurable rectal cancer—A systematic review. *Acta Oncol.* **2013**, *53*, 164–173. [CrossRef]
39. Cirocchi, R.; Trastulli, S.; Abraha, I.; Vettoretto, N.; Boselli, C.; Montedori, A.; Parisi, A.; Noya, G.; Platell, C. Non-resection versus resection for an asymptomatic primary tumour in patients with unresectable Stage IV colorectal cancer. *Cochrane Database Syst. Rev.* **2012**, *8*, CD008997. [CrossRef] [PubMed]
40. Mun, J.-Y.; Kim, J.-E.; Yoo, N.; Cho, H.-M.; Kim, H.; An, H.-J.; Kye, B.-H. Survival Outcomes after Elective or Emergency Surgery for Synchronous Stage IV Colorectal Cancer. *Biomedicines* **2022**, *10*, 3114. [CrossRef] [PubMed]
41. Fiori, E.; Lamazza, A.; Schillaci, A.; Femia, S.; DeMasi, E.; DeCesare, A.; Sterpetti, A.V. Palliative management for patients with subacute obstruction and stage IV unresectable rectosigmoid cancer: Colostomy versus endoscopic stenting: Final results of a prospective randomized trial. *Am. J. Surg.* **2012**, *204*, 321–326. [CrossRef]
42. Gianotti, L.; Tamini, N.; Nespoli, L.; Rota, M.; Bolzonaro, E.; Frego, R.; Redaelli, A.; Antolini, L.; Ardito, A.; Nespoli, A.; et al. A prospective evaluation of short-term and long-term results from colonic stenting for palliation or as a bridge to elective operation versus immediate surgery for large-bowel obstruction. *Surg. Endosc.* **2012**, *27*, 832–842. [CrossRef]
43. Urgorri, A.S.; Saperas, E.; Castella, E.O.; Román, M.P.; Pons, F.R.; Priego, L.B.; Cusco, J.M.D.; Sánchez, M.P.; Caserras, X.B.; Álvarez-González, M.A. Colonic stent vs surgical resection of the primary tumor. Effect on survival from stage-IV obstructive colorectal cancer. *Rev. Esp. Enferm. Dig.* **2020**, *112*, 694–700. [CrossRef]
44. Daniels, M.; Merkel, S.; Agaimy, A.; Hohenberger, W. Treatment of perforated colon carcinomas—Outcomes of radical surgery. *Int. J. Color. Dis.* **2015**, *30*, 1505–1513. [CrossRef]
45. Bs, J.K.L.; Huber, K.E.; DiPetrillo, T.A.; Wazer, D.E.; Leonard, K.L. Patterns of care of radiation therapy in patients with stage IV rectal cancer: A Surveillance, Epidemiology, and End Results analysis of patients from 2004 to 2009. *Cancer* **2013**, *120*, 731–737. [CrossRef]
46. Horn, S.R.; Stoltzfus, K.C.; Lehrer, E.J.; Dawson, L.A.; Tchelebi, L.; Gusani, N.J.; Sharma, N.K.; Chen, H.; Trifiletti, D.M.; Zaorsky, N.G. Epidemiology of liver metastases. *Cancer Epidemiol.* **2020**, *67*, 101760. [CrossRef]
47. Akgül, Ö.; Çetinkaya, E.; Ersöz, Ş.; Tez, M. Role of surgery in colorectal cancer liver metastases. *World J. Gastroenterol.* **2014**, *20*, 6113. [CrossRef]
48. Nordlinger, B.; Van Cutsem, E.; Rougier, P.; Köhne, C.-H.; Ychou, M.; Sobrero, A.; Adam, R.; Arvidsson, D.; Carrato, A.; Georgoulias, V.; et al. Does chemotherapy prior to liver resection increase the potential for cure in patients with metastatic colorectal cancer? A report from the European Colorectal Metastases Treatment Group. *Eur. J. Cancer* **2007**, *43*, 2037–2045. [CrossRef]
49. Engstrand, J.; Nilsson, H.; Strömberg, C.; Jonas, E.; Freedman, J. Colorectal cancer liver metastases—A population-based study on incidence, management and survival. *BMC Cancer* **2018**, *18*, 78. [CrossRef] [PubMed]
50. Nordlinger, B.; Sorbye, H.; Glimelius, B.; Poston, G.J.; Schlag, P.M.; Rougier, P.; Bechstein, W.O.; Primrose, J.N.; Walpole, E.T.; Finch-Jones, M.; et al. Perioperative FOLFOX4 chemotherapy and surgery versus surgery alone for resectable liver metastases from colorectal cancer (EORTC 40983): Long-term results of a randomised, controlled, phase 3 trial. *Lancet Oncol.* **2013**, *14*, 1208–1215. [CrossRef] [PubMed]
51. Chun, Y.J.; Kim, S.-G.; Lee, K.-W.; Cho, S.H.; Kim, T.W.; Baek, J.Y.; Park, Y.S.; Hong, S.; Chu, C.W.; Beom, S.-H.; et al. A Randomized Phase II Study of Perioperative Chemotherapy Plus Bevacizumab Versus Postoperative Chemotherapy Plus Bevacizumab in Patients With Upfront Resectable Hepatic Colorectal Metastases. *Clin. Color. Cancer* **2020**, *19*, e140–e150. [CrossRef]

52. Park, E.J.; Baik, S.H. Recent Advance in the Surgical Treatment of Metastatic Colorectal Cancer-An English Version. *J. Anus Rectum Colon* **2022**, *6*, 213–220. [CrossRef] [PubMed]
53. Ghiasloo, M.; Pavlenko, D.; Verhaeghe, M.; Van Langenhove, Z.; Uyttebroek, O.; Berardi, G.; Troisi, R.I.; Ceelen, W. Surgical treatment of stage IV colorectal cancer with synchronous liver metastases: A systematic review and network meta-analysis. *Eur. J. Surg. Oncol. (EJSO)* **2020**, *46*, 1203–1213. [CrossRef]
54. Mahmoud, N.; Dunn, K.B. Metastasectomy for Stage IV Colorectal Cancer. *Dis. Colon Rectum* **2010**, *53*, 1080–1092. [CrossRef]
55. de Jong, M.C.; Pulitano, C.; Ribero, D.; Strub, J.; Mentha, G.; Schulick, R.D.; Choti, M.A.; Aldrighetti, L.; Capussotti, L.; Pawlik, T.M. Rates and Patterns of Recurrence Following Curative Intent Surgery for Colorectal Liver Metastasis: An international multi-institutional analysis of 1669 patients. *Ann. Surg.* **2009**, *250*, 440–448. [CrossRef] [PubMed]
56. Folprecht, G.; Gruenberger, T.; Bechstein, W.; Raab, H.-R.; Weitz, J.; Lordick, F.; Hartmann, J.; Stoehlmacher-Williams, J.; Lang, H.; Trarbach, T.; et al. Survival of patients with initially unresectable colorectal liver metastases treated with FOLFOX/cetuximab or FOLFIRI/cetuximab in a multidisciplinary concept (CELIM study). *Ann. Oncol.* **2014**, *25*, 1018–1025. [CrossRef] [PubMed]
57. Stewart, C.L.; Warner, S.; Ito, K.; Raoof, M.; Wu, G.X.; Lu, W.P.; Kessler, J.; Kim, J.Y.; Fong, Y. Cytoreduction for colorectal metastases: Liver, lung, peritoneum, lymph nodes, bone, brain. When does it palliate, prolong survival, and potentially cure? *Curr. Probl. Surg.* **2018**, *55*, 330–379. [CrossRef] [PubMed]
58. Deng, G.; Li, H.; Jia, G.-Q.; Fang, D.; Tang, Y.-Y.; Xie, J.; Chen, K.-F.; Chen, Z.-Y. Parenchymal-sparing versus extended hepatectomy for colorectal liver metastases: A systematic review and meta-analysis. *Cancer Med.* **2019**, *8*, 6165–6175. [CrossRef]
59. Moris, D.; Ronnekleiv-Kelly, S.; Rahnemai-Azar, A.A.; Felekouras, E.; Dillhoff, M.; Schmidt, C.; Pawlik, T.M. Parenchymal-Sparing Versus Anatomic Liver Resection for Colorectal Liver Metastases: A Systematic Review. *J. Gastrointest. Surg.* **2017**, *21*, 1076–1085. [CrossRef] [PubMed]
60. Torzilli, G.; Donadon, M.; Marconi, M.; Botea, F.; Palmisano, A.; Del Fabbro, D.; Procopio, F.; Montorsi, M. Systematic Extended Right Posterior Sectionectomy. *Ann. Surg.* **2008**, *247*, 603–611. [CrossRef]
61. Chouillard, E.; Cherqui, D.; Tayar, C.; Brunetti, F.; Fagniez, P.-L. Anatomical Bi- and Trisegmentectomies as Alternatives to Extensive Liver Resections. *Ann. Surg.* **2003**, *238*, 29–34. [CrossRef]
62. Margonis, G.A.; Buettner, S.; Andreatos, N.; Sasaki, K.; Ijzermans, J.N.M.; van Vugt, J.L.A.; Pawlik, T.M.; Choti, M.A.; Cameron, J.L.; He, J.; et al. Anatomical Resections Improve Disease-free Survival in Patients With KRAS-mutated Colorectal Liver Metastases. *Ann. Surg.* **2017**, *266*, 641–649. [CrossRef]
63. Keck, J.; Gaedcke, J.; Ghadimi, M.; Lorf, T. Surgical Therapy in Patients with Colorectal Liver Metastases. *Digestion* **2022**, *103*, 245–252. [CrossRef]
64. Mentha, G.; Majno, P.E.; Andres, A.; Rubbia-Brandt, L.; Morel, P.; Roth, A.D. Neoadjuvant chemotherapy and resection of advanced synchronous liver metastases before treatment of the colorectal primary. *Br. J. Surg.* **2006**, *93*, 872–878. [CrossRef]
65. Frühling, P.; Strömberg, C.; Isaksson, B.; Urdzik, J. A comparison of the simultaneous, liver-first, and colorectal-first strategies for surgical treatment of synchronous colorectal liver metastases at two major liver-surgery institutions in Sweden. *HPB* **2022**, *25*, 26–36. [CrossRef]
66. Boudjema, K.; Locher, C.; Sabbagh, C.; Ortega-Deballon, P.; Heyd, B.; Bachellier, P.; Métairie, S.; Paye, F.; Bourlier, P.; Adam, R.; et al. Simultaneous Versus Delayed Resection for Initially Resectable Synchronous Colorectal Cancer Liver Metastases: A Prospective, Open-label, Randomized, Controlled Trial. *Ann. Surg.* **2021**, *273*, 49–56. [CrossRef] [PubMed]
67. Wang, S.-H.; Song, L.; Tang, J.-Y.; Sun, W.-P.; Li, Z. Safety and long-term prognosis of simultaneous versus staged resection in synchronous colorectal cancer with liver metastasis: A systematic review and meta-analysis. *Eur. J. Med. Res.* **2022**, *27*, 297. [CrossRef]
68. Adam, R.; Miller, R.; Pitombo, M.; Wicherts, D.A.; de Haas, R.J.; Bitsakou, G.; Aloia, T. Two-stage Hepatectomy Approach for Initially Unresectable Colorectal Hepatic Metastases. *Surg. Oncol. Clin. N. Am.* **2007**, *16*, 525–536. [CrossRef] [PubMed]
69. Jaeck, D.; Oussoultzoglou, E.; Rosso, E.; Greget, M.; Weber, J.-C.; Bachellier, P. A Two-Stage Hepatectomy Procedure Combined With Portal Vein Embolization to Achieve Curative Resection for Initially Unresectable Multiple and Bilobar Colorectal Liver Metastases. *Ann. Surg.* **2004**, *240*, 1037–1051. [CrossRef]
70. Del Basso, C.; Gaillard, M.; Lainas, P.; Zervaki, S.; Perlemuter, G.; Chagué, P.; Rocher, L.; Voican, C.S.; Dagher, I.; Tranchart, H. Current strategies to induce liver remnant hypertrophy before major liver resection. *World J. Hepatol.* **2021**, *13*, 1629–1641. [CrossRef]
71. Imai, K.; Benitez, C.C.; Allard, M.-A.; Vibert, E.; Cunha, A.S.; Cherqui, D.; Castaing, D.; Bismuth, H.; Baba, H.; Adam, R. Failure to Achieve a 2-Stage Hepatectomy for Colorectal Liver Metastases: How to Prevent It? *Ann. Surg.* **2015**, *262*, 772–779. [CrossRef]
72. Brouquet, A.; Abdalla, E.K.; Kopetz, S.; Garrett, C.R.; Overman, M.J.; Eng, C.; Andreou, A.; Loyer, E.M.; Madoff, D.C.; Curley, S.A.; et al. High Survival Rate After Two-Stage Resection of Advanced Colorectal Liver Metastases: Response-Based Selection and Complete Resection Define Outcome. *J. Clin. Oncol.* **2011**, *29*, 1083–1090. [CrossRef]
73. Yi, F.; Zhang, W.; Feng, L. Efficacy and safety of different options for liver regeneration of future liver remnant in patients with liver malignancies: A systematic review and network meta-analysis. *World J. Surg. Oncol.* **2022**, *20*, 399. [CrossRef]
74. Moris, D.; Ronnekleiv-Kelly, S.; Kostakis, I.D.; Tsilimigras, D.I.; Beal, E.W.; Papalampros, A.; Dimitroulis, D.; Felekouras, E.; Pawlik, T.M. Operative Results and Oncologic Outcomes of Associating Liver Partition and Portal Vein Ligation for Staged Hepatectomy (ALPPS) Versus Two-Stage Hepatectomy (TSH) in Patients with Unresectable Colorectal Liver Metastases: A Systematic Review and Meta-Analysis. *World J. Surg.* **2017**, *42*, 806–815. [CrossRef]

75. Sandström, P.; Røsok, B.I.; Sparrelid, E.; Larsen, P.N.; Larsson, A.L.; Lindell, G.; Schultz, N.A.; Bjørnbeth, B.A.; Isaksson, B.; Rizell, M.; et al. ALPPS Improves Resectability Compared With Conventional Two-stage Hepatectomy in Patients With Advanced Colorectal Liver Metastasis: Results From a Scandinavian Multicenter Randomized Controlled Trial (LIGRO Trial). *Ann. Surg.* **2018**, *267*, 833–840. [CrossRef] [PubMed]
76. Zhang, L.; Yang, Z.; Zhang, S.; Wang, W.; Zheng, S. Conventional Two-Stage Hepatectomy or Associating Liver Partitioning and Portal Vein Ligation for Staged Hepatectomy for Colorectal Liver Metastases? A Systematic Review and Meta-Analysis. *Front. Oncol.* **2020**, *10*, 1391. [CrossRef] [PubMed]
77. Bednarsch, J.; Czigany, Z.; Sharmeen, S.; Van Der Kroft, G.; Strnad, P.; Ulmer, T.F.; Isfort, P.; Bruners, P.; Lurje, G.; Neumann, U.P. ALPPS versus two-stage hepatectomy for colorectal liver metastases—A comparative retrospective cohort study. *World J. Surg. Oncol.* **2020**, *18*, 140. [CrossRef] [PubMed]
78. Vico, T.D.; Castro, P.G.; Navarro, L.A.; Sánchez, A.S.; Góngora, L.M.; Orón, E.M.M.; Ibáñez, J.M.; Alonso, N.T.; Arrillaga, I.G.-P.; Trancón, J.E.G. Two stage hepatectomy (TSH) versus ALPPS for initially unresectable colorectal liver metastasis: A systematic review and meta-analysis. *Eur. J. Surg. Oncol. (EJSO)* **2023**, *49*, 550–559. [CrossRef] [PubMed]
79. Meijerink, M.R.; Puijk, R.S.; Van Tilborg, A.A.J.M.; Henningsen, K.H.; Fernandez, L.G.; Neyt, M.; Heymans, J.; Frankema, J.S.; De Jong, K.P.; Richel, D.J.; et al. Radiofrequency and Microwave Ablation Compared to Systemic Chemotherapy and to Partial Hepatectomy in the Treatment of Colorectal Liver Metastases: A Systematic Review and Meta-Analysis. *Cardiovasc. Interv. Radiol.* **2018**, *41*, 1189–1204. [CrossRef]
80. Engstrand, J.; Nilsson, H.; Jansson, A.; Isaksson, B.; Freedman, J.; Lundell, L.; Jonas, E. A multiple microwave ablation strategy in patients with initially unresectable colorectal cancer liver metastases—A safety and feasibility study of a new concept. *Eur. J. Surg. Oncol. (EJSO)* **2014**, *40*, 1488–1493. [CrossRef]
81. Di Martino, M.; Rompianesi, G.; Mora-Guzmán, I.; Martín-Pérez, E.; Montalti, R.; Troisi, R.I. Systematic review and meta-analysis of local ablative therapies for resectable colorectal liver metastases. *Eur. J. Surg. Oncol. (EJSO)* **2019**, *46*, 772–781. [CrossRef] [PubMed]
82. Guadagni, S.; Marmorino, F.; Furbetta, N.; Carullo, M.; Gianardi, D.; Palmeri, M.; Di Franco, G.; Comandatore, A.; Moretto, R.; Cecilia, E.; et al. Surgery combined with intra-operative microwaves ablation for the management of colorectal cancer liver metastasis: A case-matched analysis and evaluation of recurrences. *Front. Oncol.* **2022**, *12*, 1023301. [CrossRef]
83. Morris, V.K.; Kennedy, E.B.; Baxter, N.N.; Benson, A.B.; Cercek, A.; Cho, M.; Ciombor, K.K.; Cremolini, C.; Davis, A.; Deming, D.A.; et al. Treatment of Metastatic Colorectal Cancer: ASCO Guideline. *J. Clin. Oncol.* **2023**, *41*, 678–700. [CrossRef]
84. Olson, R.; Jiang, W.; Liu, M.; Bergman, A.; Schellenberg, D.; Mou, B.; Alexander, A.; Carolan, H.; Hsu, F.; Miller, S.; et al. Treatment With Stereotactic Ablative Radiotherapy for Up to 5 Oligometastases in Patients With Cancer: Primary Toxic Effect Results of the Nonrandomized Phase 2 SABR-5 Clinical Trial. *JAMA Oncol.* **2022**, *8*, 1644. [CrossRef]
85. Mühlbacher, F.; Huk, I.; Steininger, R.; Gnant, M.; Götzinger, P.; Wamser, P.; Banhegyi, C.; Piza, F. Is orthotopic liver transplantation a feasible treatment for secondary cancer of the liver? *Transplant Proc.* **1991**, *23 Pt 2*, 1567–1568. [PubMed]
86. Hagness, M.; Foss, A.; Line, P.-D.; Scholz, T.; Jørgensen, P.F.; Fosby, B.; Boberg, K.M.; Mathisen, Ø.; Gladhaug, I.P.; Egge, T.S.; et al. Liver Transplantation for Nonresectable Liver Metastases From Colorectal Cancer. *Ann. Surg.* **2013**, *257*, 800–806. [CrossRef] [PubMed]
87. Dueland, S.; Syversveen, T.; Solheim, J.M.; Solberg, S.; Grut, H.; Bjørnbeth, B.A.; Hagness, M.; Line, P.-D. Survival Following Liver Transplantation for Patients With Nonresectable Liver-only Colorectal Metastases. *Ann. Surg.* **2020**, *271*, 212–218. [CrossRef] [PubMed]
88. Mitry, E.; Guiu, B.; Cosconea, S.; Jooste, V.; Faivre, J.; Bouvier, A.-M. Epidemiology, management and prognosis of colorectal cancer with lung metastases: A 30-year population-based study. *Gut* **2010**, *59*, 1383–1388. [CrossRef] [PubMed]
89. Meimarakis, G.; Spelsberg, F.; Angele, M.; Preissler, G.; Fertmann, J.; Crispin, A.; Reu, S.; Kalaitzis, N.; Stemmler, M.; Giessen, C.; et al. Resection of Pulmonary Metastases from Colon and Rectal Cancer: Factors to Predict Survival Differ Regarding to the Origin of the Primary Tumor. *Ann. Surg. Oncol.* **2014**, *21*, 2563–2572. [CrossRef]
90. Li, J.; Yuan, Y.; Yang, F.; Wang, Y.; Zhu, X.; Wang, Z.; Zheng, S.; Wan, D.; He, J.; Wang, J.; et al. Expert consensus on multidisciplinary therapy of colorectal cancer with lung metastases (2019 edition). *J. Hematol. Oncol.* **2019**, *12*, 16. [CrossRef]
91. Nanji, S.; Karim, S.; Tang, E.; Brennan, K.; McGuire, A.; Pramesh, C.; Booth, C.M. Pulmonary Metastasectomy for Colorectal Cancer: Predictors of Survival in Routine Surgical Practice. *Ann. Thorac. Surg.* **2018**, *105*, 1605–1612. [CrossRef]
92. Handy, J.R.; Bremner, R.M.; Crocenzi, T.S.; Detterbeck, F.C.; Fernando, H.C.; Fidias, P.M.; Firestone, S.; Johnstone, C.A.; Lanuti, M.; Litle, V.R.; et al. Expert Consensus Document on Pulmonary Metastasectomy. *Ann. Thorac. Surg.* **2019**, *107*, 631–649. [CrossRef]
93. Mangiameli, G.; Cioffi, U.; Alloisio, M.; Testori, A. *Pulmonary Metastases: Surgical Principles, Surgical Indications, and Innovations*; Sergi, C.M., Ed.; Exon Publications: Brisbane, Australia, 3 May 2022.
94. Cerfolio, R.J.; Mccarty, T.; Bryant, A. Non-imaged pulmonary nodules discovered during thoracotomy for metastasectomy by lung palpation. *Eur. J. Cardio-Thorac.Surg.* **2009**, *35*, 786–791. [CrossRef]
95. Hamaji, M.; Cassivi, S.D.; Shen, K.R.; Allen, M.S.; Nichols, F.C.; Deschamps, C.; Wigle, D.A. Is Lymph Node Dissection Required in Pulmonary Metastasectomy for Colorectal Adenocarcinoma? *Ann. Thorac. Surg.* **2012**, *94*, 1796–1800. [CrossRef]
96. Wolf, F.J.; Grand, D.J.; Machan, J.T.; DiPetrillo, T.A.; Mayo-Smith, W.W.; Dupuy, D.E. Microwave Ablation of Lung Malignancies: Effectiveness, CT Findings, and Safety in 50 Patients. *Radiology* **2008**, *247*, 871–879. [CrossRef] [PubMed]

97. Ibrahim, T.; Tselikas, L.; Yazbeck, C.; Kattan, J. Systemic Versus Local Therapies for Colorectal Cancer Pulmonary Metastasis: What to Choose and When? *J. Gastrointest. Cancer* **2016**, *47*, 223–231. [CrossRef] [PubMed]
98. Flood, M.; Das, A.; Soucisse, M.; Kong, J.; Ramsay, R.; Michael, M.; Loveday, B.; Warrier, S.; Heriot, A. Synchronous Liver Resection, Cytoreductive Surgery and Hyperthermic Intraperitoneal Chemotherapy for Colorectal Liver and Peritoneal Metastases: A Systematic Review and Meta-analysis. *Dis. Colon Rectum* **2021**, *64*, 754–764. [CrossRef]
99. Vassos, N.; Piso, P. Metastatic Colorectal Cancer to the Peritoneum: Current Treatment Options. *Curr. Treat. Options Oncol.* **2018**, *19*, 49. [CrossRef] [PubMed]
100. Ren, K.; Xie, X.; Min, T.; Sun, T.; Wang, H.; Zhang, Y.; Dang, C.; Zhang, H. Development of the Peritoneal Metastasis: A Review of Back-Grounds, Mechanisms, Treatments and Prospects. *J. Clin. Med.* **2022**, *12*, 103. [CrossRef]
101. Sato, H.; Kotake, K.; Sugihara, K.; Takahashi, H.; Maeda, K.; Uyama, I. Clinicopathological Factors Associated with Recurrence and Prognosis after R0 Resection for Stage IV Colorectal Cancer with Peritoneal Metastasis. *Dig. Surg.* **2016**, *33*, 382–391. [CrossRef]
102. Verwaal, V.J.; Van Ruth, S.; De Bree, E.; Van Slooten, G.W.; Van Tinteren, H.; Boot, H.; Zoetmulder, F.A. Randomized Trial of Cytoreduction and Hyperthermic Intraperitoneal Chemotherapy Versus Systemic Chemotherapy and Palliative Surgery in Patients With Peritoneal Carcinomatosis of Colorectal Cancer. *J. Clin. Oncol.* **2003**, *21*, 3737–3743. [CrossRef]
103. Cashin, P.; Mahteme, H.; Spång, N.; Syk, I.; Frödin, J.; Torkzad, M.; Glimelius, B.; Graf, W. Cytoreductive surgery and intraperitoneal chemotherapy versus systemic chemotherapy for colorectal peritoneal metastases: A randomised trial. *Eur. J. Cancer* **2016**, *53*, 155–162. [CrossRef]
104. Narasimhan, V.; Tan, S.; Kong, J.; Pham, T.; Michael, M.; Ramsay, R.; Warrier, S.; Heriot, A. Prognostic factors influencing survival in patients undergoing cytoreductive surgery with hyperthermic intraperitoneal chemotherapy for isolated colorectal peritoneal metastases: A systematic review and meta-analysis. *Color. Dis.* **2020**, *22*, 1482–1495. [CrossRef]
105. Quénet, F.; Elias, D.; Roca, L.; Goéré, D.; Ghouti, L.; Pocard, M.; Facy, O.; Arvieux, C.; Lorimier, G.; Pezet, D.; et al. Cytoreductive surgery plus hyperthermic intraperitoneal chemotherapy versus cytoreductive surgery alone for colorectal peritoneal metastases (PRODIGE 7): A multicentre, randomised, open-label, phase 3 trial. *Lancet Oncol.* **2021**, *22*, 256–266. [CrossRef]
106. Brind'Amour, A.; Dubé, P.; Tremblay, J.; Soucisse, M.; Mack, L.; Bouchard-Fortier, A.; McCart, J.; Govindarajan, A.; Bischof, D.; Haase, E.; et al. Canadian Guidelines on the Management of Colorectal Peritoneal Metastases. *Curr. Oncol.* **2020**, *27*, 621–631. [CrossRef] [PubMed]
107. Di Carlo, S.; Cavallaro, G.; La Rovere, F.; Usai, V.; Siragusa, L.; Izzo, P.; Izzo, L.; Fassari, A.; Izzo, S.; Franceschilli, M.; et al. Synchronous liver and peritoneal metastases from colorectal cancer: Is cytoreductive surgery and hyperthermic intraperitoneal chemotherapy combined with liver resection a feasible option? *Front. Surg.* **2022**, *9*, 1006591. [CrossRef]
108. Zou, Y.; Chen, X.; Zhang, X.; Shen, Z.; Cai, J.; Tan, Y.; Weng, J.; Rong, Y.; Lin, X. Clinical outcomes of curative treatment for colorectal liver metastases combined with cytoreductive surgery and intraperitoneal chemotherapy for peritoneal metastases: A systematic review and meta-analysis of current evidence. *Int. J. Hyperth.* **2020**, *37*, 944–954. [CrossRef] [PubMed]
109. Ganesh, K.; Shah, R.H.; Vakiani, E.; Nash, G.M.; Skottowe, H.P.; Yaeger, R.; Cercek, A.; Lincoln, A.; Tran, C.; Segal, N.H.; et al. Clinical and genetic determinants of ovarian metastases from colorectal cancer. *Cancer* **2016**, *123*, 1134–1143. [CrossRef]
110. Chen, Z.; Liu, Z.; Yang, J.; Sun, J.; Wang, P. The clinicopathological characteristics, prognosis, and CT features of ovary metastasis from colorectal carcinoma. *Transl. Cancer Res.* **2021**, *10*, 3248–3258. [CrossRef]
111. Van der Meer, R.; de Hingh, I.H.J.T.; Bloemen, J.G.; Janssen, L.; Roumen, R.M.H. Role Of Ovarian Metastases In Colorectal Cancer (ROMIC): A Dutch study protocol to evaluate the effect of prophylactic salpingo-oophorectomy in postmenopausal women. *BMC Women's Health* **2022**, *22*, 441. [CrossRef]
112. Li, X.; Hu, W.; Sun, H.; Gou, H. Survival outcome and prognostic factors for colorectal cancer with synchronous bone metastasis: A population-based study. *Clin. Exp. Metastasis* **2021**, *38*, 89–95. [CrossRef]
113. Tsao, M.N.; Xu, W.; Wong, R.K.; Lloyd, N.; Laperriere, N.; Sahgal, A.; Rakovitch, E.; Chow, E. Whole brain radiotherapy for the treatment of newly diagnosed multiple brain metastases. *Cochrane Database Syst. Rev.* **2018**, *1*, CD003869. [CrossRef]
114. Zhao, P.; Yang, X.; Yan, Y.; Yang, J.; Li, S.; Du, X. Effect of radical lymphadenectomy in colorectal cancer with para-aortic lymph node metastasis: A systematic review and meta-analysis. *BMC Surg.* **2022**, *22*, 181. [CrossRef]
115. Kwon, J.; Kim, J.-S.; Kim, B.H. Is There a Role for Perioperative Pelvic Radiotherapy in Surgically Resected Stage IV Rectal Cancer? A Propensity Score-matched Analysis. *Am. J. Clin. Oncol.* **2021**, *44*, 308–314. [CrossRef] [PubMed]
116. Frykholm, G.J.; Glimelius, B.; Påhlman, L. Preoperative or postoperative irradiation in adenocarcinoma of the rectum: Final treatment results of a randomized trial and an evaluation of late secondary effects. *Dis. Colon Rectum* **1993**, *36*, 564–572. [CrossRef] [PubMed]
117. Sebag-Montefiore, D.; Stephens, R.J.; Steele, R.; Monson, J.; Grieve, R.; Khanna, S.; Quirke, P.; Couture, J.; de Metz, C.; Myint, A.S.; et al. Preoperative radiotherapy versus selective postoperative chemoradiotherapy in patients with rectal cancer (MRC CR07 and NCIC-CTG C016): A multicentre, randomised trial. *Lancet* **2009**, *373*, 811–820. [CrossRef] [PubMed]
118. Renz, P.; Wegner, R.E.; Hasan, S.; Brookover, R.; Finley, G.; Monga, D.; Raj, M.; McCormick, J.; Kirichenko, A. Survival Outcomes After Surgical Management of the Primary Tumor With and Without Radiotherapy for Metastatic Rectal Adenocarcinoma: A National Cancer Database (NCDB) Analysis. *Clin. Color. Cancer* **2019**, *18*, e237–e243. [CrossRef] [PubMed]

119. Custers, P.A.; Hupkens, B.J.P.; Grotenhuis, B.A.; Kuhlmann, K.F.D.; Breukink, S.O.; Beets, G.L.; Melenhorst, J.; Beets-Tan, R.G.H.; Buijsen, J.; Festen, S.; et al. Selected stage IV rectal cancer patients managed by the watch-and-wait approach after pelvic radiotherapy: A good alternative to total mesorectal excision surgery? *Color. Dis.* **2022**, *24*, 401–410. [CrossRef] [PubMed]
120. Erlandsson, J.; Holm, T.; Pettersson, D.; Berglund, A.; Cedermark, B.; Radu, C.; Johansson, H.; Machado, M.; Hjern, F.; Hallböök, O.; et al. Optimal fractionation of preoperative radiotherapy and timing to surgery for rectal cancer (Stockholm III): A multicentre, randomised, non-blinded, phase 3, non-inferiority trial. *Lancet Oncol.* **2017**, *18*, 336–346. [CrossRef]
121. van Gestel, Y.R.; de Hingh, I.H.; van Herk-Sukel, M.P.; van Erning, F.N.; Beerepoot, L.V.; Wijsman, J.H.; Slooter, G.D.; Rutten, H.J.; Creemers, G.-J.M.; Lemmens, V.E. Patterns of metachronous metastases after curative treatment of colorectal cancer. *Cancer Epidemiol.* **2014**, *38*, 448–454. [CrossRef]
122. Reboux, N.; Jooste, V.; Goungounga, J.; Robaszkiewicz, M.; Nousbaum, J.-B.; Bouvier, A.-M. Incidence and Survival in Synchronous and Metachronous Liver Metastases from Colorectal Cancer. *JAMA Netw. Open* **2022**, *5*, e2236666. [CrossRef]
123. Guo, Y.; Xiong, B.-H.; Zhang, T.; Cheng, Y.; Ma, L. XELOX *vs.* FOLFOX in metastatic colorectal cancer: An updated meta-analysis. *Cancer Investig.* **2016**, *34*, 94–104. [CrossRef]
124. Tournigand, C.; André, T.; Achille, E.; Lledo, G.; Flesh, M.; Mery-Mignard, D.; Quinaux, E.; Couteau, C.; Buyse, M.; Ganem, G.; et al. FOLFIRI Followed by FOLFOX6 or the Reverse Sequence in Advanced Colorectal Cancer: A Randomized GERCOR Study. *J. Clin. Oncol.* **2004**, *22*, 229–237. [CrossRef]
125. Colucci, G.; Gebbia, V.; Paoletti, G.; Giuliani, F.; Caruso, M.; Gebbia, N.; Cartenì, G.; Agostara, B.; Pezzella, G.; Manzione, L.; et al. Phase III Randomized Trial of FOLFIRI Versus FOLFOX4 in the Treatment of Advanced Colorectal Cancer: A Multicenter Study of the Gruppo Oncologico Dell'Italia Meridionale. *J. Clin. Oncol.* **2005**, *23*, 4866–4875. [CrossRef]
126. Guo, Y.; Shi, M.; Shen, X.; Yang, C.; Yang, L.; Zhang, J. Capecitabine Plus Irinotecan Versus 5-FU/Leucovorin Plus Irinotecan in the Treatment of Colorectal Cancer: A Meta-analysis. *Clin. Color. Cancer* **2013**, *13*, 110–118. [CrossRef] [PubMed]
127. Hurwitz, H.; Fehrenbacher, L.; Novotny, W.; Cartwright, T.; Hainsworth, J.; Heim, W.; Berlin, J.; Baron, A.; Griffing, S.; Holmgren, E.; et al. Bevacizumab plus Irinotecan, Fluorouracil, and Leucovorin for Metastatic Colorectal Cancer. *N. Engl. J. Med.* **2004**, *350*, 2335–2342. [CrossRef]
128. Food and Drug Administration. U.S. Food & Drug Administration. Package Insert. AVASTIN® (bevacizumab) Injection, for Intravenous Use. Available online: https://www.accessdata.fda.gov/drugsatfda_docs/label/2011/125085s225lbl.pdf (accessed on 27 January 2023).
129. Cunningham, D.; Lang, I.; Marcuello, E.; Lorusso, V.; Ocvirk, J.; Shin, D.B.; Jonker, D.; Osborne, S.; Andre, N.; Waterkamp, D.; et al. Bevacizumab plus capecitabine versus capecitabine alone in elderly patients with previously untreated metastatic colorectal cancer (AVEX): An open-label, randomised phase 3 trial. *Lancet Oncol.* **2013**, *14*, 1077–1085. [CrossRef]
130. Kabbinavar, F.F.; Schulz, J.; McCleod, M.; Patel, T.; Hamm, J.T.; Hecht, J.R.; Mass, R.; Perrou, B.; Nelson, B.; Novotny, W.F. Addition of Bevacizumab to Bolus Fluorouracil and Leucovorin in First-Line Metastatic Colorectal Cancer: Results of a Randomized Phase II Trial. *J. Clin. Oncol.* **2005**, *23*, 3697–3705. [CrossRef] [PubMed]
131. Buchler, T.; Pavlík, T.; Melichar, B.; Bortlíček, Z.; Usiakova, Z.; Dušek, L.; Kiss, I.; Kohoutek, M.; Benešová, V.; Vyzula, R.; et al. Bevacizumab with 5-fluorouracil, leucovorin, and oxaliplatin versus bevacizumab with capecitabine and oxaliplatin for metastatic colorectal carcinoma: Results of a large registry-based cohort analysis. *BMC Cancer* **2014**, *14*, 323. [CrossRef] [PubMed]
132. Saltz, L.B.; Clarke, S.; Diaz-Rubio, E.; Scheithauer, W.; Figer, A.; Wong, R.; Koski, S.; Lichinitser, M.; Yang, T.-S.; Rivera, F.; et al. Bevacizumab in Combination With Oxaliplatin-Based Chemotherapy As First-Line Therapy in Metastatic Colorectal Cancer: A Randomized Phase III Study. *J. Clin. Oncol.* **2008**, *26*, 2013–2019. [CrossRef]
133. Hochster, H.S.; Hart, L.L.; Ramanathan, R.K.; Childs, B.H.; Hainsworth, J.D.; Cohn, A.L.; Wong, L.; Fehrenbacher, L.; Abubakr, Y.; Saif, M.W.; et al. Safety and Efficacy of Oxaliplatin and Fluoropyrimidine Regimens With or Without Bevacizumab As First-Line Treatment of Metastatic Colorectal Cancer: Results of the TREE Study. *J. Clin. Oncol.* **2008**, *26*, 3523–3529. [CrossRef] [PubMed]
134. Reddy, S.K.; Morse, M.A.; Hurwitz, H.I.; Bendell, J.C.; Gan, T.J.; Hill, S.E.; Clary, B.M. Addition of Bevacizumab to Irinotecan- and Oxaliplatin-Based Preoperative Chemotherapy Regimens Does Not Increase Morbidity after Resection of Colorectal Liver Metastases. *J. Am. Coll. Surg.* **2008**, *206*, 96–106. [CrossRef]
135. Scappaticci, F.A.; Fehrenbacher, L.; Cartwright, T.; Hainsworth, J.D.; Heim, W.; Berlin, J.; Kabbinavar, F.; Novotny, W.; Sarkar, S.; Hurwitz, H. Surgical wound healing complications in metastatic colorectal cancer patients treated with bevacizumab. *J. Surg. Oncol.* **2005**, *91*, 173–180. [CrossRef]
136. Cremolini, C.; Antoniotti, C.; Stein, A.; Bendell, J.; Gruenberger, T.; Rossini, D.; Masi, G.; Ongaro, E.; Hurwitz, H.; Falcone, A.; et al. Individual Patient Data Meta-Analysis of FOLFOXIRI Plus Bevacizumab Versus Doublets Plus Bevacizumab as Initial Therapy of Unresectable Metastatic Colorectal Cancer. *J. Clin. Oncol.* **2020**, *38*, 3314–3324. [CrossRef]
137. Cremolini, C.; Rossini, D.; Lonardi, S.; Antoniotti, C.; Pietrantonio, F.; Marmorino, F.; Antonuzzo, L.; Boccaccino, A.; Randon, G.; Giommoni, E.; et al. Modified FOLFOXIRI plus panitumumab (mFOLFOXIRI/PAN) versus mFOLFOX6/PAN as initial treatment of patients with unresectable *RAS* and *BRAF* wild-type metastatic colorectal cancer (mCRC): Results of the phase III randomized TRIPLETE study by GONO. *J. Clin. Oncol.* **2022**, *40*, LBA3505. [CrossRef]
138. Venderbosch, S.; Nagtegaal, I.D.; Maughan, T.S.; Smith, C.G.; Cheadle, J.P.; Fisher, D.; Kaplan, R.; Quirke, P.; Seymour, M.T.; Richman, S.D.; et al. Mismatch Repair Status and *BRAF* Mutation Status in Metastatic Colorectal Cancer Patients: A Pooled Analysis of the CAIRO, CAIRO2, COIN, and FOCUS Studies. *Clin. Cancer Res.* **2014**, *20*, 5322–5330. [CrossRef] [PubMed]

139. Lenz, H.-J.; Van Cutsem, E.; Limon, M.L.; Wong, K.Y.M.; Hendlisz, A.; Aglietta, M.; García-Alfonso, P.; Neyns, B.; Luppi, G.; Cardin, D.B.; et al. First-Line Nivolumab Plus Low-Dose Ipilimumab for Microsatellite Instability-High/Mismatch Repair-Deficient Metastatic Colorectal Cancer: The Phase II CheckMate 142 Study. *J. Clin. Oncol.* **2022**, *40*, 161–170. [CrossRef]
140. André, T.; Shiu, K.-K.; Kim, T.W.; Jensen, B.V.; Jensen, L.H.; Punt, C.; Smith, D.; Garcia-Carbonero, R.; Benavides, M.; Gibbs, P.; et al. Pembrolizumab in Microsatellite-Instability–High Advanced Colorectal Cancer. *N. Engl. J. Med.* **2020**, *383*, 2207–2218. [CrossRef] [PubMed]
141. A Diaz, L.; Shiu, K.-K.; Kim, T.-W.; Jensen, B.V.; Jensen, L.H.; Punt, C.; Smith, D.; Garcia-Carbonero, R.; Benavides, M.; Gibbs, P.; et al. Pembrolizumab versus chemotherapy for microsatellite instability-high or mismatch repair-deficient metastatic colorectal cancer (KEYNOTE-177): Final analysis of a randomised, open-label, phase 3 study. *Lancet Oncol.* **2022**, *23*, 659–670. [CrossRef]
142. Patelli, G.; Tosi, F.; Amatu, A.; Mauri, G.; Curaba, A.; Patanè, D.; Pani, A.; Scaglione, F.; Siena, S.; Sartore-Bianchi, A. Strategies to tackle RAS-mutated metastatic colorectal cancer. *ESMO Open* **2021**, *6*, 100156. [CrossRef]
143. Rowland, A.; Dias, M.M.; Wiese, M.D.; Kichenadasse, G.; McKinnon, R.A.; Karapetis, C.S.; Sorich, M.J. Meta-analysis comparing the efficacy of anti-EGFR monoclonal antibody therapy between KRAS G13D and other KRAS mutant metastatic colorectal cancer tumours. *Eur. J. Cancer* **2016**, *55*, 122–130. [CrossRef]
144. Douillard, J.-Y.; Oliner, K.S.; Siena, S.; Tabernero, J.; Burkes, R. Panitumumab–FOLFOX4 Treatment and RAS Mutations in Colorectal Cancer. *N. Engl. J. Med.* **2013**, *369*, 1023–1034. [CrossRef]
145. Brulé, S.; Jonker, D.; Karapetis, C.; O'Callaghan, C.; Moore, M.; Wong, R.; Tebbutt, N.; Underhill, C.; Yip, D.; Zalcberg, J.; et al. Location of colon cancer (right-sided versus left-sided) as a prognostic factor and a predictor of benefit from cetuximab in NCIC CO.17. *Eur. J. Cancer* **2015**, *51*, 1405–1414. [CrossRef]
146. Moretto, R.; Cremolini, C.; Rossini, D.; Pietrantonio, F.; Battaglin, F.; Mennitto, A.; Bergamo, F.; Loupakis, F.; Marmorino, F.; Berenato, R.; et al. Location of Primary Tumor and Benefit From Anti-Epidermal Growth Factor Receptor Monoclonal Antibodies in Patients With *RAS* and *BRAF* Wild-Type Metastatic Colorectal Cancer. *Oncology* **2016**, *21*, 988–994. [CrossRef]
147. Venook, A.P.; Niedzwiecki, D.; Innocenti, F.; Fruth, B.; Greene, C.; O'Neil, B.H.; Shaw, J.E.; Atkins, J.N.; Horvath, L.E.; Polite, B.N.; et al. Impact of primary (1°) tumor location on overall survival (OS) and progression-free survival (PFS) in patients (pts) with metastatic colorectal cancer (mCRC): Analysis of CALGB/SWOG 80405 (Alliance). *J. Clin. Oncol.* **2016**, *34*, 3504. [CrossRef]
148. Alavi, K.M.; Poylin, V.M.; Davids, J.S.M.; Patel, S.V.M.; Felder, S.M.; Valente, M.A.D.; Paquette, I.M.M.; Feingold, D.L.M. The American Society of Colon and Rectal Surgeons Clinical Practice Guidelines for the Management of Colonic Volvulus and Acute Colonic Pseudo-Obstruction. *Dis. Colon Rectum* **2021**, *64*, 1046–1057. [CrossRef] [PubMed]
149. Rowland, A.; Dias, M.M.; Wiese, M.; Kichenadasse, G.; McKinnon, R.; Karapetis, C.; Sorich, M. Meta-analysis of BRAF mutation as a predictive biomarker of benefit from anti-EGFR monoclonal antibody therapy for RAS wild-type metastatic colorectal cancer. *Br. J. Cancer* **2015**, *112*, 1888–1894. [CrossRef]
150. Pietrantonio, F.; Petrelli, F.; Coinu, A.; Di Bartolomeo, M.; Borgonovo, K.; Maggi, C.; Cabiddu, M.; Iacovelli, R.; Bossi, I.; Lonati, V.; et al. Predictive role of BRAF mutations in patients with advanced colorectal cancer receiving cetuximab and panitumumab: A meta-analysis. *Eur. J. Cancer* **2015**, *51*, 587–594. [CrossRef] [PubMed]
151. Kopetz, S.; Grothey, A.; Yaeger, R.; Cutsem, E.V.; Desai, J. Encorafenib, Binimetinib, and Cetuximab in BRAF V600E–Mutated Colorectal Cancer. *N. Engl. J. Med.* **2019**, *381*, 1632–1643. [CrossRef] [PubMed]
152. Tabernero, J.; Grothey, A.; Van Cutsem, E.; Yaeger, R.; Wasan, H.; Yoshino, T.; Desai, J.; Ciardiello, F.; Loupakis, F.; Hong, Y.S.; et al. Encorafenib Plus Cetuximab as a New Standard of Care for Previously Treated *BRAF* V600E–Mutant Metastatic Colorectal Cancer: Updated Survival Results and Subgroup Analyses from the BEACON Study. *J. Clin. Oncol.* **2021**, *39*, 273–284. [CrossRef] [PubMed]
153. Van Cutsem, E.; Köhne, C.-H.; Láng, I.; Folprecht, G.; Nowacki, M.P.; Cascinu, S.; Shchepotin, I.; Maurel, J.; Cunningham, D.; Tejpar, S.; et al. Cetuximab Plus Irinotecan, Fluorouracil, and Leucovorin As First-Line Treatment for Metastatic Colorectal Cancer: Updated Analysis of Overall Survival According to Tumor *KRAS* and *BRAF* Mutation Status. *J. Clin. Oncol.* **2011**, *29*, 2011–2019. [CrossRef]
154. Ross, J.S.; Fakih, M.; Ali, S.M.; Elvin, J.A.; Schrock, A.B.; Suh, J.; Vergilio, J.-A.; Ramkissoon, S.; Severson, E.; Daniel, S.; et al. Targeting HER2 in colorectal cancer: The landscape of amplification and short variant mutations in *ERBB2* and *ERBB3*. *Cancer* **2018**, *124*, 1358–1373. [CrossRef]
155. Wang, X.-Y.; Zheng, Z.-X.; Sun, Y.; Bai, Y.-H.; Shi, Y.-F.; Zhou, L.-X.; Yao, Y.-F.; Wu, A.-W.; Cao, D.-F. Significance of HER2 protein expression and *HER2* gene amplification in colorectal adenocarcinomas. *World J. Gastrointest. Oncol.* **2019**, *11*, 335–347. [CrossRef]
156. Sartore-Bianchi, A.; Trusolino, L.; Martino, C.; Bencardino, K.; Lonardi, S.; Bergamo, F.; Zagonel, V.; Leone, F.; Depetris, I.; Martinelli, E.; et al. Dual-targeted therapy with trastuzumab and lapatinib in treatment-refractory, KRAS codon 12/13 wild-type, HER2-positive metastatic colorectal cancer (HERACLES): A proof-of-concept, multicentre, open-label, phase 2 trial. *Lancet Oncol.* **2016**, *17*, 738–746. [CrossRef]
157. Hainsworth, J.D.; Meric-Bernstam, F.; Swanton, C.; Hurwitz, H. Targeted Therapy for Advanced Solid Tumors on the Basis of Molecular Pro-files: Results From MyPathway, an Open-Label, Phase IIa Multiple Basket Study. *J. Clin. Oncol.* **2018**, *6*, 536–542. [CrossRef] [PubMed]
158. Gatalica, Z.; Xiu, J.; Swensen, J.; Vranic, S. Molecular characterization of cancers with NTRK gene fusions. *Mod. Pathol.* **2019**, *32*, 147–153. [CrossRef] [PubMed]

159. Doebele, R.C.; Drilon, A.; Paz-Ares, L.; Siena, S.; Shaw, A.T.; Farago, A.F.; Blakely, C.M.; Seto, T.; Cho, B.C.; Tosi, D.; et al. Entrectinib in patients with advanced or metastatic NTRK fusion-positive solid tumours: Integrated analysis of three phase 1–2 trials. *Lancet Oncol.* **2020**, *21*, 271–282. [CrossRef] [PubMed]
160. Hong, D.S.; DuBois, S.G.; Kummar, S.; Farago, A.F.; Albert, C.M.; Rohrberg, K.S.; van Tilburg, C.M.; Nagasubramanian, R.; Berlin, J.D.; Federman, N.; et al. Larotrectinib in patients with TRK fusion-positive solid tumours: A pooled analysis of three phase 1/2 clinical trials. *Lancet Oncol.* **2020**, *21*, 531–540. [CrossRef]
161. Sonbol, M.B.; Mountjoy, L.J.; Firwana, B.; Liu, A.J.; Almader-Douglas, D.; Mody, K.; Hubbard, J.; Borad, M.; Ahn, D.H.; Murad, M.H.; et al. The Role of Maintenance Strategies in Metastatic Colorectal Cancer. *JAMA Oncol.* **2020**, *6*, e194489. [CrossRef]
162. Chibaudel, B.; Maindrault-Goebel, F.; Lledo, G.; Mineur, L.; André, T.; Bennamoun, M.; Mabro, M.; Artru, P.; Carola, E.; Flesch, M.; et al. Can Chemotherapy Be Discontinued in Unresectable Metastatic Colorectal Cancer? The GERCOR OPTIMOX2 Study. *J. Clin. Oncol.* **2009**, *27*, 5727–5733. [CrossRef]
163. Hegewisch-Becker, S.; Graeven, U.; A Lerchenmüller, C.; Killing, B.; Depenbusch, R.; Steffens, C.-C.; Al-Batran, S.-E.; Lange, T.; Dietrich, G.; Stoehlmacher, J.; et al. Maintenance strategies after first-line oxaliplatin plus fluoropyrimidine plus bevacizumab for patients with metastatic colorectal cancer (AIO 0207): A randomised, non-inferiority, open-label, phase 3 trial. *Lancet Oncol.* **2015**, *16*, 1355–1369. [CrossRef]
164. Koeberle, D.; Betticher, D.C.; von Moos, R.; Dietrich, D.; Brauchli, P.; Baertschi, D.; Matter, K.; Winterhalder, R.; Borner, M.; Anchisi, S.; et al. Bevacizumab continuation versus no continuation after first-line chemotherapy plus bevacizumab in patients with metastatic colorectal cancer: A randomized phase III non-inferiority trial (SAKK 41/06). *Ann. Oncol.* **2015**, *26*, 709–714. [CrossRef]
165. Simkens, L.H.J.; van Tinteren, H.; May, A.; Tije, A.J.T.; Creemers, G.-J.M.; Loosveld, O.J.L.; E de Jongh, F.; Erdkamp, F.L.G.; Erjavec, Z.; E van der Torren, A.M.; et al. Maintenance treatment with capecitabine and bevacizumab in metastatic colorectal cancer (CAIRO3): A phase 3 randomised controlled trial of the Dutch Colorectal Cancer Group. *Lancet* **2015**, *385*, 1843–1852. [CrossRef]
166. Luo, H.; Li, Y.; Wang, W.; Wang, Z.; Yuan, X.; Ma, D.; Wang, F.; Zhang, D.; Lin, D.; Lin, Y.; et al. Single-agent capecitabine as maintenance therapy after induction of XELOX (or FOLFOX) in first-line treatment of metastatic colorectal cancer: Randomized clinical trial of efficacy and safety. *Ann. Oncol.* **2016**, *27*, 1074–1081. [CrossRef]
167. Aparicio, T.; Ghiringhelli, F.; Boige, V.; Le Malicot, K.; Taieb, J.; Bouché, O.; Phelip, J.-M.; François, E.; Borel, C.; Faroux, R.; et al. Bevacizumab Maintenance Versus No Maintenance During Chemotherapy-Free Intervals in Metastatic Colorectal Cancer: A Randomized Phase III Trial (PRODIGE 9). *J. Clin. Oncol.* **2018**, *36*, 674–681. [CrossRef]
168. Díaz-Rubio, E.; Gómez-España, A.; Massutí, B.; Sastre, J.; Abad, A.; Valladares, M.; Rivera, F.; Safont, M.J.; de Prado, P.M.; Gallén, M.; et al. First-Line XELOX Plus Bevacizumab Followed by XELOX Plus Bevacizumab or Single-Agent Bevacizumab as Maintenance Therapy in Patients with Metastatic Colorectal Cancer: The Phase III MACRO TTD Study. *Oncology* **2012**, *17*, 15–25. [CrossRef]
169. Yalcin, S.; Uslu, R.; Dane, F.; Yilmaz, U.; Zengin, N.; Buyukunal, E.; Buyukberber, S.; Camci, C.; Sencan, O.; Kilickap, S.; et al. Bevacizumab + Capecitabine as Maintenance Therapy after Initial Bevacizumab + XELOX Treatment in Previously Untreated Patients with Metastatic Colorectal Cancer: Phase III 'Stop and Go' Study Results—A Turkish Oncology Group Trial. *Oncology* **2013**, *85*, 328–335. [CrossRef] [PubMed]
170. Hagman, H.; Frödin, J.-E.; Berglund, Å.; Sundberg, J.; Vestermark, L.; Albertsson, M.; Fernebro, E.; Johnsson, A. A randomized study of KRAS-guided maintenance therapy with bevacizumab, erlotinib or metronomic capecitabine after first-line induction treatment of metastatic colorectal cancer: The Nordic ACT2 trial. *Ann. Oncol.* **2016**, *27*, 140–147. [CrossRef] [PubMed]
171. Cremolini, C.; Antoniotti, C.; Lonardi, S.; Aprile, G.; Bergamo, F.; Masi, G.; Grande, R.; Tonini, G.; Mescoli, C.; Cardellino, G.G.; et al. Activity and Safety of Cetuximab Plus Modified FOLFOXIRI Followed by Maintenance With Cetuximab or Bevacizumab for *RAS* and *BRAF* Wild-type Metastatic Colorectal Cancer. *JAMA Oncol.* **2018**, *4*, 529–536. [CrossRef] [PubMed]
172. Pietrantonio, F.; Morano, F.; Corallo, S.; Miceli, R.; Lonardi, S.; Raimondi, A.; Cremolini, C.; Rimassa, L.; Bergamo, F.; Sartore-Bianchi, A.; et al. Maintenance Therapy With Panitumumab Alone vs Panitumumab Plus Fluorouracil-Leucovorin in Patients With *RAS* Wild-Type Metastatic Colorectal Cancer. *JAMA Oncol.* **2019**, *5*, 1268–1275. [CrossRef] [PubMed]
173. Modest, D.P.; Karthaus, M.; Fruehauf, S.; Graeven, U.; Müller, L.; König, A.O.; von Weikersthal, L.F.; Caca, K.; Kretzschmar, A.; Goekkurt, E.; et al. Panitumumab Plus Fluorouracil and Folinic Acid Versus Fluorouracil and Folinic Acid Alone as Maintenance Therapy in *RAS* Wild-Type Metastatic Colorectal Cancer: The Randomized PANAMA Trial (AIO KRK 0212). *J. Clin. Oncol.* **2022**, *40*, 72–82. [CrossRef]
174. Giantonio, B.J.; Catalano, P.J.; Meropol, N.J.; O'Dwyer, P.J.; Mitchell, E.P.; Alberts, S.R.; Schwartz, M.A.; Benson, A.B., III. Bevacizumab in Combination with Oxaliplatin, Fluorouracil, and Leucovorin (FOLFOX4) for Previously Treated Metastatic Colorectal Cancer: Results From the Eastern Cooperative Oncology Group Study E3200. *J. Clin. Oncol.* **2007**, *25*, 1539–1544. [CrossRef]
175. Van Cutsem, E.; Tabernero, J.; Lakomy, R.; Prenen, H.; Prausová, J.; Macarulla, T.; Ruff, P.; van Hazel, G.A.; Moiseyenko, V.; Ferry, D.; et al. Addition of Aflibercept to Fluorouracil, Leucovorin, and Irinotecan Improves Survival in a Phase III Randomized Trial in Patients With Metastatic Colorectal Cancer Previously Treated With an Oxaliplatin-Based Regimen. *J. Clin. Oncol.* **2012**, *30*, 3499–3506. [CrossRef]
176. Tabernero, J.; Yoshino, T.; Cohn, A.L.; Obermannova, R.; Bodoky, G.; Garcia-Carbonero, R.; Ciuleanu, T.-E.; Portnoy, D.C.; Van Cutsem, E.; Grothey, A.; et al. Ramucirumab versus placebo in combination with second-line FOLFIRI in patients with metastatic

colorectal carcinoma that progressed during or after first-line therapy with bevacizumab, oxaliplatin, and a fluoropyrimidine (RAISE): A randomised, double-blind, multicentre, phase 3 study. *Lancet Oncol.* **2015**, *16*, 499–508. [CrossRef]
177. Grothey, A.; Van Cutsem, E.; Sobrero, A.; Siena, S.; Falcone, A.; Ychou, M.; Humblet, Y.; Bouché, O.; Mineur, L.; Barone, C.; et al. Regorafenib monotherapy for previously treated metastatic colorectal cancer (CORRECT): An international, multicentre, randomised, placebo-controlled, phase 3 trial. *Lancet* **2013**, *381*, 303–312. [CrossRef] [PubMed]
178. Mayer, R.J.; Van Cutsem, E.; Falcone, A.; Yoshino, T.; Garcia-Carbonero, R.; Mizunuma, N.; Yamazaki, K.; Shimada, Y.; Tabernero, J.; Komatsu, Y.; et al. Randomized Trial of TAS-102 for Refractory Metastatic Colorectal Cancer. *N. Engl. J. Med.* **2015**, *372*, 1909–1919. [CrossRef]
179. Sargent, D.; Sobrero, A.; Grothey, A.; O'Connell, M.J.; Buyse, M.; André, T.; Zheng, Y.; Green, E.; Labianca, R.; O'Callaghan, C.; et al. Evidence for Cure by Adjuvant Therapy in Colon Cancer: Observations Based on Individual Patient Data From 20,898 Patients on 18 Randomized Trials. *J. Clin. Oncol.* **2009**, *27*, 872–877. [CrossRef] [PubMed]
180. Seo, S.I.; Lim, S.-B.; Yoon, Y.S.; Kim, C.W.; Yu, C.S.; Kim, T.W.; Kim, J.H.; Kim, J.C. Comparison of recurrence patterns between ≤5 years and >5 years after curative operations in colorectal cancer patients. *J. Surg. Oncol.* **2013**, *108*, 9–13. [CrossRef]
181. Butte, J.M.; Gönen, M.; Allen, P.J.; Kingham, T.P.; Sofocleous, C.T.; DeMatteo, R.P.; Fong, Y.; Kemeny, N.E.; Jarnagin, W.R.; D'Angelica, M.I. Recurrence After Partial Hepatectomy for Metastatic Colorectal Cancer: Potentially Curative Role of Salvage Repeat Resection. *Ann. Surg. Oncol.* **2015**, *22*, 2761–2771. [CrossRef] [PubMed]
182. Kennedy, E.; Zwaal, C.; Asmis, T.; Cho, C.; Galica, J.; Ginty, A.; Govindarajan, A. An Evidence-Based Guideline for Surveillance of Patients after Curative Treatment for Colon and Rectal Cancer. *Curr. Oncol.* **2022**, *29*, 724–740. [CrossRef]
183. Verberne, C.J.; Zhan, Z.; Heuvel, E.R.V.D.; Oppers, F.; de Jong, A.M.; Grossmann, I.; Klaase, J.M.; de Bock, G.H.; Wiggers, T. Survival analysis of the CEAwatch multicentre clustered randomized trial. *Br. J. Surg.* **2017**, *104*, 1069–1077. [CrossRef]
184. Desch, C.E.; Benson, A.B.; Somerfield, M.R.; Flynn, P.J.; Krause, C.; Loprinzi, C.L.; Minsky, B.D.; Pfister, D.G.; Virgo, K.S.; Petrelli, N.J. Colorectal Cancer Surveillance: 2005 Update of an American Society of Clinical Oncology Practice Guideline. *J. Clin. Oncol.* **2005**, *23*, 8512–8519. [CrossRef]
185. Hardiman, K.M.M.; Felder, S.I.M.; Friedman, G.M.; Migaly, J.M.; Paquette, I.M.M.; Feingold, D.L.M. The American Society of Colon and Rectal Surgeons Clinical Practice Guidelines for the Surveillance and Survivorship Care of Patients After Curative Treatment of Colon and Rectal Cancer. *Dis. Colon Rectum* **2021**, *64*, 517–533. [CrossRef]
186. Hyder, O.; Dodson, R.M.; Mayo, S.C.; Schneider, E.B.; Weiss, M.J.; Herman, J.M.; Wolfgang, C.L.; Pawlik, T.M. Post-treatment surveillance of patients with colorectal cancer with surgically treated liver metastases. *Surgery* **2013**, *154*, 256–265. [CrossRef]
187. Sobhani, I.; Itti, E.; Luciani, A.; Baumgaertner, I.; Layese, R.; André, T.; Ducreux, M.; Gornet, J.-M.; Goujon, G.; Aparicio, T.; et al. Colorectal cancer (CRC) monitoring by 6-monthly 18FDG-PET/CT: An open-label multicentre randomised trial. *Ann. Oncol.* **2018**, *29*, 931–937. [CrossRef]
188. Kotani, D.; Oki, E.; Nakamura, Y.; Yukami, H.; Mishima, S.; Bando, H.; Shirasu, H.; Yamazaki, K.; Watanabe, J.; Kotaka, M.; et al. Molecular residual disease and efficacy of adjuvant chemotherapy in patients with colorectal cancer. *Nat. Med.* **2023**, *29*, 127–134. [CrossRef] [PubMed]
189. Hervieu, C.; Christou, N.; Battu, S.; Mathonnet, M. The Role of Cancer Stem Cells in Colorectal Cancer: From the Basics to Novel Clinical Trials. *Cancers* **2021**, *13*, 1092. [CrossRef] [PubMed]
190. Munro, M.; Wickremesekera, S.K.; Peng, L.; Tan, S.T.; Itinteang, T. Cancer stem cells in colorectal cancer: A review. *J. Clin. Pathol.* **2017**, *71*, 110–116. [CrossRef]
191. Nenkov, M.; Ma, Y.; Gaßler, N.; Chen, Y. Metabolic Reprogramming of Colorectal Cancer Cells and the Microenvironment: Implication for Therapy. *Int. J. Mol. Sci.* **2021**, *22*, 6262. [CrossRef] [PubMed]

Disclaimer/Publisher's Note: The statements, opinions and data contained in all publications are solely those of the individual author(s) and contributor(s) and not of MDPI and/or the editor(s). MDPI and/or the editor(s) disclaim responsibility for any injury to people or property resulting from any ideas, methods, instructions or products referred to in the content.

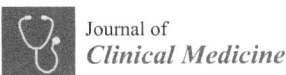

Article

The Effects of Primary Tumor Location on Survival after Liver Resection for Colorectal Liver Metastasis in the Mediterranean Population

Ahmad Mahamid [1,2], Omar Abu-Zaydeh [1], Esther Kazlow [1,2], Dvir Froylich [1,2], Muneer Sawaied [1], Natalia Goldberg [2,3], Yael Berger [4,5], Wissam Khoury [1,2], Eran Sadot [4,5] and Riad Haddad [1,2,*]

1. Department of Surgery, Carmel Medical Center, Haifa 3436212, Israel; mahamidam@yahoo.com (A.M.); oabuzaydeh@gmail.com (O.A.-Z.); ekazlow@gmail.com (E.K.); dvirfr7@gmail.com (D.F.); moneerswaed@gmail.com (M.S.); wekhoury@gmail.com (W.K.)
2. The Ruth and Bruce Rappaport Faculty of Medicine, Technion-Israel Institute of Technology, Haifa 3200003, Israel; natalia.goldberg@gmail.com
3. Department of Radiology, Carmel Medical Center, Haifa 3436212, Israel
4. Department of Surgery, Rabin Medical Center, Petch Tiqvah 4941492, Israel; yaelberger1@gmail.com (Y.B.); eransadot@gmail.com (E.S.)
5. Sackler School of Medicine, Tel Aviv University, Tel Aviv 6139001, Israel
* Correspondence: dr.riad.haddad@gmail.com

Abstract: (1) Background: There is an abundance of literature available on predictors of survival for patients with colorectal liver metastases (CRLM) but minimal information available on the relationship between the primary tumor location and CRLM survival. The studies that focus on the primary tumor location and CRLM survival exhibit a great deal of controversy and inconsistency with regard to their results (some studies show statistically significant connections between the primary tumor location and prognosis versus other studies that find no significant relationship between these two factors). Furthermore, the majority of these studies have been conducted in the West and have studied more diverse and heterogenous populations, which may be a contributing factor to the conflicting results. (2) Methods: We included patients who underwent liver resection for CRLM between December 2004 and January 2019 at two university-affiliated medical centers in Israel: Carmel Medical Center (Haifa) and Rabin Medical Center (Petach Tiqvah). Primary tumors located from the cecum up to and including the splenic flexure were labeled as right-sided primary tumors, whereas tumors located from the splenic flexure down to the anal verge were labeled as left-sided primary tumors. (3) Results: We identified a total of 501 patients. Of these patients, 225 had right-sided primary tumors and 276 had left-sided primary tumors. Patients with right-sided tumors were significantly older at the time of liver surgery compared to those with left-sided tumors (66.1 + 12.7 vs. 62 + 13.1, $p = 0.002$). Patients with left-sided tumors had slightly better overall survival rates than those with right-sided tumors. However, the differences were not statistically significant (57 vs. 50 months, $p = 0.37$ after liver surgery). (4) Conclusions: The primary tumor location does not significantly affect patient survival after liver resection for colorectal liver metastasis in the Mediterranean population.

Keywords: colorectal liver metastasis; survival; colon cancer; tumor side

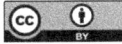

1. Introduction

Colorectal cancer with liver metastasis (CRLM) is a major health concern worldwide. CRLM occurs in almost half of all patients with colorectal cancer, with an estimated 20–25% of newly diagnosed colorectal cancer patients presenting with liver metastases at the time of diagnosis [1].

According to the Israeli Health Ministry, colorectal cancer has become the second most prevalent malignancy in Jewish and Arab Israeli women, closely following breast cancer. It is the second most common malignancy in Arab Israeli men following lung cancer, and the third most prevalent malignancy in Jewish Israeli men following prostate and lung cancers. According to an international comparison, the incidence rate of colorectal cancer is slightly higher in Israel in comparison to the world average [2]. There are various factors that influence the prognosis of patients with CRLM. A largely understudied factor is the relationship between the primary tumor location (right colon versus left colon) and prognosis in patients with CRLM. The literature available on this association has provided conflicting and inconsistent results.

A previous study identified seven factors as significant and independent predictors of poor long-term outcomes. These included a positive margin, extrahepatic disease, node-positive primary disease, a disease-free interval from primary to metastasis < 12 months, a number of hepatic tumors > 1, the largest hepatic tumor > 5 cm, and a carcinoembryonic antigen level > 200 ng/mL. A preoperative scoring system was developed using the last five criteria, assigning one point for each criterion. The total score was highly predictive of outcomes ($p < 0.0001$). No patient with a score of 5 or above was a long-term survivor [3]. Other studies have identified reliable prognostic biomarkers in patients with resectable CRLM. In a 2013 study, Umeda et al. analyzed genomic DNA obtained from CRLM tissue from patients undergoing curative hepatic resection. The results showed that KRAS and BRAF mutations were poor prognostic factors in CRLM and that microsatellite instability (MSIH) cancer rarely revealed metastatic potential [4].

A 2015 retrospective study investigated the prognostic impact of the primary tumor location in metastatic colorectal cancer (mCRC) in patients receiving first-line chemotherapy ± bevacizumab in three independent cohorts: a prospective pharmacogenetic study (PROVETTA) and two randomized phase III trials, AVF2107g and NO16966. The study found that patients with left-sided primary tumors had superior OS ($p < 0.001$) and progression-free survival ($p < 0.001$) in comparison to patients with right-sided primary tumors [5].

Recent studies also found that patients with CRLM with right-sided primary tumors had a significantly worse prognosis compared to those with left-sided primary tumors [6,7]. Moreover, other studies have suggested that right-sided colon cancers are more likely to have specific genetic mutations that may contribute to their more aggressive behavior. One such mutation is the BRAF mutation, which has been found to be more common in right-sided colon cancers compared to left-sided colon cancers [8].

However, other studies have reported conflicting results. For example, a 2011 study analyzed the relationship between the colon cancer location (right versus left side) and tumor stage and their effects on 5-year mortality. The study found that there was no major difference in mortality between right- and left-sided cancers for all stages. Stage II right-sided cancers had lower mortality than left-sided cancers, while stage III right-sided cancers had higher mortality than left-sided tumors [9]. Furthermore, a 2017 study investigated the impact of the primary tumor location on overall survival (OS), recurrence-free survival (RFS), and long-term outcomes in patients undergoing potentially curative resection of colorectal liver metastases (CRLM). The analysis was based on data from a single-institution database of 907 patients who underwent initial resections for CRLM. The results showed that patients with left-sided primary tumors had a significantly improved median OS compared to those with right-sided primaries (5.2 years vs. 3.6 years, $p = 0.004$). However, there was no significant difference in median RFS stratified by primary location (1.3 vs. 1.7 years, $p = 0.065$) and the association of the primary location with RFS was not statistically significant in a multivariable analysis ($p = 0.105$) [10].

It is important to note that most of the current data on the differences between right- and left-sided colon cancers come from studies conducted in the Western world. There are limited data available on the differences between these tumors in the Mediterranean population, and it is unclear whether the same differences exist in this population. The aim of our study was to investigate, for the first time, this largely understudied association with a geographically specific population with the aim of improving the interpretability and validity of this association so that it can be further extrapolated to the population at large.

By studying this homogenous population, we hoped to gain a better understanding of the genetic and environmental factors that contribute to the differences in prognosis between right- and left-sided colon cancers. This may ultimately lead to more personalized and effective treatments for patients with CRLM.

2. Materials and Methods

Patients who underwent liver resection for CRLM between December 2004 and January 2019 were identified from the surgical databases at Carmel Medical Center (Haifa, Israel) and Rabin Medical Center (Petach Tikvah, Israel). Clinical indicators of these patients' perioperative courses were retrospectively examined, including their demographics, detailed surgical history, pathology results, and oncologic follow-up records. The study was conducted in accordance with the Declaration of Helsinki and Good Clinical Practice Guidelines and was approved by the institutional review boards (IRBs) of the Carmel and Rabin Medical Centers. Indications for surgery were determined during a weekly multidisciplinary conference. The pre-operative workup included blood tests, tumor markers, imaging modalities (computed tomography (CT), positron emission CT (PET-CT), and magnetic resonance imaging (MRI)), and characterization of the specific tumor (number, location, size, and relation to intrahepatic vascular or biliary structures). All patients underwent standard evaluation for surgery by an attending anesthesiologist. Patients were informed in detail about the procedure, including the risks and benefits, and written consent was obtained before surgery.

Metastasis was defined as the occurrence of a liver tumor, during follow-up or at diagnosis, in patients with colorectal cancer. Tumors located from the cecum up to and including the splenic flexure were labeled as right-sided primary tumors. Tumors located from the splenic flexure down to the anal verge were labeled as left-sided primary tumors. Based on previous studies, rectal cancer patients were treated as left-sided primary tumors in our study [5]. Blood loss was estimated using the volume of blood lost from the abdominal cavity during the procedure. Operative time was defined as the time elapsed from the initial incision until closure. Postoperative hospital stay was defined as the number of hospitalized days from the day of operation until the day of discharge, inclusive. We used the Clavien–Dindo grading system to characterize any post-operative complications occurring within 30 days of surgery [11]. Tumor size and resection margins were determined according to the pathological reports from the permanent sections of tissue samples. R0 was defined as no cancer cells seen microscopically at the resection margin.

After discharge, the patients were followed by our multidisciplinary team during the first month post-surgery, every 4 months for the first 2 years thereafter, and subsequently twice a year. Follow-up examinations included blood work (including CBC, chemistries, liver function tests, and carcinoembryonic antigens) and a spiral CT of the chest–abdomen or PET-CT as indicated.

Statistical Analysis

All statistical analyses were performed using IBM statistics (SPSS) vs. 24. Continuous variables were summarized with the mean ± SD or median and IQR, as appropriate. Categorical variables were presented as numbers and proportions Disease-free (DFS) and overall survival (OS) were estimated using Kaplan–Meier curves and compared between groups by log-rank test. $p < 0.05$ was considered statistically significant.

3. Results

The data from Tables 1–3 and Figures 1 and 2 provide a detailed analysis of the differences and similarities between patients who underwent liver surgery for CRLM, as categorized by the primary tumor location.

Table 1. Baseline demographic, liver, and colorectal characteristics, and perioperative and histological outcomes.

	Right-Sided Primary (Total = 225) n (%)	Left-Sided Primary (Total = 276) n (%)	p
Age (liver surgery)	66.1 ± 12.7	62 ± 13.1	0.002
Gender			
Male	129 (57.3%)	155 (56.2%)	0.43
Female	96 (42.7%)	121 (43.8%)	
T			
1	1 (0.4%)	3 (1.1%)	
2	7 (3.1%)	14 (5.1%)	
3	157 (69.8%)	144 (52.2%)	0.19
4	8 (3.6%)	13 (4.7%)	
unknown	52 (23.1%)	102 (36.9%)	
N			
N0	61 (27.1%)	75 (27.2%)	
N1	72 (32%)	64 (23.2%)	0.20
N2	43 (19.1%)	34 (12.4%)	
unknown	49 (21.8)	103 (37.3%)	
DFS (liver mets)			
<12 months	126 (56%)	142 (51.4%)	
>12 months	89 (39.6%)	110 (38.9%)	0.35
unknown	10 (4.4%)	24 (8.7%)	
Clinical risk factor			
0–2	156 (69.4%)	154 (55.8%)	
3–5	48 (21.3%)	41 (14.9%)	0.31
unknown	22 (9.3%)	81 (29.3%)	
Size of largest liver tumor			
<5 cm	201 (89.3%)	223 (80.8%)	0.08
>5 cm	24 (10.7%)	53 (19.2%)	
Number of liver mets			
1	117 (52%)	152 (55.1%)	0.24
>1	108 (48%0	124 (44.9%)	
R status			
Negative	207 (92%)	245 (88.7%)	0.16
Positive	18 (8%)	31 (11.3%)	
Peri-operative chemotherapy			
Yes	155 (68.9%)	197 (71.4%)	0.27
No	70 (31.1%)	79 (28.6%)	
Blood transfusion			
Yes	41 (18.2)	67 (24.3%)	
No	176 (78.2%)	178 (64.5%)	0.02
unknown	8 (3.6%)	31 (11.2%)	
Liver resection			
Anatomical	43 (19.1%)	67 (24.4%)	0.37
Non-anatomical	182 (80.1%)	208 (75.6%)	
Complication			
Yes	100 (44.4%)	100 (36.2%)	0.053
No	125 (55.6%)	176 (63.8%)	
Sequence of resection			
Liver first	9 (3.6%)	19 (6.6%)	
Colon first	181 (80.7%)	213 (77.2%)	0.31
Combined	35 (15.7%)	44 (16.2%)	

Table 2. Short- and long-term outcomes after liver surgery.

	Right-Sided Primary (Total = 225)	Left-Sided Primary (Total = 276)	p
12 months	88.4%	91.6%	
24 months	74.9%	76.2%	
36 months	62.3%	66.5%	
60 months	42.8%	45.8%	
120 months	30.6%	29.6%	
Median (95% CI) months	50 (41:60)	57 (47:58)	0.37

Table 3. Short- and long-term outcomes after colon surgery.

	Right-Sided Primary (Total = 225)	Left-Sided Primary (Total = 276)	p
12 months	96.4%	96.7%	
24 months	86.8%	87.3%	
36 months	74.7%	77.3%	
60 months	51.3%	57.8%	
120 months	32%	34.2%	
Median (95% CI) months	63 (49:77)	76 (63:89)	0.19

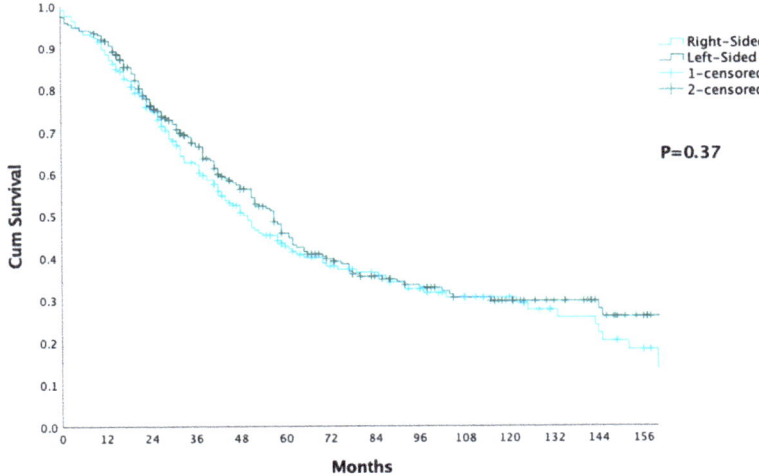

Figure 1. Overall survival after liver surgery.

Table 1 shows that patients with right-sided primary tumors were significantly older (mean age 66.1 ± 12.7 years) than those with left-sided primary tumors (mean age 62 ± 13.1 years) ($p = 0.002$). The gender distribution was similar between the two groups ($p = 0.43$). In terms of T stage, there were no significant differences between the groups ($p = 0.19$). The distribution of n stages was also similar between the two groups, with no major differences observed ($p = 0.20$). The percentage of patients who had disease-free survival (DFS) for liver metastases of more than 12 months was not appreciably different between the two groups ($p = 0.35$).

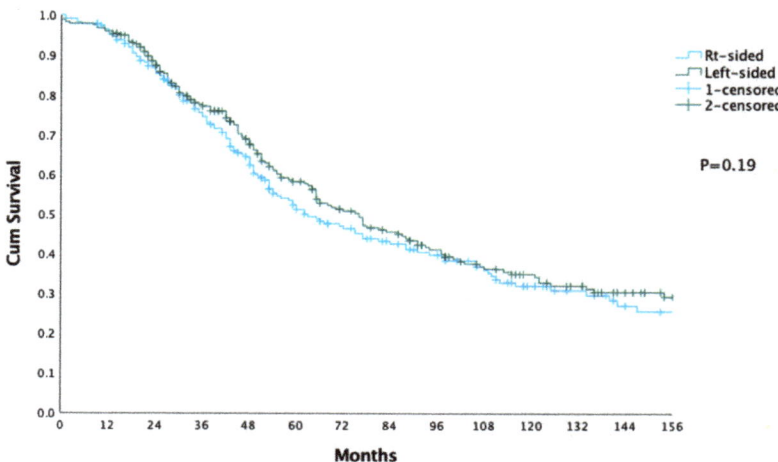

Figure 2. Overall survival after colon surgery.

Clinical risk factors (Fong), the size of the largest liver tumor, and the number of liver metastases were not significantly different between the two groups ($p = 0.31$, $p = 0.08$, $p = 0.24$, respectively). There was no noteworthy difference in R status between the two groups ($p = 0.16$). The proportion of patients who received perioperative chemotherapy was not significantly different between the two groups ($p = 0.27$). However, more patients in the right-sided group received blood transfusions ($p = 0.02$) and experienced complications after surgery ($p = 0.053$). The distribution of liver resection types (anatomical and non-anatomical) and the sequence of resection were also not significantly different between the two groups ($p = 0.37$ and $p = 0.31$, respectively).

Table 2 and Figure 1 show the short- and long-term outcomes after liver surgery, comparing the survival between the groups at different time points (12, 24, 36, 60, 120 months). The median survival time for the right-sided group was 50 months (95% CI 41:60), and for the left-sided group, it was 57 months (95% CI 47:58). There were no major differences in survival rates between the two groups ($p = 0.37$).

Table 3 and Figure 2 show the short- and long-term outcomes after colon surgery. Comparing the survival between the groups at different time points (12, 24, 36, 60, 120 months), the median survival time for the right-sided group was 63 months (95% CI 49:77), and for the left-sided group, it was 76 months (95% CI 63:89). There were no significant differences in survival rates between the two groups ($p = 0.19$).

4. Discussion

Our study suggests that the primary tumor location does not significantly affect patient survival after liver resection for colorectal liver metastasis in the Mediterranean population.

There has been a great deal of controversy with regard to the primary tumor location and the ultimate prognosis of patients with CRLM available in the literature to date. The majority of these studies have been conducted in the West and focused on heterogenous populations, which may be a contributing factor to the conflicting results. The aim of our study was to investigate, for the first time, this relationship (primary tumor location and prognosis) in a Mediterranean population. Our goal was to study a more homogenous population in an attempt to minimize the potential for false-positive or false-negative results related to genetic confounding.

A 2017 systematic review and meta-analysis aimed to determine the prognostic role of the primary tumor location in patients with colon cancer. The review included 66 studies with a total of 1,437,846 patients and concluded that a left-sided primary tumor location was associated with a significantly reduced risk of death independently of stage, race, adjuvant chemotherapy, year of study, number of participants, and quality of included studies. The study suggested that the colon cancer location should be acknowledged as a criterion in establishing prognosis at all stages of the disease and should be considered when deciding on a treatment in metastatic settings [12].

Furthermore, a 2020 review discussed the impact of the primary tumor location on the prognosis of patients after the local treatment of CRLM. The authors reviewed and analyzed 10 studies that examined the association between right- and left-sided colorectal cancer on overall survival (OS) and recurrence-free survival (RFS) after local treatment (resection and/or ablation) of CRLM. The results showed that patients with right-sided tumors had a significantly decreased OS ($p < 0.001$) and RFS ($p = 0.03$) compared to patients with left-sided tumors [6].

Another study conducted in 2019 investigated the impact of the location of the primary tumor on the long-term survival outcomes of colorectal liver metastases following hepatic resection. The review analyzed 12 studies with 6387 patients and found that primary right-sided colorectal liver metastases following hepatic resection had significantly worse overall survival compared to left-sided tumors. However, the analysis did not find a significant difference in disease-free survival [7].

The role of tumor genetics in relation to the primary tumor location and prognosis is a potential confounding variable. A study on data from twins in Sweden, Denmark, and Finland analyzed the role of genetic and environmental factors in the development of cancer. The study found that genetic factors play a minor role in the development of most types of cancer and that environmental factors have the primary role in causing sporadic cancer. However, the study also revealed that genetics play a significant role in the development and prognosis of prostate and colorectal cancer [13].

Tsilimigras et al. conducted a systematic review of the literature in 2018, which analyzed the clinical significance and prognostic relevance of genetic mutations of KRAS for resectable and unresectable CRLM. The review included 78 studies that reported mutation data for patients with resectable and unresectable CRLM. The review found that KRAS mutation was a negative prognostic factor for overall and recurrence-free survival [14] Studies have also shown that the BRAF mutation is associated with worse prognosis and an increased risk of recurrence in patients with CRLM [8,14,15]. Furthermore, Yaeger et al. found that BRAF-mutant CRLM cases were associated with a right-sided location [8]. Interestingly, the BRAF mutation has been found to be more common in Western populations [16]. Therefore, the lower prevalence of BRAF mutations in the Mediterranean population may contribute to the lack of significant differences in survival between right- and left-sided primary tumors in our study.

The reason for these conflicting results is not entirely clear, but one possible explanation is that the studies used different definitions of the primary tumor location, leading to inconsistent results. Another possible explanation is that the studies included heterogenous patient populations with varying characteristics, such as age, gender, and disease stage, which may have contributed to the differences in the results. In addition, genetic differences between populations may also contribute to the conflicting results on the impact of the primary tumor location and the prognosis of patients with CRLM. The Mediterranean population differs from Western populations in many genetic and environmental factors, such as a high degree of endogamy, climate, and diet, which may play a role in the differences in tumor biology and clinical outcomes.

The impact of the primary tumor location on the prognosis of patients with colorectal liver metastasis (CRLM) remains controversial. While several studies have investigated the relationship between the primary tumor location and patient outcomes, the results have been inconsistent. In this study, we investigated the effects of the primary tumor location on the survival of patients who underwent liver resection for CRLM in the Mediterranean population. Our findings showed no statistically significant differences between patients who had right-sided and left-sided primary tumors in terms of overall survival after liver resection for CRLM. Our results are consistent with previous studies that have reported no significant differences in long-term survival and recurrence-free survival between right- and left-sided primary tumors in patients with CRLM.

Our study has several limitations that should be considered when interpreting the results. Firstly, the retrospective nature of the study may have introduced selection bias, as only patients who underwent liver resection for CRLM were included in the analysis. Furthermore, we did not analyze the genetic differences between right and left colon cancers in our study, which may have contributed to our findings. Additionally, our study focused on the Mediterranean population, and the results may not be applicable to other populations. Lastly, another potential confounding variable is age. In our study, patients with right-sided tumors were significantly older at the time of liver surgery compared to those with left-sided tumors. Despite these limitations, our study has several strengths, including the analysis of a homogeneous population of patients from the Mediterranean region, which reduces the confounding effects of genetic and environmental factors that may vary across different populations. In addition, our study provides evidence of the impact of the primary tumor location on the prognosis of patients with CRLM, which is a topic of ongoing debate in the literature. Lastly, our study adds to the growing body of literature on the differences between right and left colon cancers, and the implications for the clinical outcomes of patients with CRLM.

5. Conclusions

Overall, our study suggests that the primary tumor location may not be a significant predictor of survival in patients who undergo liver resection for CRLM in the Mediterranean population. However, further research is needed to better understand the genetic and environmental factors that contribute to the differences in prognosis between right- and left-sided colon cancers across different populations, and to develop personalized treatment strategies for patients with CRLM based on their tumor characteristics.

Author Contributions: Conceptualization, A.M. and R.H.; methodology, A.M.; formal analysis, R.H. and N.G.; data curation, O.A.-Z., M.S. and Y.B. writing—original draft preparation, A.M.; writing—review and editing, A.M., O.A.-Z., E.K., D.F., M.S., N.G., W.K., E.S. and R.H. All authors have read and agreed to the published version of the manuscript.

Funding: This research received no external funding.

Institutional Review Board Statement: The study was conducted according to the guidelines of the Declaration of Helsinki and approved by the Institutional Review Board (or Ethics Committee) of Carmel Medical Center (protocol code 0117-20-CMC and date of approval 19 July 2020) and Rabin Medical Center (protocol code RMC-0709-16, and date of approval 14 November 2016).

Informed Consent Statement: Not applicable—a retrospective study.

Data Availability Statement: The data presented in this study are available on request from the corresponding author.

Conflicts of Interest: The authors declare no conflict of interest.

References

1. Van Cutsem, E.; Cervantes, A.; Adam, R.; Sobrero, A.; Van Krieken, J.H.; Aderka, D.; Aranda Aguilar, D.; Bardelli, A.; Benson, A.; Bodoky, G.; et al. ESMO consensus guidelines for the management of patients with metastatic colorectal cancer. *Ann. Oncol.* **2016**, *27*, 1386–1422. [PubMed]
2. Itzhaki, M. Knowledge and feelings about colorectal cancer among the Jewish adult population in Israel: A mixed methods study. *Appl. Nurs. Res.* **2018**, *43*, 64–68. [CrossRef] [PubMed]
3. Fong, Y.; Fortner, J.; Sun, R.L.; Brennan, M.F.; Blumgart, L.H. Clinical score for predicting recurrence after hepatic resection for metastatic colorectal cancer: Analysis of 1001 consecutive cases. *Ann. Surg.* **1999**, *230*, 309–318; discussion 318. [CrossRef] [PubMed]
4. Umeda, Y.; Nagasaka, T.; Mori, Y.; Sadamori, H.; Sun, D.-S.; Shinoura, S.; Yoshida, R.; Satoh, D.; Nobuoka, D.; Utsimi, M.; et al. Poor prognosis of KRAS or BRAF mutant colorectal liver metastasis without microsatellite instability. *J. Hepatobiliary Pancreat. Sci.* **2013**, *20*, 223–233. [CrossRef] [PubMed]

5. Loupakis, F.; Yang, D.; Yau, L.; Feng, S.; Cremolini, C.; Zhang, W.; Maus, M.K.H.; Antoniotti, C.; Lagner, C.; Scherer, S.J.; et al. Primary tumor location as a prognostic factor in metastatic colorectal cancer. *J. Natl. Cancer Inst.* **2015**, *107*, dju427. [CrossRef]
6. Buisman, F.E.; Galjart, B.; Buettner, S.; Groot Koerkamp, B.; Grünhagen, D.J.; Verhoef, C. Primary tumor location and the prognosis of patients after local treatment of colorectal liver metastases: A systematic review and meta-analysis. *HPB* **2020**, *22*, 351–357. [CrossRef] [PubMed]
7. Liu, W.; Wang, H.-W.; Wang, K.; Xing, B.-C. The primary tumor location impacts survival outcome of colorectal liver metastases after hepatic resection: A systematic review and meta-analysis. *Eur. J. Surg. Oncol.* **2019**, *45*, 1349–1356. [CrossRef]
8. Yaeger, R.; Cercek, A.; Chou, J.F.; Sylvester, B.E.; Kemeny, N.E.; Hechtman, J.F.; Ladanyi, M.; Rosen, N.; Weiser, M.R.; Capanu, M.; et al. BRAF mutation predicts for poor outcomes after metastasectomy in patients with metastatic colorectal cancer. *Cancer* **2014**, *120*, 2316–2324. [CrossRef]
9. Weiss, J.M.; Pfau, P.R.; O'Connor, E.S.; King, J.; LoConte, N.; Kennedy, G.; Smith, M.A. Mortality by stage for right- versus left-sided colon cancer: Analysis of surveillance, epidemiology, and end results—Medicare data. *J. Clin. Oncol.* **2011**, *29*, 4401–4409. [CrossRef] [PubMed]
10. Creasy, J.M.; Sadot, E.; Koerkamp, B.G.; Chou, J.F.; Gonen, M.; Kemeny, N.E.; Saltz, L.B.; Balachandran, V.P.; Kingham, T.P.; DeMatteo, R.P.; et al. The Impact of Primary Tumor Location on Long-Term Survival in Patients Undergoing Hepatic Resection for Metastatic Colon Cancer. *Ann. Surg. Oncol.* **2018**, *25*, 431–438. [CrossRef] [PubMed]
11. Dindo, D.; Demartines, N.; Clavien, P.-A. Classification of surgical complications: A new proposal with evaluation in a cohort of 6336 patients and results of a survey. *Ann. Surg.* **2004**, *240*, 205–213. [CrossRef] [PubMed]
12. Petrelli, F.; Tomasello, G.; Borgonovo, K.; Ghidini, M.; Turati, L.; Dallera, P.; Passalacqua, R.; Sgroi, G.; Barni, S. Prognostic Survival Associated with Left-Sided vs Right-Sided Colon Cancer: A Systematic Review and Meta-analysis. *JAMA Oncol.* **2017**, *3*, 211–219. [CrossRef] [PubMed]
13. Lichtenstein, P.; Holm, N.V.; Verkasalo, P.K.; Iliadou, A.; Kaprio, J.; Koskenvuo, M.; Pukkala, E.; Skytthe, A.; Hemminki, K. Environmental and heritable factors in the causation of cancer—Analyses of cohorts of twins from Sweden, Denmark, and Finland. *N. Engl. J. Med.* **2000**, *343*, 78–85. [CrossRef] [PubMed]
14. Tsilimigras, D.I.; Ntanasis-Stathopoulos, I.; Bagante, F.; Moris, D.; Cloyd, J.; Spartalis, E.; Pawlik, T.M. Clinical significance and prognostic relevance of KRAS, BRAF, PI3K and TP53 genetic mutation analysis for resectable and unresectable colorectal liver metastases: A systematic review of the current evidence. *Surg. Oncol.* **2018**, *27*, 280–288. [CrossRef] [PubMed]
15. Margonis, G.A.; Buettner, S.; Andreatos, N.; Kim, Y.; Wagner, D.; Sasaki, K.; Beer, A.; Schwarz, C.; Løes, I.M.; Smolle, M.; et al. Association of BRAF mutations with survival and recurrence in surgically treated patients with metastatic colorectal liver cancer. *JAMA Surg.* **2018**, *153*, e180996. [CrossRef] [PubMed]
16. Ibrahim, T.; Saer-Ghorra, C.; Trak-Smayra, V.; Nadiri, S.; Yazbeck, C.; Baz, M.; Kattan, J.G. Molecular characteristics of colorectal cancer in a Middle Eastern population in a single institution. *Ann. Saudi Med.* **2018**, *38*, 251–259. [CrossRef]

Disclaimer/Publisher's Note: The statements, opinions and data contained in all publications are solely those of the individual author(s) and contributor(s) and not of MDPI and/or the editor(s). MDPI and/or the editor(s) disclaim responsibility for any injury to people or property resulting from any ideas, methods, instructions or products referred to in the content.

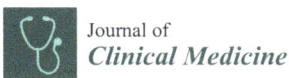

Article

Emergency Colectomies in the Elderly Population—Perioperative Mortality Risk-Factors and Long-Term Outcomes

Ilan Kent [1,2,*], Amandeep Ghuman [3], Luna Sadran [1,2], Adi Rov [1,2], Guy Lifschitz [1,2], Yaron Rudnicki [1,2], Ian White [1,2], Nitzan Goldberg [1,2] and Shmuel Avital [1,2]

1 Department of Surgery, Meir Medical Center, Kfar Saba 4428164, Israel
2 Sackler Faculty of Medicine, Tel Aviv University, Tel Aviv 6139001, Israel
3 Department of Surgery, University of British Columbia, Vancouver, BC V6T 1Z4, Canada
* Correspondence: ilankent@gmail.com; Tel.: +972-9-7472164; Fax: +972-9-7471305

Abstract: Background: As the population ages emergency surgeries among the elderly population, including colonic resections, is also increasing. Data regarding the short- and long-term outcomes in this population is scarce. Methods: A retrospective study was performed to investigate mortality and mortality risk factors associated with emergent colectomies in older compared to younger patients in a single university affiliated tertiary hospital. Patients with metastatic disease, colectomy due to trauma or index colectomy within 30 days prior to emergent surgery were excluded. Results: Operative outcomes compared among age groups, included 30-day mortality, mortality risk-factors and long-term survival. 613 eligible patients were included in the cohort. Mean age was 69.4 years, 45.1% were female. Patients were divided into four age groups: 18–59, 60–69, 70–79 and ≥80-years. Thirty-day mortality rates were 3.2%, 11%, 29.3% and 37.8%, respectively and 22% for the entire cohort. Risk-factors for perioperative death in the younger group were related to severity of ASA score and WBC count. In groups 60–69, 70–79, main risk-factors were ADL dependency and ASA score. In the ≥80 group, risk-factors affecting perioperative mortality, included ASA score, pre-operative albumin, creatinine, WBC levels, cancer etiology, ADL dependency, and dementia. Long-term survival differed significantly between age groups. Conclusion: Perioperative mortality with emergency colectomy increases with patients' age. Patients older than eighty-years undergoing urgent colectomies have extremely high mortality rates, leading to a huge burden on medical services. Evaluating risk-factors for mortality and pre-operative discussion with patients and families is important. Screening the elderly population for colonic pathologies can result in early diagnosis potentially leading to elective surgeries with decreased mortality.

Keywords: emergent colectomy; elderly; geriatric; mortality; dementia; bedridden

Citation: Kent, I.; Ghuman, A.; Sadran, L.; Rov, A.; Lifschitz, G.; Rudnicki, Y.; White, I.; Goldberg, N.; Avital, S. Emergency Colectomies in the Elderly Population—Perioperative Mortality Risk-Factors and Long-Term Outcomes. *J. Clin. Med.* **2023**, *12*, 2465. https://doi.org/10.3390/jcm12072465

Academic Editors: Maria Elena Riccioni and Toshio Uraoka

Received: 17 January 2023
Revised: 5 March 2023
Accepted: 13 March 2023
Published: 23 March 2023

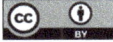

Copyright: © 2023 by the authors. Licensee MDPI, Basel, Switzerland. This article is an open access article distributed under the terms and conditions of the Creative Commons Attribution (CC BY) license (https:// creativecommons.org/licenses/by/ 4.0/).

1. Introduction

The elderly population in the western world is growing rapidly. It is estimated that by 2030, the world is likely to have 1 billion people older than age 65, accounting for 13% of the world population [1]. In the United States, more than 35 million Americans are 65 years or older, which represents more than 12% of the population [2]. This segment of the population is expected to increase very quickly in the near future [3]. General surgery, like many other fields of medicine, is facing a tremendous shift, with accommodations made to treat patients in this age group. It is estimated that more than half of the operations performed in the United States involve patients 65 or older [4]; although they comprise only 15% of the population. Many colonic pathologies requiring surgery, including colorectal cancer, diverticulitis and ischemic colitis, are diseases of aging [5–7]. The number of abdominal surgeries performed on elderly patients is expected to increase, including emergent surgeries. Emergent surgery in any population, even more so among the elderly and specifically emergent colorectal surgery, all have higher rates of morbidity and mortality and poorer outcomes [8]. Therefore, it is becoming imperative to investigate modifiable risk-factors, to improve patient outcomes among the elderly. This study evaluated 30-day mortality after emergency colorectal surgery in elderly patients to identify risk-factors for mortality and to evaluate their long-term survival compared to younger patients.

2. Methods

2.1. Study Design

This retrospective study included all patients ≥18 years of age who underwent an emergent colectomy at a university-affiliated tertiary medical center from 2005 to 2017. Patients were identified from the institutional database. Exclusion criteria were patients who underwent a colostomy as primary surgery, patients with metastatic disease, colonic injury secondary to trauma or a colectomy performed within 30-days secondary to a previous operation. Patients with metastatic disease, including oligometastatic disease, were excluded from this cohort in order to try to investigate the impact of the emergent surgery disregarding the background of potentially terminal disease and its associated significant risk factors such as malnourishment, immunologic deficiency and other related conditions. As we also tried to evaluate long term survival after surgery (up to 12 years) related mainly to the traumatic event of the emergent surgery and not to a metastatic disease.

2.2. Study Rationale, Variables, and Outcome Measures

First, we analyzed the primary outcome of 30-day mortality to compare overall survival across the groups, to determine a cut-off value of a meaningful decrease in 30-day survival. A sharp increase in 30-day mortality was observed in the groups older than 60 years. We than aimed to determine risk-factors for 30-day mortality. The cohort was subdivided into four age categories 18–59, 60–69, 70–79 and ≥80-years. Factors assessed for inclusion in the models included gender, body mass index (BMI), etiology for resection, stoma creation, being bed ridden (ADL dependency) diagnosis of dementia, Charlson comorbidity index, blood transfusion, hemoglobin level, white blood cell count (WBC), American Society of Anesthesiologists physical status score (ASA) and creatinine level. Main outcome measures were 30-day mortality and post-operative complications.

2.3. Statistical Analysis

Descriptive statistical analysis was performed on patient characteristics, including demographics and operative variables and compared between the various groups using student t-test for continuous data and chi squared for categorical data. A p-value < 0.05 was considered significant. Univariate logistic regression was performed to identify predictors of 30-day mortality in each age group. Factors with p-values < 0.05 were considered significant and included in a multivariable logistic regression analysis. A p-value < 0.05 was considered significant in multivariable analysis to determine adjusted odds ratios of risk-factors for 30-day mortality in the four age categories. Statistical analyses were performed using IBM SPSS Statistics for Windows, version 21.0 (IBM Corp., Armonk, NY, USA).

3. Results

A total of 784 patients who underwent an emergent colectomy from January 2005 to December 2017 were initially identified for chart review. Of these, 613 met the inclusion criteria and were included in the analysis (Figure 1). The cohort included 336 (55%) men and 277 (45%) women. Operation for cancer as an etiology was performed in 408 (66.5%) patients. A diversion with an ostomy was performed in 230 (37.5%) patients. The Average length of stay was 14.4 days (1–107 Days). The median follow-up for the entire cohort was 77 months. The number of emergency operations increased with age, with the largest group of patients ≥80 years (Figure 2). The two most common surgeries performed were right colectomy (n = 178) and Hartmann's procedure (n = 178). All procedures performed on the cohort are shown in Table 1. The overall 30-day mortality rate was 22% for the entire cohort. The 30-day mortality in the four age groups was 3.2%, 11%, 29.3% and 37.8%, respectively (Figure 3). In the youngest patient group, perioperative mortality was related to illness status when arriving to surgery, as reflected by ASA scores and WBC counts (Tables 2 and 3). In the intermediate age groups (69–69, 70–79), there was an incremental increase in mortality rate that was associated with ASA score and ADL dependency (Tables 2 and 3). The high mortality rate (37.8%) in patients older than 80 years was associated, in a univariate analysis, with ASA score and ADL dependency like in the younger age groups. However, many other risk-factors, including, WBC, creatinine, albumin levels prior to surgery, dementia, cancer etiology and blood transfusion were found to be associated with perioperative mortality in this age group (Table 2). Interestingly, these factors did not reach statistical significance in multivariate analysis. This could be because these factors are much more prevalent in patients older than 80 in general and their combination together leads to a substantial increase in perioperative mortality in this specific age group. Long-term overall survival was also in accordance with the age group (Figure 4). Patients ≥80 years who survived the operation had a 22% mortality rate one year after surgery.

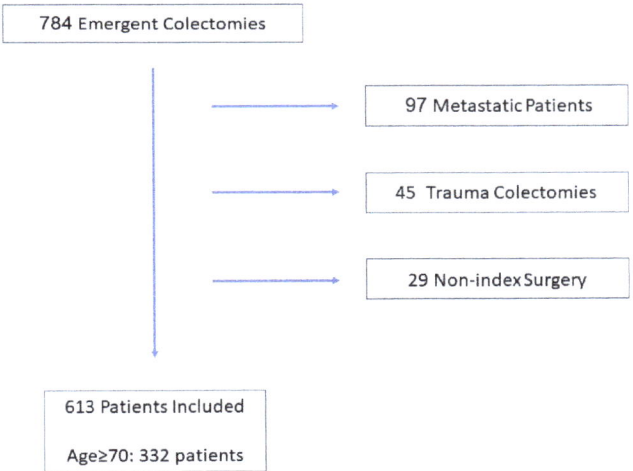

Figure 1. Flow diagram of patient inclusion.

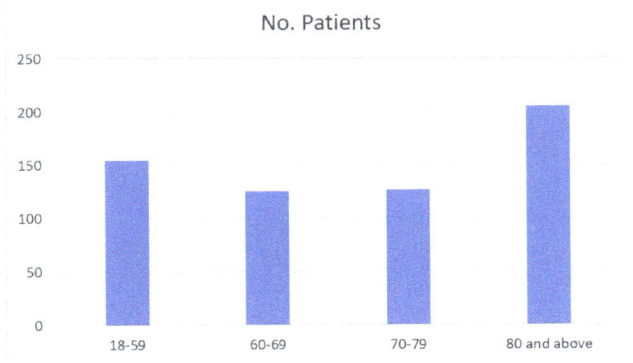

Figure 2. Surgeries in each age group.

Table 1. Total procedures performed.

Procedure	Total Cohort $n = 613$
Right colectomy, n (%)	178 (29)
Hartmann's procedure, n (%)	178 (29)
Left colectomy, n (%)	71 (11.5)
Sub-total colectomy, n (%)	54 (9)
Cecectomy, n (%)	53 (8)
Sigmoidectomy, n (%)	29 (4.7)
Subtotal colectomy with ileostomy, n (%)	25 (4)
Total colectomy, n (%)	15 (2.4)
Anterior resection, n (%)	9 (1.4)
Abdominoperineal resection, n (%)	1 (0.1)

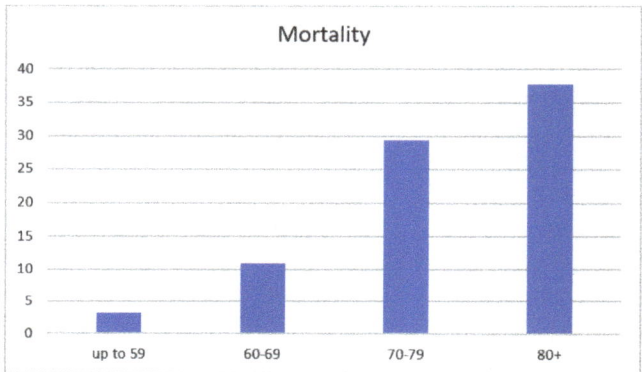

Figure 3. 30-day mortality rates in each age group.

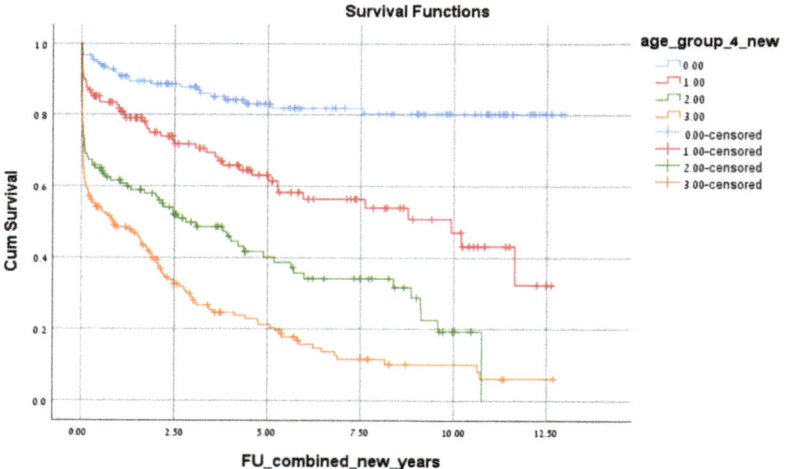

Figure 4. Overall Kaplan-Meier survival curve.

Table 2. Risk-factors for 30-day mortality according to age groups- univariate analysis.

	18–59			60–69			70–79			80+		
	Survive n=150 (96.8%)	30d Death n=5 (3.2%)	p Value	Survive n=113 (89%)	30d Death n=14 (11%)	p Value	Survive n=87 (70.7%)	30d Death n=36 (29.3%)	p Value	Survive n=130 (62.2%)	30d Death n=79 (37.8%)	p Value
Gender n (%)			1.000			0.392			0.877			0.107
Male	98 (65.3)	3 (60)		71 (62.8)	7 (50)		47 (54.0)	20 (55.6)		51 (39.2)	40 (50.6)	
Female	52 (34.7)	2 (40)		42 (37.2)	7 (50)		40 (46.0)	16 (44.4)		79 (60.8)	39 (49.4)	
BMI mean ± SD	–	–		28.62 ± 5.36	31.72 ± 6.98	0.162	27.23 ± 4.17	27.92 ± 7.53	0.766	25.49 ± 4.55	26.23 ± 6.32	0.787
ADL-dependent n (%)	10 (6.7)	1 (20)	0.311	12 (10.6)	8 (57.1)	**0.000**	7 (8.0)	12 (33.3)	**0.000**	30 (23.1)	37 (47.4)	**0.000**
Dementia n (%)	3 (2)	1 (20)	0.124	4 (3.5)	2 (14.3)	0.131	3 (3.4)	8 (22.2)	**0.002**	21 (16.2)	29 (37.2)	**0.001**
Cancer n (%)	121 (80.7)	4 (80)	1.000	73 (64.6)	12 (85.7)	0.141	58 (66.7)	24 (66.7)	1.000	63 (48.5)	53 (67.1)	**0.009**
ASA score n (%)			**0.008**			**0.000**			**0.032**			**0.001**
1	68 (45.3)	1 (20)		19 (16.8)	0 (0)		6 (6.9)	2 (5.6)		8 (6.2)	5 (6.3)	
2	54 (36.0)	2 (40)		53 (46.9)	5 (35.7)		39 (44.8)	10 (27.8)		54 (41.5)	13 (16.5)	
3	21 (14)	0 (0)		36 (31.9)	4 (28.6)		36 (41.4)	15 (41.7)		64 (49.2)	50 (63.3)	
4	7 (4.7)	2 (40)		5 (4.4)	5 (35.7)		6 (6.9)	9 (25.0)		4 (3.1)	10 (12.7)	
5	0 (0)	0 (0)		0 (0)	0 (0)		0 (0)	0 (0)		0	1 (1.3)	
Charlson score mean ± SD	1.26 ± 2.52	2.60 ± 3.209	0.182	2.16 ± 2.52	2.64 ± 2.24	0.173	2.77 ± 2.69	2.97 ± 2.75	0.650	3.10 ± 3.23	3.33 ± 2.79	0.128
LOS mean ± SD	13.81 ± 12.54	7.00 ± 5.38	0.087	17.23 ± 16.34	11.43 ± 8.76	0.195	14.86 ± 12.30	7.25 ± 8.54	**0.001**	18.01 ± 16.43	9.41 ± 8.68	**0.000**
Blood transfusion n (%)	16 (10.7)	2 (40)	0.103	16 (14.2)	4 (28.6)	0.234	12 (13.8)	8 (22.2)	0.249	25 (19.2)	16 (20.3)	0.857
Hemoglobin mean ± SD	13.08 ± 2.21	12.54 ± 2.87	0.594	13.05 ± 2.16	12.01 ± 1.98	0.101	12.21 ± 2.05	12.10 ± 2.54	0.818	11.81 ± 1.89	13.38 ± 12.43	0.385
WBC mean ± SD	13.09 ± 5.46	19.15 ± 6.50	**0.017**	12.32 ± 5.25	17.68 ± 16.65	0.270	12.75 ± 4.57	14.54 ± 8.04	0.247	12.13 ± 5.27	14.83 ± 8.33	**0.035**
Creatinine mean ± SD	1.19 ± 1.43	2.75 ± 3.50	0.441	1.21 ± 0.91	1.9 ± 1.71	0.217	1.306 ± 0.927	1.946 ± 1.56	0.058	1.25 ± 0.52	1.83 ± 1.60	**0.000**
Albumin mean ± SD	–	–		3.03 ± 0.83	2.45 ± 0.49	0.375	2.87 ± 0.55	2.83 ± 0.66	0.901	2.95 ± 0.69	2.34 ± 0.72	**0.017**
Surgery specific cause			0.084			0.259			0.074			0.286
Obstruction, n (%)	39 (29.9)	3 (60)		50 (44.2)	4 (28.6)		43 (51.8)	10 (30.3)		75 (58.1)	37 (48.1)	
Perforation, n (%)	65 (44.8)	1 (20)		40 (35.4)	5 (35.7)		28 (33.7)	18 (54.5)		37 (28.7)	22 (28.6)	
Ischemia, n (%)	3 (2.1)	1 (20)		9 (8.0)	4 (28.6)		5 (6.0)	5 (15.2)		11 (8.5)	11 (14.3)	
Infection, n (%)	16 (11.0)	0 (0)		9 (8.0)	1 (7.1)		4 (4.8)	0 (0)		5 (3.9)	4 (5.7)	
Inflammation, n (%)	21 (14.5)	0 (0)		3 (2.7)	0 (0)		1 (1.2)	0 (0)		0 (0)	0 (0)	
Bleeding, n (%)	1 (0.7)	0 (0)		2 (1.8)	0 (0)		2 (2.4)	0 (0)		1 (0.8)	3 (3.9)	

Statistical significant values are in bold.

Table 3. Multivariable regression analysis for risk-factors for 30-day mortality.

Variables in the Model	18-59			Variables in the Model	60-69			Variables in the Model	70-79			Variables in the Model	≥80		
	Adjusted OR	95% CI	p Value		Adjusted OR	95% CI	p Value		Adjusted OR	95% CI	p Value		Adjusted OR	95% CI	p Value
WBC	1.215	1.040–1.421	**0.014**	WBC	2.459	1.057–5.72	**0.037**	ASA	2.428	1.085–5.43	**0.031**	ASA	1.503	0.139–16.29	0.738
ASA	2.675	0.943–7.584	0.064	ADL	6.773	1.652–27.76	**0.008**	ADL	9.664	1.536–60.79	**0.016**	ADL	2.030	0.119–34.49	0.624
Blood transfusion	2.156	0.219–21.194	0.510	Dementia	1.113	0.123–10.08	0.924	Dementia	0.848	0.089–8.04	0.886	Dementia	3.988	0.150–105.78	0.408
Specific cause	0.258	0.052–1.270	0.096	Hemoglobin	0.841	0.612–1.15	0.288	Creatinine	1.344	0.894–2.02	0.155	Cancer	2.370	0.083–67.309	0.613
Dementia	13.164	0.722–240.149	0.082									WBC	1.285	0.982–1.681	0.068
												Creatinine	4.169	0.617–28.16	0.143
												Albumin	0.050	0.002–1.112	0.058

CI, confidence interval; OR, odds ratio; WBC, white blood cell count; ASA, American Society of Anesthesiologists; ADL, activities of daily living. Statistically significant variables and values are in bold.

4. Discussion

The number of emergency colectomies performed increases as the population ages. As shown in our cohort, these surgeries entail higher mortality rates. This is a growing healthcare concern and a major economic and social burden that will likely intensify as the fraction of the aging population continues to increase.

This study evaluated 30-day mortality rates and risk-factors after emergent colectomies in different age groups. We found an increase in emergent colectomies performed in patients over the age of 80. We also found a substantial, gradual increase in perioperative mortality in patients above 60 years old, reaching to almost 40% among patients 80 or older. These findings are in contrast to younger patient populations where morbidity and mortality rates are similar between elective colorectal resections and emergency colectomies [3,9] and also potentially in contrast to elective colorectal surgery in the elderly were 30 days mortality rates were also lower [10].

The mortality rates in our cohort are slightly higher than those reported in a retrospective review of emergent colorectal surgeries by McGillicuddy and co-workers [11]. Their study revealed a 15% in-hospital mortality in an elderly cohort. However, they defined elderly as patients older than 65. Modini and colleagues reported a 30% mortality rate among 93 patients over 80 years old [12]. This is comparable to the rates in our cohort. In addition, in a review of 1245 patients undergoing colorectal resection, Klima et al. reported a 1.32 times greater likelihood of mortality for each 10 year age increase [13].

The observed high mortality rates after emergency surgery in elderly patients may be due to pre-existing comorbidities and impairments reflected in our study, with a high prevalence of as ADL dependency and dementia. This results in poor candidates for emergency surgery. Furthermore, lower physiological reserve may decrease their ability to cope with surgical stress and lead to more complications. Frailty scores are often used to assess surgical risk in the elderly population [14]. 30% of older people with frailty die within a year after having an emergency surgery compared to older patients who are not frail [12]. In our study that specifically evaluated perioperative outcomes following emergency colectomy, the mortality rate one year after surgery in patients ≥80 years who survived the operation was 22%; much higher than among younger patients.

This study identified several risk-factors for perioperative mortality that varied across age groups. In the below 60 age group, perioperative mortality was directly associated with the level of the severity of their condition in which surgery was performed, reflected by the ASA score and WBC count. In patients up to 79 years, ADL dependency became significant which is more common in this age group. In the oldest group (≥80 years) additional risk-factors were identified in univariate analysis, including dementia. However, did not reach statistical significance in multivariate analysis. This may be because these factors are generally more prevalent in patients older than 80 and that the combination of all these factors and not a specific single factor leads to a substantial increase in perioperative mortality in this age group.

Previous studies in elderly patients undergoing emergent and elective general surgery, trauma surgery, vascular surgery or orthopedic surgery for hip fractures, have reported higher mortality rates when dementia was present [15–18]. ASA score, another non-modifiable risk factor, has been linked to higher mortality after acute surgery in the elderly [19,20]. This factor could account for the multiple co-morbidities often seen in the elderly population.

To the best of our knowledge, this is the first study that specifically examined ADL dependency as a risk-factor for mortality after colorectal surgery. Other studies have shown frailty to be associated with mortality, but not specifically ADL dependence [21,22]. ADL dependence is a risk factor for 30-day mortality probably because these patients are less physically active, have worse preconditioning and are less likely to adhere to recovery activities such as early mobilization, and physical and respiratory therapy. This makes them potentially more prone to life-threatening complications such as venous thromboembolism, and pulmonary and urinary tract complications.

Several studies evaluated patients who underwent emergency surgery and identified sepsis as a risk-factor for 30 day-mortality [23,24]. These findings may imply it is important to appropriately resuscitate patients prior to surgery with timely antibiotics and fluids prior to surgery in septic patients. These recommendations are in line with the Surviving Sepsis campaign, which has outlined the importance of these interventions and should be generalized to include patients with underlying sepsis requiring emergency colectomies [25].

The limitations of this study include its retrospective nature and single academic center setting with general surgeons of varying levels of colorectal surgery training performing emergency colonic resections. A previous study on emergent colectomies showed lower rates of postoperative morbidity and mortality when performed by a trained colorectal surgeon [26]. Thus, these results may not apply to institutions where emergent colonic resections are performed by dedicated colorectal surgeons.

Furthermore, the retrospective nature of this study precluded calculation of objective scores such as a frailty score or Katz index of independence in ADL. Calculation of these scores requires data which is not routinely collected in the medical records of acutely admitted patients. Despite these limitations, this study confirms high mortality rates after emergent colonic resections in older patients and identifies potential the risk-factors that could be applicable to any practice performing emergency colectomies in the elderly. Larger scale and possibly multi-center studies may further elucidate mortality rates and other risk-factors for mortality in this growing population.

Our findings may encourage colorectal cancer screening in the elderly population, which can lead to early diagnosis and treatment with elective surgery and potentially lower mortality. Furthermore, physicians and healthcare workers caring for this population should be familiar with the signs and symptoms of large bowel pathologies that can lead to prompt diagnosis and timely transfer to emergency healthcare facilities.

Surgeons are increasingly consulted on elderly patients with acute surgical pathologies, often requiring surgery with large bowel resection. When considering the potential risks of surgery, the surgeon must consider the patient's age, general status, comorbidities, and surgical problems, to name a few. This information may be valuable for the surgeon and critical surgical teams preparing a patient for acute care surgery and when discussing expectations regarding surgical outcomes with patients and their families.

5. Conclusions

Increasing life expectancy coupled with the high prevalence of colorectal pathologies have led to a dramatic rise in the number of elderly patients undergoing emergency colorectal surgery. Perioperative mortality increases gradually from the age of 60, reaching a high percentage in patients over 80 years old. In this age group, the mortality rate is extremely high and is believed to be associated with a combination of risk-factors related to the severity of their presentation and pre-existing conditions typical of the elderly population. Surgeons treating the older population should be aware of higher mortality risks and try to address modifiable risk-factors prior to undertaking emergent colorectal resections, when applicable. Screening of the elderly population for colonic pathologies can result in early diagnosis that would lead to elective surgeries with decreased mortality.

Author Contributions: Conceptualization, I.K., I.W. and S.A.; methodology, I.K., A.G., I.W. and S.A.; formal analysis, A.G., N.G. and S.A.; data curation, L.S., A.R., G.L. and Y.R.; writing—original draft, I.K. and A.G.; writing—review & editing, S.A. All authors have read and agreed to the published version of the manuscript.

Funding: This research received no external funding.

Institutional Review Board Statement: The study was conducted in accordance with the Declaration of Helsinki, and approved by the Institutional Review Board of Meir Medical center (protocol code MMC-0121-18, and date of approval 9 April 2018).

Informed Consent Statement: Patient consent was waived due to the retrospective nature of the study and the analysis used anonymous clinical data.

Data Availability Statement: The data presented in this study are available on request from the corresponding author.

Conflicts of Interest: The authors declare no conflict of interest.

References

1. National Institute on Aging (NIA). Why Population Aging Matters: A Global Perspective. Report by the National Institute on Aging, Summit on Global Aging. 2007. Available online: http://www.nia.nih.gov/ResearchInformation/ExtramuralPrograms/BehavioralAndSocialResearch/GlobalAging.htm (accessed on 2 March 2023).
2. Rix, T.E.; Bates, T. Pre-operative risk scores for the prediction of outcome in elderly people who require emergency surgery. *World J. Emerg. Surg.* **2007**, *2*, 16–18. [CrossRef] [PubMed]
3. Biondi, A.; Vacante, M.; Ambrosino, I.; Cristaldi, E.; Pietrapertosa, G.; Basile, F. Role of surgery for colorectal cancer in the elderly. *World J. Gastrointest. Surg.* **2016**, *8*, 606–613. [CrossRef] [PubMed]
4. Etzioni, D.A.; Liu, J.H.; Maggard, M.A.; Ko, C.Y. The Aging Population and Its Impact on the Surgery Workforce. *Ann. Surg.* **2003**, *238*, 170–177. [CrossRef] [PubMed]
5. Siegel, R.; Naishadham, D.; Jemal, A. Cancer statistics, 2013. *CA Cancer J. Clin.* **2013**, *63*, 11–30. [CrossRef] [PubMed]
6. Hupfeld, L.; Pommergaard, H.-C.; Burcharth, J.; Rosenberg, J. Emergency admissions for complicated colonic diverticulitis are increasing: A nationwide register-based cohort study. *Int. J. Colorectal. Dis.* **2018**, *33*, 879–886. [CrossRef]
7. Brandt, L.J.; Feuerstadt, P.; Longstreth, G.F.; Boley, S.J. American College of Gastroenterology. ACG clinical guideline: Epidemiology, risk factors, patterns of presentation, diagnosis, and management of colon ischemia (CI). *Am. J. Gastroenterol.* **2015**, *110*, 18–44. [CrossRef]
8. McArdle, C.S.; Hole, D.J. Emergency presentation of colorectal cancer is associated with poor 5-year survival. *Br. J. Surg.* **2004**, *91*, 605–609. [CrossRef]
9. Basili, G.; Lorenzetti, L.; Biondi, G.; Preziuso, E.; Angrisano, C.; Carnesecchi, P.; Roberto, E.; Goletti, O. Colorectal cancer in the elderly. Is there a role for safe and curative surgery? *ANZ J. Surg.* **2008**, *78*, 466–470. [CrossRef]
10. Fagard, K.; Casaer, J.; Wolthuis, A.; Flamaing, J.; Milisen, K.; Lobelle, J.P.; Wildiers, H.; Kenis, C. Postoperative complications in individuals aged 70 and over undergoing elective surgery for colorectal cancer. *Color. Dis.* **2017**, *19*, O329–O338. [CrossRef]
11. McGillicuddy, E.A.; Schuster, K.M.; Davis, K.A.; Longo, W.E. Factors predicting morbidity and mortality in emergency colorectal procedures in elderly patients. *Arch Surg.* **2009**, *144*, 1157–1162. [CrossRef]
12. Modini, C.; Romagnoli, F.; De Milito, R.; Romeo, V.; Petroni, R.; La Torre, F.; Catani, M. Octogenarians: An increasing challenge for acute care and colorectal surgeons. An outcomes analysis of emergency colorectal surgery in the elderly. *Colorectal. Dis.* **2012**, *14*, e312–e318. [CrossRef]
13. Klima, D.A.; Brintzenhoff, R.A.; Agee, N.; Walters, A.; Heniford, B.T.; Mostafa, G. A Review of Factors that Affect Mortality Following Colectomy. *J. Surg. Res.* **2012**, *174*, 192–199. [CrossRef]
14. Lin, H.-S.; Watts, J.N.; Peel, N.M.; Hubbard, R.E. Frailty and post-operative outcomes in older surgical patients: A systematic review. *BMC Geriatr.* **2016**, *16*, 157. [CrossRef]
15. Kassahun, W.T. The effects of pre-existing dementia on surgical outcomes in emergent and nonemergent general surgical procedures: Assessing differences in surgical risk with dementia. *BMC Geriatr.* **2018**, *18*, 153. [CrossRef]
16. Mehaffey, J.H.; Hawkins, R.; Tracci, M.C.; Robinson, W.P.; Cherry, K.J.; Kern, J.A.; Upchurch, G.R. Preoperative dementia is associated with increased cost and complications after vascular surgery. *J. Vasc. Surg.* **2018**, *68*, 1203–1208. [CrossRef]
17. Bai, J.; Zhang, P.; Liang, X.; Wu, Z.; Wang, J.; Liang, Y. Association between dementia and mortality in the elderly patients undergoing hip fracture surgery: A meta-analysis. *J. Orthop. Surg. Res.* **2018**, *13*, 298. [CrossRef]
18. Jordan, B.C.; Brungardt, J.; Reyes, J.; Helmer, S.D.; Haan, J.M. Dementia as a predictor of mortality in adult trauma patients. *Am. J. Surg.* **2018**, *215*, 48–52. [CrossRef]
19. Davis, P.; Hayden, J.; Springer, J.; Bailey, J.; Molinari, M.; Johnson, P. Prognostic factors for morbidity and mortality in elderly patients undergoing acute gastrointestinal surgery: A systematic review. *Can J. Surg.* **2014**, *57*, E44–E52. [CrossRef]
20. Arenal, J.J.; Bengoechea-Beeby, M. Mortality associated with emergency abdominal surgery in the elderly. *Can. J. Surg.* **2003**, *46*, 111–116.
21. McIsaac, D.I.; Taljaard, M.; Bryson, G.L.; Beaulé, P.E.; Gagné, S.; Hamilton, G.; Hladkowicz, E.; Huang, A.; Joanisse, J.A.; Lavallée, L.T.; et al. Frailty as a Predictor of Death or New Disability After Surgery: A Prospective Cohort Study. *Ann. Surg.* **2020**, *271*, 283–289. [CrossRef]

22. Shah, R.; Attwood, K.; Arya, S.; Hall, D.E.; Johanning, J.M.; Gabriel, E.; Visioni, A.; Nurkin, S.; Kukar, M.; Hochwald, S.; et al. Association of Frailty with Failure to Rescue After Low-Risk and High-Risk Inpatient Surgery. *JAMA Surg.* **2018**, *153*, e180214. [CrossRef] [PubMed]
23. Moore, L.J.; Moore, F.A.; Jones, S.L.; Xu, J.; Bass, B.L. Sepsis in general surgery: A deadly complication. *Am. J. Surg.* **2009**, *198*, 868–874. [CrossRef] [PubMed]
24. Mačiulienė, A.; Maleckas, A.; Kriščiukaitis, A.; Mačiulis, V.; Vencius, J.; Macas, A. Predictors of 30-Day In-Hospital Mortality in Patients Undergoing Urgent Abdominal Surgery Due to Acute Peritonitis Complicated with Sepsis. *Med. Sci. Monit.* **2019**, *25*, 6331–6340. [CrossRef] [PubMed]
25. Rhodes, A.; Evans, L.E.; Alhazzani, W.; Levy, M.M.; Antonelli, M.; Ferrer, R.; Kumar, A.; Sevransky, J.E.; Sprung, C.L.; Nunnally, M.E.; et al. Surviving Sepsis Campaign: International Guidelines for Management of Sepsis and Septic Shock: 2016. *Intensive Care Med.* **2017**, *43*, 304–377. [CrossRef]
26. Kulaylat, A.S.; Pappou, E.; Philp, M.M.; Kuritzkes, B.A.; Ortenzi, G.; Hollenbeak, C.S.; Choi, C.; Messaris, E. Emergent Colon Resections. *Dis. Colon. Rectum.* **2019**, *62*, 79–87. [CrossRef]

Disclaimer/Publisher's Note: The statements, opinions and data contained in all publications are solely those of the individual author(s) and contributor(s) and not of MDPI and/or the editor(s). MDPI and/or the editor(s) disclaim responsibility for any injury to people or property resulting from any ideas, methods, instructions or products referred to in the content.

Article

Developing a Robotic Surgical Platform Is Beneficial to the Implementation of the ERAS Program for Colorectal Surgery: An Outcome and Learning Curve Analysis

Chun-Yen Hung [1], Chun-Yu Lin [1], Ming-Cheng Chen [1], Teng-Yi Chiu [1], Tzu-Wei Chiang [1] and Feng-Fan Chiang [1,2,*]

[1] Division of Colorectal Surgery, Department of Surgery, Taichung Veterans General Hospital, 1650 Taiwan Boulevard Sect. 4, Taichung 40705, Taiwan

[2] Department of Food and Nutrition, Providence University, Taichung 43301, Taiwan

* Correspondence: hankel.chiang@gmail.com; Tel.: +886-4-2359-2525 or +886-915-710-446; Fax: +886-4-2359-5046

Abstract: Background: Robotic surgery and ERAS protocol care are both prominent developments and have each become global trends. However, the effects and learning curves of combining robotic surgery and ERAS care in colorectal resection have not yet been well validated. This study aimed to present our real-world experience and establish the learning curves necessary for the implementation of an ERAS program in minimally-invasive surgery for colorectal resection, while also evaluating the impact that the development of the robotic technique has on ERAS outcomes. Methods: A total of 155 patients who received elective, minimally-invasive surgery, including laparoscopic and robotic surgery for colorectal resection, with ERAS care during the period June 2019 to September 2021 were included in this retrospective analysis. Patients were divided chronologically into five groups (31 cases per quintile). Patient demographics, tumor characteristics, perioperative data, ERAS compliance, and surgical outcomes were all compared among the quintiles. Learning curves were evaluated based on ERAS compliance and optimal recovery, which are composed of an absence of major complications, postoperative length of stay (LOS) of no more than five days, and no readmission within 30 days. A multivariable logistic regression model was used to assess factors associated with postoperative LOS. Results: There were no statistically significant differences seen overall or between the quintile groups in regards to demographic and tumor characteristic parameters. A total of 79 patients (51%) received robotic surgery, with the ratio of robotic groups rising chronologically from zero in the first quintile to 90.3% in the fifth quintile ($p < 0.001$). The median compliance rate of total ERAS protocol was 83.3% overall, 72.2% in the first quintile and 83.3% in the 2nd–5th quintiles ($p < 0.001$). A total of 85 patients underwent optimal recovery after surgery, four patients in the first quintile, 11 patients in the second quintile, and 21, 24, 25 patients in the 3rd–5th quintiles respectively ($p < 0.001$). There were significant improvements from early to later groups upon postoperative LOS ($p < 0.001$). In addition, the surgical outcomes including first oral intake within 24 hours after surgery, time to first stool and early termination of intravenous fluid administration showed significant improvement among the quintiles. A multivariable logistic regression model demonstrated that robotic surgery was superior to laparoscopic surgery upon postoperative LOS (odds ratio = 5.029, 95% confidence interval [CI] = 1.321 to 19.142; $p = 0.018$). Conclusions: Our experience demonstrated that an effective implementation of the ERAS program in minimally-invasive colorectal surgery requires 31 patients to accomplish the higher compliance and requires more cases to reach the maturation phase for optimal recovery. We believe that developing a robotic platform would have no impact on the learning curve of ERAS implementation. Moreover, there is a beneficial effect on the postoperative length of surgery provided through the combination of ERAS care and robotic surgery for patients undergoing colorectal resection.

Keywords: enhanced recovery after surgery; ERAS; colorectal surgery; minimally-invasive; laparoscopic; robotic; learning curve; outcome; compliance

1. Introduction

Enhanced recovery after surgery (ERAS) protocols are multimodal perioperative care pathways designed to achieve early recovery for patients after surgical procedures through maintaining preoperative organ function and reducing any profound stress response following surgery. In the past two decades, ERAS protocol has been widely accepted worldwide and has been proved effective in bringing about shorter lengths of hospital stays, decreased postoperative pain and need for analgesia, decreased complications and readmission rates, and increased patient satisfaction. However, the effective implementation of ERAS requires close multidisciplinary teamwork and learning curves in order to best adjust the protocols into daily practice.

In Taiwan, promotion of the ERAS program has exploded over the past three years. The *Taiwan Chapter, ERAS Society* was established in July 2019, with more and more medical providers developing their tailored ERAS protocols on a diverse array of surgical procedures. In our institution, the implementation of ERAS programs for colorectal surgery patients began in June 2019. It is worth noting that a growing trend in the adoption of robotic surgery as a minimally-invasive technique for colorectal surgery has been happening since 2020 in our institution, while we have also carried out ERAS protocols for robotic surgery during its early stages of development.

The primary objective of this retrospective study was to present our real-world experience and establish the learning curves necessary for the implementation of an ERAS program for patients undergoing minimally-invasive surgery for colorectal resection, while also evaluating the impact that the development of robotic surgery has on the outcomes of ERAS.

2. Materials and Method

We collected 176 adult patients who had received elective, minimally-invasive surgery, including laparoscopic and robotic surgery for colorectal resection with ERAS care during the period June 2019 to September 2021. Nineteen patients required conversion to open surgery due to severe adhesion or anatomic difficulty, while two patients required immediate postoperative intensive care due to unstable vital signs during surgery, and in turn were all excluded. Overall, a total of 155 patients were ultimately included in the retrospective analysis.

All patients had received the same ERAS programs and equivalent forms of treatment from the same multidisciplinary team. Our ERAS protocol was revised according to the ERAS Society Guidelines [1] and consisted of 18 core elements, including 4 preadmission items, 4 preoperative items, 3 intraoperative items and 7 postoperative items, as summarized in Table 1.

Table 1. Tailored ERAS protocol.

Preadmission	1.	Dedicated preoperative counselling
	2.	Cessation of smoking
	3.	Screening and treatment of anemia before surgery
	4.	Nutritional assessment and support as needed
Preoperative	5.	Prevention of nausea and vomiting
	6.	Avoidance of routine sedative medication
	7.	Antimicrobial prophylaxis and skin preparation
	8.	Preoperative fasting and carbohydrate treatment
Intraoperative	9.	Standard anesthetic protocol
	10.	Prevention of intraoperative hypothermia
	11.	Avoidance of intra-abdominal or pelvic drain

Table 1. Cont.

Postoperative	12.	Avoidance of nasogastric intubation
	13.	Multimodal postoperative analgesia
	14.	Near-zero fluid balance therapy
	15.	Early oral intake within 24 h after surgery
	16.	Termination of intravenous fluid administration by *POD 3
	17.	Removal of urinary catheter by *POD 3
	18.	Early mobilization by *POD 3

*POD = Postoperative Day.

Patients were divided into 5 groups chronologically (31 cases per quintile). Patient demographics, perioperative data, tumor characteristics, surgical outcomes, and ERAS compliance were all compared among the quintiles. Learning curves of effective ERAS implementation were evaluated based on ERAS compliance and optimal recovery, which are composed of an absence of major complications, postoperative LOS of no more than 5 days, and no readmission within 30 days. We compared the outcomes between the laparoscopic and robotic groups and carried out multivariable logistic regression analysis to figure out significant direct correlations.

All statistical analyses were performed using PASW Statistics software (SPSS version 22.0). Continuous variables were expressed as mean (SD) or median (Q1–Q3) and were compared among groups using either one-way analysis of variance (ANOVA) or Kruskal–Wallis test or Mann–Whitney U test. Categorical data were expressed as numbers (percentage) and were compared using either Pearson's Chi-square test or Fisher's exact probability test or Yates' Correction for Continuity. A p-value of <0.05 was considered statistically significant. This retrospective study was approved by the Institutional Review Board of Taichung Veterans General Hospital (No: CE21319A) and written informed consent was obtained from each patient.

3. Results

3.1. Patients' Demographics and Tumor Characteristics

Overall, 155 patients were included in this analysis (Table 2) Among these patients, 85 (54.8%) were male, the mean age was 61.3 years, and the mean BMI was 24.9 kg/m^2, with 117 of the patients (75.5%) having an ASA ≤ 2, and 35 patients (22.6%) citing previous cigarette use. There were 94 patients (60.6%) diagnosed with any type of comorbidity, including hypertension (45.2%), diabetes (25.2%), and cardiovascular events (9.7%), with two or more having primary cancer (4.5%). Median preoperative hemoglobin was 13.1 gm/dL. There were 32 patients (20.6%) who had undergone previous abdominopelvic surgery, and 22 (14.2%) with neoadjuvant CCRT. Among all the above demographic parameters, there were no statistically significant differences seen between the overall patients and each quintile group. In total, 29 patients (18.7%) experienced a right-sided colon tumor, 65 (41.9%) had a left-sided colon tumor and 61 (39.4%) had a rectal tumor. There were 136 patients (87.7%) having malignant tumors, of whom 16 experienced a T4 lesion (10.3%).

Table 2. Demographic analysis of patient groups.

Parameters	Overall	Group 1	Group 2	Group 3	Group 4	Group 5	p Value
Number of patients, n	155	31	31	31	31	31	
Males, n (%)	85 (54.8%)	22 (71%)	17 (54.8%)	17 (54.8%)	16 (51.6%)	13 (41.9%)	0.242 ^{P}
Mean age, years ± SD	61.3 ± 14.2	61.4 ± 13.6	64.4 ± 16.0	63.8 ± 13.4	60.4 ± 12.8	56.4 ± 14.3	0.176 ^{A}
BMI, kg/m^2 ± SD	24.9 ± 4.2	25.3 ± 4.0	24.4 ± 5.1	25.3 ± 3.6	24.4 ± 3.2	24.9 ± 4.9	0.577 ^{K}
ASA ≤ 2, n (%)	117 (75.5%)	26 (83.9%)	23 (74.2%)	24 (77.4%)	23 (74.2%)	21 (67.7%)	0.681 ^{P}
Cigarette use, n (%)	35 (22.6%)	12 (38.7%)	5 (16.1%)	6 (19.4%)	7 (22.6%)	5 (16.1%)	0.180 ^{P}
Any comorbidity, n (%)	94 (60.6%)	19 (61.3%)	19 (61.3%)	22 (71.0%)	18 (58.1%)	16 (51.6%)	0.637 ^{P}
Hypertension, n (%)	70 (45.2%)	13 (41.9%)	15 (48.4%)	16 (51.6%)	14 (45.2%)	12 (38.7%)	0.861 ^{P}
Diabetes, n (%)	39 (25.2%)	7 (22.6%)	5 (16.1%)	9 (29.0%)	9 (29.0%)	9 (29.0%)	0.700 ^{P}
Cardiovascular, n (%)	15 (9.7%)	1 (3.2%)	4 (12.9%)	6 (19.4%)	1 (3.2%)	3 (9.7%)	0.156 ^{P}
Multiple primary cancers, n (%)	7 (4.5%)	3 (9.7%)	1 (3.2%)	1 (3.2%)	1 (3.2%)	1 (3.2%)	0.664 ^{P}
Median preop hemoglobin, gm/dl (IQR)	13.1 (11.8–14.5)	13.4 (11.9–14.8)	13.5 (11.5–14.9)	13.1 (11.9–13.8)	13.5 (12.0–14.5)	13.0 (11.6–14.1)	0.290 ^{A}

Table 2. Cont.

Parameters	Overall	Group 1	Group 2	Group 3	Group 4	Group 5	p Value
Previous abdominopelvic surgery, n (%)	32 (20.6%)	5 (16.1%)	6 (19.4%)	8 (25.8%)	6 (19.4%)	7 (22.6%)	0.906 [P]
Neoadjuvant CCRT, n (%)	22 (14.2%)	6 (19.4%)	2 (6.5%)	2 (6.5%)	8 (25.8%)	4 (12.9%)	0.125 [P]

SD: standard deviation; IQR: interquartile range; CCRT: Concurrent Chemo-radiotherapy. [K] Kruskal Wallis test. [P] chi-squared test. [A] ANOVA test.

The tumor characteristics, including tumor location, malignancy, tumor stage, safe margin, and residual tumor after neoadjuvant CCRT, among the quintile groups, were all comparable (Table 3). Group 5 showed a higher percentage of rectal tumors than Group 1, which may be explained due to the use of robotic surgery on a higher percentage of patients in Group 5 than in Group 1.

Table 3. Tumor histopathological characteristics.

Parameters	Overall (n = 155)	Group 1 (n = 31)	Group 2 (n = 31)	Group 3 (n = 31)	Group4 (n = 31)	Group 5 (n = 31)	p Value
Tumor location							0.313 [P]
Right-sided colon, n (%)	29 (18.7%)	5 (16.1%)	8 (25.8%)	9 (29.0%)	2 (6.5%)	5 (16.1%)	
Left-sided colon, n (%)	65 (41.9%)	14 (45.2%)	14 (45.2%)	11 (35.5%)	16 (51.6%)	10 (32.3%)	
Rectum, n (%)	61 (39.4%)	12 (38.7%)	9 (29.0%)	11 (35.5%)	13 (41.9%)	16 (51.6%)	
Malignant tumor, n (%)	136 (87.7%)	28 (90.3%)	25 (80.6%)	27 (87.1%)	29 (93.5%)	27 (87.1%)	0.620 [P]
T4 lesion	16 (10.3%)	1 (3.2%)	4 (12.9%)	4 (12.9%)	3 (9.7%)	4 (12.9%)	0.668 [P]
Stage							0.462 [P]
* Stage 0	10 (6.5%)	3 (9.7%)	1 (3.2%)	2 (6.5%)	2 (6.5%)	2 (6.5%)	
Stage I	26 (16.8%)	6 (19.4%)	1 (3.2%)	5 (16.1%)	5 (16.1%)	9 (29.0%)	
Stage II	33 (21.3%)	9 (29.0%)	7 (22.6%)	8 (25.8%)	3 (9.7%)	6 (19.4%)	
Stage III	49 (31.6%)	5 (16.1%)	13 (41.9%)	10 (32.3%)	12 (38.7%)	9 (29.0%)	
Stage IV	9 (5.8%)	3 (9.7%)	2 (6.5%)	1 (3.2%)	2 (6.5%)	1 (3.2%)	
Median length of safe margin, cm (IQR)	2.4 (1.5–4.0)	2.3 (1.9–4.1)	4.0 (1.8–4.5)	2.2 (1.0–4.0)	2.8 (2.0–3.5)	2.0 (1.0–3.0)	0.173 [K]
No residual tumor after neoadjuvant therapy	28 (18.1%)	5 (16.1%)	7 (22.6%)	5 (16.1%)	7 (22.6%)	4 (12.9%)	0.814 [P]

* Stage 0 = pTisN0M0, [K] Kruskal–Wallis test, [P] chi-squared test.

3.2. Compliance of ERAS Program

The median compliance rate for total ERAS protocol was 83.3% overall, 72.2% in Group 1, and 83.3% in Groups 2, 3, 4 and 5 (Table 4). In subgroup analysis, the median compliance rate for postoperative items was only 71.4%, while other items were 100%. The compliance with the ERAS program between the quintile groups demonstrated a statistically significant difference in total protocol, intraoperative, and postoperative items. The overall compliance rate for individual ERAS elements is shown in Supplementary Figure S1.

Table 4. ERAS compliance rate.

Parameters	Overall (n = 155)	Group 1 (n = 31)	Group 2 (n = 31)	Group 3 (n = 31)	Group4 (n = 31)	Group 5 (n = 31)	p Value
Total ERAS protocol, % (Median, range)	83.3% (50.0–94.4)	72.2% (50.0–88.9)	83.3% (66.7–94.4)	83.3% (72.2–88.9)	83.3% (72.2–94.4)	83.3% (72.2–94.4)	<0.001 [K]
Preadmission items	100% (50.0–100)	75.0% (75.0–100)	100% (50.0–100)	100% (50.0–100)	100% (50.0–100)	100% (50.0–100)	0.486 [K]
Preoperative items	100% (75.0–100)	100% (75.0–100)	100% (75.0–100)	100% (75.0–100)	100% (75.0–100)	100% (75.0–100)	0.161 [K]
Intraoperative items	100% (33.3–100)	66.7% (33.3–100)	66.7% (33.3–100)	100% (66.7–100)	100% (66.7–100)	100% (66.7–100)	<0.001 [K]
Postoperative items	71.4% (14.3–100)	57.1% (14.3–85.7)	71.4% (28.6–100)	71.4% (28.6–100)	71.4% (42.9–100)	71.4% (42.9–100)	<0.001 [K]

[K] Kruskal–Wallis test.

3.3. Perioperative Data and Clinical Outcome Analysis

Perioperative data and clinical outcome analysis of the patient groups are listed in Table 5. In total, we included 76 patients (49%) in the laparoscopic group and 79 patients (51%) in the robotic group. It is worth noting that the ratio of robotic groups rises chronologically, with zero being seen in Group 1, 42% in Group 2, 48.4% in Group 3, and 74.2% and 90.3% in Groups 4 and 5, respectively ($p < 0.001$). Mean operative time overall was 250.3 minutes, with the later groups having a relatively longer time than the earlier groups, but with no statistical significance. A total of 85 patients underwent optimal recovery after surgery, with four patients in Group 1, 11 patients in Group 2, and 21, 24, 25 patients in Group 3 to Group 5 respectively ($p < 0.001$). The median length of stay after surgery was 5 days overall, 8 days in Group 1, 7 days in the Group 2, 5 days in Group 3, and 4 days in the Group 4 and 5 ($p < 0.001$). Both absence of major complications and readmission within 30 days showed no statistically significant differences among the quintile group. Bowel functional outcomes including first oral intake within 24 hours after surgery ($p = 0.001$), time to first stool ($p < 0.001$), and early termination of intravenous fluid administration by POD-3 ($p < 0.001$) showed significant advancement among the quintiles.

Table 5. Perioperative data and clinical outcomes analysis of patient groups.

Parameters	Overall ($n = 155$)	Group 1 ($n = 31$)	Group 2 ($n = 31$)	Group 3 ($n = 31$)	Group 4 ($n = 31$)	Group 5 ($n = 31$)	p Value
Robotic method, n (%)	79 (51%)	0	13 (42%)	15 (48.4%)	23 (74.2%)	28 (90.3%)	<0.001 [P]
Operative time, minutes							0.088 [K]
Mean (SD)	250.3 (83.3)	229.3 (92.6)	242.7 (96.0)	258.1 (75.3)	262.7 (87.0)	258.9 (61.5)	
Median (IQR)	235 (195–297.5)	220 (182.5–232.5)	225 (169–285)	250 (210–310)	242 (195.5–315.5)	255 (207–282.5)	
Minimal blood loss, n (%)	129 (83.2%)	22 (71%)	25 (80.6%)	28 (90.3%)	25 (80.6%)	29 (93.5%)	0.130 [P]
Stoma construction, n (%)	29 (18.7%)	5 (16.1%)	2 (6.5%)	5 (16.1%)	11 (35.5%)	6 (19.4%)	0.059 [P]
Drainage tube placement, n (%)	73 (47.1%)	29 (93.5%)	28 (90.3%)	5 (16.1%)	5 (16.1%)	6 (19.4%)	<0.001 [P]
Visual analog scale ≤ 3, n (%)	127 (81.9%)	25 (80.6%)	24 (77.4%)	23 (74.2%)	29 (93.5%)	26 (83.9%)	0.329 [P]
First oral intake within 24 h, n (%)	137 (88.4%)	26 (83.9%)	21 (67.7%)	30 (96.8%)	30 (96.8%)	30 (96.8%)	0.001 [P]
Mean time to first stool *, day ± SD	2.5 ± 1.8	3.9 ± 1.8	2.8 ± 2.0	2.1 ± 1.2	2.0 ± 2.0	1.6 ± 1.0	<0.001 [K]
Mean IV amount, ml (SD)							
POD-0	1573.4 (810.3)	1145.4 (555.6)	1822.9 (738.4)	1658.1 (929.6)	1511.3 (707.1)	1729.3 (928.7)	0.005 [K]
POD-1	1478.5 (728.3)	1533.4 (822.1)	1811.8 (1013.4)	1277.6 (638.6)	1312.3 (390.6)	1457.2 (520.3)	0.230 [K]
POD-2	927.3 (904.8)	1198.1 (905.2)	1448.4 (1104.0)	551.6 (680.1)	782.1 (852.5)	656.5 (613.0)	0.001 [K]
POD-3	644.3 (945.9)	1034.6 (935.7)	1461.7 (1045.5)	304.0 (640.4)	275.8 (738.6)	145.5 (551.0)	<0.001 [K]
Mean urine amount, ml (SD)							
POD-1	1771.5 (884.6)	1714.8 (794.9)	2029.2 (1065.1)	1410.8 (764.1)	1662.7 (739.0)	2046.6 (912.7)	0.029 [K]
POD-2	2019.9 (902.0)	2253.8 (1069.7)	2109.6 (958.7)	1621.0 (593.9)	2010.7 (852.3)	2115.4 (902.4)	0.139 [K]
POD-3	2039.5 (879.6)	2178.6 (916.9)	2104.1 (894.5)	1837.9 (672.4)	1978.7 (711.4)	2139.7 (1232.0)	0.663 [K]
** Optimal recovery, n (%)	85 (54.8%)	4 (12.9%)	11 (35.5%)	21 (67.7%)	24 (77.4%)	25 (80.6%)	<0.001 [P]
$ Any complications, n (%)	24 (15.5%)	9 (29.0%)	7 (22.6%)	4 (12.9%)	1 (3.2%)	3 (9.7%)	0.078 [P]
Major (grade 3–5)	8 (5.2%)	5 (16.1%)	2 (6.5%)	1 (3.2%)	0	0	
Minor (grade 1–2)	16 (10.3%)	4 (12.9%)	5 (16.1%)	3 (9.7%)	1 (3.2%)	3 (9.7%)	
Postoperative LOS							
Day, median (Q1–Q3)	5 (4–7)	8 (6–9)	7 (5–10)	5 (4–6)	4 (4–5)	4 (4–5)	<0.001 [K]
More than 5 days, n (%)	67 (43.2%)	26 (83.9%)	20 (64.5%)	9 (29%)	7 (22.6%)	5 (16.1%)	<0.001 [P]
Readmission within 30 days, n (%)	7 (4.5%)	3 (9.7%)	2 (6.5%)	1 (3.2%)	0	1 (3.2%)	0.421 [P]

VAS: Visual Analogue Scale; * Patient with stoma construction were excluded. ** Optimal recovery was defined as absence of major complications, LOS no more than 5 days and no readmission within 30 days. $ Complications were graded by Calvin–Dindo classification. [K] Kruskal–Wallis test, [P] chi-squared test.

3.4. Comparison of Laparoscopic Surgery and Robotic Surgery

The first case in the laparoscopic group and that in the robotic group were separated by a period of 12 months. The case numbers in the robotic group equaled those in the laparoscopic group during the period of 14 months (Figure 1). The median compliance of total ERAS protocol was 88.9% in the robotic group and 83.3% in the laparoscopic group ($p < 0.001$). The median postoperative LOS was 4.1 days in the robotic group and 6 days in the laparoscopic group ($p = 0.016$) (Table 6). A multivariable logistic regression model demonstrated that robotics was superior to laparoscopic surgery upon postoperative LOS with statistically significant differences after adjustment for confounding variables (odds ratio = 5.029, 95% confidence interval [CI] = 1.321 to 19.142; $p = 0.018$) (Table 7).

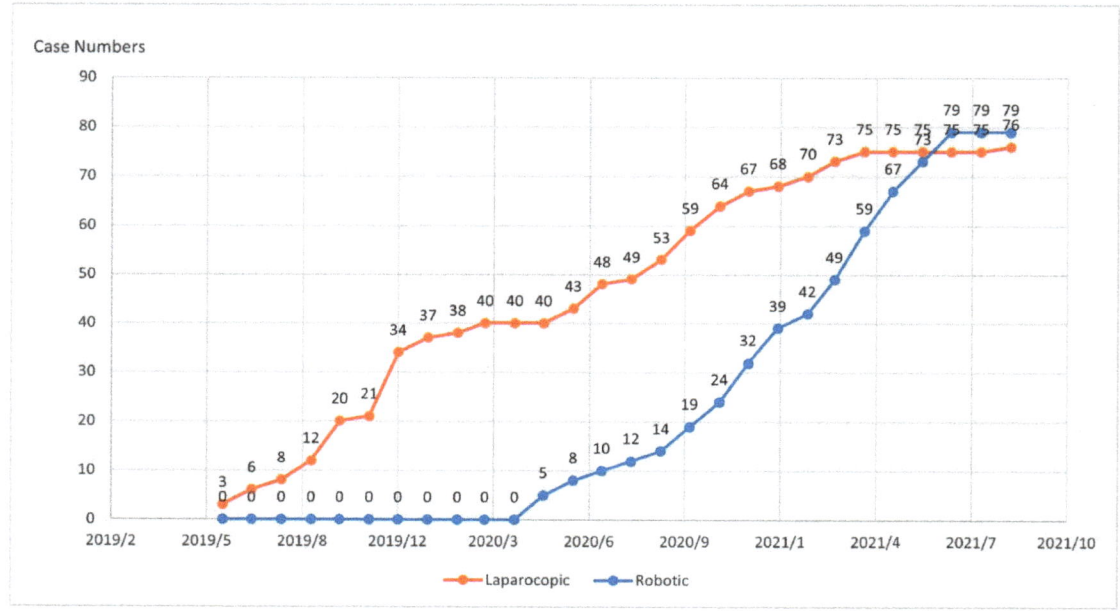

Figure 1. Cumulative numbers between Laparoscopic and Robotic group.

Table 6. Comparison of ERAS compliance and LOS between laparoscopic and robotic surgery.

Parameters	Overall (N = 155)	Laparoscopic (N = 76)	Robotic (N = 79)	p Value
Total ERAS protocol, % (Median, range)	88.9 (55.6–100.0)	83.3 (55.6–94.4)	88.9 (72.2–100.0)	<0.001 m
Preadmission items	100.0 (50.0–100.0)	87.5 (50.00–100.0)	100.0 (50.0–100.0)	0.14 m
Preoperative items	100.0 (75.0–100.0)	100.0 (75.00–100.0)	100.0 (75.0–100.0)	0.100 m
Intraoperative items	100.0 (33.3–100.0)	66.7 (33.33–100.0)	100.0 (33.3–100.0)	<0.001 m
Postoperative items	85.7 (28.8–100.0)	71.4 (28.8–100.0)	85.7 (42.9–100.0)	<0.001 m
Postoperative LOS				
Day, median (Q1–Q3)	5 (4–7)	6 (5–9)	4.1 (3.8–5.0)	0.016 m
More than 5 days, n (%)	67 (43.2%)	48 (63.1%)	19 (24%)	<0.001 y

m Mann–Whitney U test, y Yates' Correction for Continuity.

Table 7. Multivariable logistic regression model of factors associated with postoperative length of stay no more than 5 days.

Factors	LOS ≤ 5d		
	OR	95% CI	p Value
Robotic surgery	5.029	1.321 to 19.412	0.018
Quintile group sequence	1.270	0.779 to 2.070	0.337
Compliance of total ERAS protocol	0.995	0.918 to 1.079	0.910
Male	0.758	0.256 to 2.244	0.617
Age	0.996	0.958 to 1.036	0.849
BMI	1.087	0.961 to 1.229	0.184
ASA ≤ 2	4.560	1.262 to 16.382	0.020
Any comorbidity	0.816	0.288 to 2.311	0.702
Pre-op hemoglobin	1.198	0.930 to 1.542	0.163
Previous abdominopelvic surgery	0.803	0.265 to 2.435	0.698
Multiple primary cancers	0.430	0.036 to 5.185	0.507

Table 7. Cont.

Factors	LOS ≤ 5d		
	OR	95% CI	p Value
Neoadjuvant CCRT	0.336	0.045 to 2.485	0.285
Cigarette use	1.773	0.458 to 6.862	0.407
Malignant disease	0.870	0.218 to 3.471	0.843
T4 lesions	1.205	0.243 to 5.981	0.819
Minimal blood loss	0.688	0.171 to 2.772	0.599
Stoma construction	1.721	0.261 to 11.356	0.573
Drainage tube placement	0.143	0.042 to 0.490	0.002
Operative time	0.989	0.980 to 0.998	0.019

4. Discussion

Many experts have indicated that rather than sticking to complete adherence to ERAS protocols, implementing a well-tailored ERAS protocol makes it easier to apply to clinical practice, while also offering equivalent benefits [2,3]. Five basic elements of care, including preoperative patient information, multimodal analgesia, avoidance of fluid overload and hypovolemia, no nasogastric tube and early oral feeding, as well as early mobilization, were demonstrated a long time ago to be the key components for ERAS in colonic surgery [4]. These five elements were also enough to secure enhanced recovery and a length of stay within 2 to 4 days after open colonic surgery. Toh et al. [5] initiated a questionnaire survey involving 300 colorectal surgeons in Australia and New Zealand learning that eight interventions, including preoperative anemia correction, minimally-invasive surgery, early in-dwelling catheter removal, preoperative smoking cessation, preoperative counselling, avoidance of drains in colon surgery, avoiding nasogastric tubes and early drain removal in rectal surgery were all considered relatively important elements towards improving ERAS programs. Our ERAS protocol adopted five key components and other generally acknowledged elements of care. On top of that, our ERAS protocol was implemented by a group of fixed, well-trained members, including surgeons, anesthesiologists, nurse practitioners (NPs), nutritionists and case managers.

We included a total of 155 patients and used the data-splitting method [6] by placing the patients into five consecutive groups of 31 each in order to better evaluate our learning curves with regards to ERAS care. A prospective review of 380 patients who underwent elective open colorectal surgery under ERAS protocol from the period 2011–2017 in a single institution indicated that a minimum of 76 patients are required in order to achieve a significantly higher rate of ERAS compliance and optimal recovery [7]. Michal, et al. concluded that introducing the ERAS protocol is a gradual process and its compliance at the level of 80% or more requires at least 30 patients and a period of approximately 6 months [8]. Having at least 30 cases is required for Phase I of the learning curve and has been a consensus for robotic colorectal surgery [9]. After analyzing previous studies, a cutting-off point at 31 cases for our study was deemed reasonable.

The compliance of ERAS protocol still plays a critical role in improving short-term outcomes [10]. A multicenter, prospective cohort study involving 2084 consecutive adult patients who had undergone elective colorectal surgery in Spain demonstrated that an increase in ERAS adherence appeared to be associated with a decrease in postoperative complications (OR, 0.33; 95% CI, 0.26–0.43; $p < 0.001$) [11]. Wei et al. [12] confirmed that an increase in ERAS protocol adherence was associated with a further decrease in hospital length of stay. The latest ERCOLE study included prospective data from 1,138 patients who had undergone minimally-invasive colorectal cancer surgery in Italy and has shown that adherence to the ERAS program of up to 75% could be considered satisfactory in order to reach the goal of functional recovery [13].

In our experience, the median compliance regarding total ERAS protocol among all groups was 83.3%, and it underwent significant progress from 72.2% in Group 1 to 83.3% in

Group 2 while staying relatively constant from Group 3 to Group 5 ($p < 0.001$). In subgroup analysis, we discovered a similar trend in median compliance regarding intraoperative and postoperative ERAS items ($p < 0.001$). In terms of clinical outcomes, the optimal recovery showed an increasing trend in the 2nd quintile and started to plateau after the third quintile. Postoperative LOS and bowel functional outcomes (early oral intake within 24 h, time to first stool and early termination of intravenous fluid administration by POD-3) had the similar trends with statistically significant differences between the quintile groups. Comprehensively, based on these finding we concluded that an effective implementation of the ERAS program in minimally-invasive colorectal surgery required 31 patients to accomplish the higher compliance and required more patients to reach the maturation phase for optimal recovery.

In general, the adherence of preadmission and preoperative items should be independent from the surgical technique adopted (open, laparoscopic, robotic methods). We speculated that robotic surgery might have benefits on adherence of intraoperative and postoperative items because a robotic surgical platform with proficient technique helps surgeons achieve a more precise dissecting tissue plane and causes less bleeding damage. For instance, this could convince surgeons of the resultant security caused by the avoidance of intra-abdominal or pelvic drain. In this study, robotic surgery was correlated with higher compliance with total ERAS protocol, intraoperative, and postoperative items in univariate analysis. However, the multivariate comparison demonstrated ERAS compliance significantly correlated to the sequence of quintile groups, rather than the robotic surgery (Supplementary Table S1). On the other hand, the fact that robotic surgery was superior to laparoscopic surgery upon postoperative LOS and statistical significance was demonstrated after adjustment for confounding factors. Consequently, we made a conservative inference that developing a robotic platform would have no impact on the learning curve of ERAS implementation and there is a beneficial effect on the postoperative length of surgery provided through the combination of ERAS care and robotic surgery for patients undergoing colorectal resection.

Depending upon the future advancements made in robotic surgery, medical personnel will be able to easily perform more complex surgical procedures such as intersphincteric resection (ISR), pelvic autonomic nerve preservation and multivisceral resections [14–16]. However, these complex operations would affect a physician's perspective of ERAS implementation as they are different from conventional laparoscopic surgery, for instance, the duration of a urinary catheter or drainage tube placement. The consequence of this limitation is that we should categorize the various types of procedures seen between laparoscopic and robotic surgery as more cases are taken on, for required study.

5. Conclusions

Robotic surgery and ERAS protocol care have each undergone their own prominent development and in turn become global trends, with rapid progress being seen in both safety and efficacy when compared to conventional surgery over the past decade. We believe that implementing a combination of the robotic surgery and ERAS care will result in a highly promising method for use in future colorectal surgeries.

Supplementary Materials: The following supporting information can be downloaded at: https://www.mdpi.com/article/10.3390/jcm12072661/s1, Figure S1: Elements of tailored ERAS protocol and overall compliance rate; Table S1: Uni- and multivariate logistic regression analysis for ERAS compliance $\geq 75\%$.

Author Contributions: Conceptualization, C.-Y.H. and F.-F.C.; Methodology, C.-Y.L.; Validation, C.-Y.H.; Formal analysis, F.-F.C.; Resources, T.-W.C., C.-Y.L., T.-Y.C. and M.-C.C.; Data curation, T.-W.C.; Writing—original draft, C.-Y.H.; Writing—review & editing, F.-F.C.; Supervision, F.-F.C. All authors have read and agreed to the published version of the manuscript.

Funding: This research received no external funding.

Institutional Review Board Statement: The study was conducted in accordance with the Declaration of Helsinki, and approved by the Institutional Review Board of Taichung Veterans General Hospital (NO: CE21319A).

Informed Consent Statement: Informed consent was obtained from all subjects involved in the study.

Data Availability Statement: The data that support the findings of this study are available from the first or/and the corresponding author upon reasonable request.

Conflicts of Interest: The authors declare no conflict of interest.

References

1. Gustafsson, U.O.; Scott, M.J.; Hubner, M.; Nygren, J.; Demartines, N.; Francis, N.; Ljungqvist, O. Guidelines for perioperative care in elective colorectal surgery: Enhanced Recovery After Surgery (ERAS®) Society recommendations: 2018. *World J. Surg.* **2019**, *43*, 659–695. [CrossRef] [PubMed]
2. Melnyk, M.; Casey, R.G.; Black, P.; Koupparis, A.J. Enhanced recovery after surgery (ERAS) protocols: Time to change practice? *Can. Urol. Assoc. J.* **2011**, *5*, 342. [CrossRef] [PubMed]
3. Kehlet, H. ERAS Implementation-Time to Move Forward. *Ann Surg.* **2018**, *267*, 998–999. [CrossRef] [PubMed]
4. Kehlet, H. Fast-track colorectal surgery. *Lancet* **2008**, *371*, 791–793. [CrossRef] [PubMed]
5. Toh, J.; Collins, G.P.; Pathma-Nathan, N.; El-Khoury, T.; Engel, A.; Smith, S.; Richardson, A.; Ctercteko, G. Attitudes towards Enhanced Recovery after Surgery (ERAS) interventions in colorectal surgery: A nationwide survey of Australia and New Zealand colorectal surgeons. *Langenbeck's Arch. Surg.* **2022**, *407*, 1637–1646. [CrossRef] [PubMed]
6. Khan, N.; Abboudi, H.; Khan, M.S.; Dasgupta, P.; Ahmed, K. Measuring the surgical 'learning curve': Methods, variables and competency. *BJU Int.* **2014**, *113*, 504–508. [CrossRef] [PubMed]
7. Lohsiriwat, V. Learning curve of enhanced recovery after surgery program in open colorectal surgery *World J. Gastrointest. Surg.* **2019**, *11*, 169–178. [CrossRef] [PubMed]
8. Pędziwiatr, M.; Kisialeuski, M.; Wierdak, M.; Stanek, M.; Natkaniec, M.; Matłok, M.; Major, P.; Małczak, P.; Budzyński, A. Early implementation of Enhanced Recovery after Surgery (ERAS®) protocol-Compliance improves outcomes: A prospective cohort study. *Int. J. Surg.* **2015**, *21*, 75–81. [CrossRef] [PubMed]
9. Jiménez-Rodríguez, R.M.; Rubio-Dorado-Manzanares, M.; Díaz-Pavón, J.M.; Reyes-Díaz, M.L.; Vazquez-Monchul, J.M.; Garcia-Cabrera, A.M.; Padillo, J.; De la Portilla, F. Learning curve in robotic rectal cancer surgery: Current state of affairs. *Int. J. Color. Dis.* **2016**, *31*, 1807–1815. [CrossRef] [PubMed]
10. Pisarska, M.; Pędziwiatr, M.; Małczak, P.; Major, P.; Ochenduszko, S.; Zub-Pokrowiecka, A.; Kulawik, J.; Budzyński, A. Do we really need the full compliance with ERAS protocol in laparoscopic colorectal surgery? A prospective cohort study. *Int. J. Surg.* **2016**, *36 Pt A*, 377–382. [CrossRef]
11. Ripollés-Melchor, J.; Ramírez-Rodríguez, J.M.; Casans-Francés, R.; Aldecoa, C.; Abad-Motos, A.; Logroño-Egea, M.; García-Erce, J.A.; Camps-Cervantes, Á.; Ferrando-Ortolá, C.; Suarez de la Rica, A.; et al. Association between Use of Enhanced Recovery After Surgery Protocol and Postoperative Complications in Colorectal Surgery: The Postoperative Outcomes Within Enhanced Recovery After Surgery Protocol (POWER) Study. *JAMA Surg.* **2019**, *154*, 725–736. [CrossRef] [PubMed]
12. Wei, I.H.; Pappou, E.P.; Smith, J.J.; Widmar, M.; Nash, G.M.; Weiser, M.R.; Paty, P.B.; Guillem, J.G.; Afonso, A.; Garcia-Aguilar, J. Monitoring an Ongoing Enhanced Recovery After Surgery (ERAS) Program: Adherence Improves Clinical Outcomes in a Comparison of Three Thousand Colorectal Cases. *Clin. Surg.* **2020**, *5*, 2909. [PubMed]
13. Milone, M.; Elmore, U.; Manigrasso, M.; Ortenzi, M.; Botteri, E.; Arezzo, A.; Silecchia, G.; Guerrieri, M.; De Palma, G.D.; Agresta, F.; et al. ERas and COLorectal endoscopic surgery: An Italian society for endoscopic surgery and new technologies (SICE) national report. *Surg. Endosc.* **2022**, *36*, 7619–7627. [CrossRef] [PubMed]
14. Lee, S.H.; Kim, D.H.; Lim, S.W. Robotic versus laparoscopic intersphincteric resection for low rectal cancer: A systematic review and meta-analysis. *Int. J. Color. Disease* **2018**, *33*, 1741–1753. [CrossRef] [PubMed]
15. Kim, N.K.; Kim, Y.W.; Cho, M.S. Total mesorectal excision for rectal cancer with emphasis on pelvic autonomic nerve preservation: Expert technical tips for robotic surgery. *Surg. Oncol.* **2015**, *24*, 172–180. [CrossRef] [PubMed]
16. Liu, G.; Zhang, S.; Zhang, Y.; Fu, X.; Liu, X. Robotic Surgery in Rectal Cancer: Potential, Challenges, and Opportunities. *Curr. Treat. Options Oncol.* **2022**, *23*, 961–979. [CrossRef] [PubMed]

Disclaimer/Publisher's Note: The statements, opinions and data contained in all publications are solely those of the individual author(s) and contributor(s) and not of MDPI and/or the editor(s). MDPI and/or the editor(s) disclaim responsibility for any injury to people or property resulting from any ideas, methods, instructions or products referred to in the content.

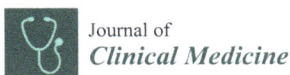

Article

A Synchronous Robotic Resection of Colorectal Cancer and Liver Metastases—Our Initial Experience

Yaron Rudnicki [1,2,*], Ron Pery [3,4], Sherief Shawki [1], Susanne Warner [3], Sean Patrick Cleary [3] and Kevin T. Behm [1]

1. Department of Surgery, Division of Colon and Rectal Surgery, Mayo Clinic, Rochester, MN 55905, USA
2. Department of Surgery, Meir Medical Center, Faculty of Medicine, Tel Aviv University, Kfar Saba 4428164, Israel
3. Department of Surgery, Division of Hepatobiliary and Pancreatic Surgery, Mayo Clinic, Rochester, MN 55905, USA
4. Department of Surgery and Transplantation, Sheba Medical Center, Faculty of Medicine, Tel Aviv University, Kfar Saba 4428164, Israel
* Correspondence: yaron217@gmail.com

Abstract: Introduction: Synchronous robotic colorectal and liver resection for metastatic colorectal cancer (mCRC) is gaining popularity. This case series describes our initial institutional experience. Methods: A retrospective study of synchronous robotic colorectal and liver resections for metastatic colorectal cancer (March 2020 to December 2021). Results: Eight patients underwent synchronous robotic resections. The median age was 59 (45–72), and the median body mass index was 29 (20–33). Seven received neoadjuvant chemotherapy, and five rectal cancers received neoadjuvant radiotherapy. One patient had a low anterior resection with major hepatectomy, two had low anterior resection with minor hepatectomy, and one had abdominoperineal resection with major hepatectomy. One patient had a left colectomy with minor hepatectomy, and two had right colectomies with minor hepatectomy. We used five robotic 8/12 mm ports in all cases. Extraction incisions were Pfannenstiel in four patients, colostomy site in two patients, one perineal incision, and one supra-umbilical incision. The median estimated blood loss was 200 mL (25–500), and the median operative time was 448 min (374–576). There were no intra-operative complications or conversions. Five patients had the liver resection first, and two of six anastomoses were performed before the liver resection. The Median length of stay was 4 days (3–14). There were two post-operative complications, prolonged ileus and DVT, with a Clavien-Dindo complication grade of I and II, respectively. There were no readmissions or reoperations. All colorectal and liver resection margins were negative. Conclusions: Synchronous robotic colorectal and liver resection can be performed effectively utilizing one port configuration with acceptable short-term outcomes and quality of oncologic resection.

Keywords: robotic surgery; metastatic colorectal cancer; colorectal surgery; liver surgery

1. Introduction

Colorectal cancer (CRC) is the third most common cancer worldwide, and the fourth most common cause of cancer mortality is primarily attributed to CRC metastases (mCRC) [1]. A quarter of newly diagnosed CRC patients are diagnosed yearly with a stage IV metastatic disease, mainly metastases to the liver [2,3]. Treatment for stage IV CRC disease is usually a combination of treatments with systemic chemotherapy, possible immunotherapy, possible chemoradiation for rectal cancer, and surgery when appropriate [4,5]. The rate of patients with CRC and liver metastasis amenable to surgery has risen substantially over the last decade, with multiple large epidemiological studies demonstrating an incidence of 14–17% of patients who present with synchronous liver metastases, which occur more frequently in male patients [6]. Most often, the surgical plan is based on a staged approach, either colorectal resection first followed by liver resection at a second stage or the other way around, most often with systemic or local treatment in between. When assessing the liver disease burden, the traditional treatment is resection when there is a resectable disease with or without perioperative systemic treatment, usually a combination of chemotherapy and molecular treatment such as Avastin. When there is a non-resectable liver disease, other forms of localized treatments can be considered, such as ablation or irradiation. In a select group of patients, a synchronous colorectal resection combined with partial liver resection is a viable and preferable surgical option. For some patients, the burden of a combined open surgery can be mitigated by a synchronous minimally invasive approach [7].

The advantages of a synchronous minimally invasive CRC and liver resection are reduced blood loss, early mobility, lower rates of surgical site infections, shorter length of stay, and reduced time interruption of systemic therapy. These peri-operative and oncologic benefits can be combined with the advantages of robotic surgery, mainly three-dimensional augmented vision, the flexibility of wristed instruments, tremor suppression, and better access to the posterosuperior segment's lesions [8,9]. Robotic colorectal resection has become prevalent in the Western world, yet not many centers perform robotic liver resection, let alone synchronous robotic colorectal and liver surgery. Although synchronous robotic colorectal and liver resection for mCRC is gaining popularity, very little was published on this approach's feasibility, safety, and manner. This case series describes our initial institutional experience with a synchronous robotic approach and offers some recommendations regarding how we do it.

2. Materials and Methods

A retrospective study was designed to identify patients that underwent a combined synchronous robotic colorectal and liver resection for metastatic colorectal cancer at the Mayo Clinic. This study was conducted in accordance with the ethical principles of the Declaration of Helsinki (Edinburgh 2000) and the approval of the Institutional Review Board. A prospectively maintained institutional database was queried for patients that underwent this procedure from March 2020 to December 2021. Data collected included demographic information such as age, gender, Body mass index (BMI), type of liver and colorectal resection, number of robotic ports used, specimen incision extraction site, length of operation, intraoperative complications, and estimated blood loss, and preoperative neoadjuvant treatment.

All cases were performed using the da Vinci XI platform. After laparoscopic exploration of the abdomen, all patients had four robotic trocars inserted, three 8 mm trocars and one 12 mm trocar, and another 8 mm AirSeal assistant trocar. The robotic port arrays and positions over the abdominal wall were mainly in a horizontal line at the level of the umbilicus for the rectal and sigmoid cases and with a slight diagonal line from the left upper quadrant to the right lower quadrant for the cases with a right colon lesion (Figure 1). Therefore, there was no need for any added ports or repositing of ports for the liver resection.

In addition, the patient's post-operative course was monitored for the length of stay, post-operative complications, and pathological reports, including resection margins. The procedures were performed by three dedicated colorectal surgeons and three dedicated hepatobiliary surgeons. The order of resection and timing of anastomosis creation was decided by each colorectal and hepatobiliary surgeon's preference. The definition of a major hepatectomy was defined as a complete resection of three or more continuous liver segments and a minor hepatectomy was defined as any resection that included less than the above.

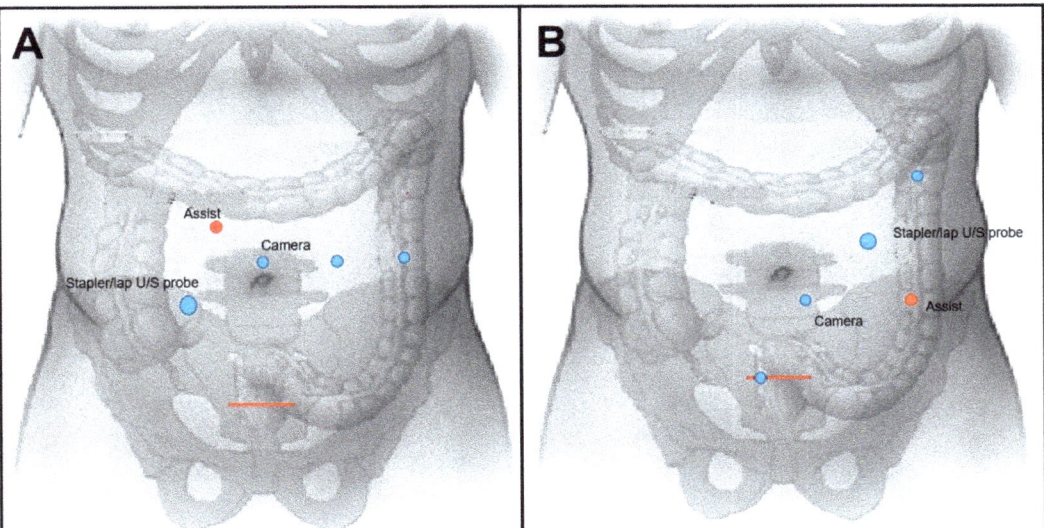

Figure 1. Diagram of two robotic port placement arrays for combined colorectal and liver resection. (**A**) Horizontal line array at the level of the umbilicus for rectal and sigmoid colon resection, red line marks a Pfannenstiel incision. (**B**) Diagonal line array from the left upper abdominal quadrant to the right lower quadrant for right colon resection.

3. Results

During a period of 22 months, eight patients with metastatic colon or rectal cancer (CRC) with liver metastasis underwent synchronous robotic resections. The patient cohort comprised four males and four females, with a median age of 59 years with a range of 45–72 and a median body mass index (BMI) of 29 kg/m^2 with a range of 20–33 kg/m^2. Five patients were diagnosed with rectal cancer, four in the mid-rectum and one in the low rectum. One patient was diagnosed with sigmoid colon cancer and two with ascending colon cancer. All patients had CRC metastases to the liver that were initially diagnosed as resectable. Five had solitary metastases, one had two bilobar metastases, one had three unilobar metastases, and one had three bilobar metastases. All liver lesions other than one were relatively peripheral, which allowed for minor hepatectomies. No metastases involved the major portal or venous pedicles. Two patients were obstructed and initially underwent loop colostomy creation before neoadjuvant treatment. Perioperatively, seven patients (87.5%) received neoadjuvant chemotherapy using a FOLFOX protocol, with three receiving Bevacizumab. All five rectal cancer patients received neoadjuvant radiotherapy, four had a short course, and one had a long course of radiotherapy. One patient with an ascending colon lesion and a solitary 4b/5 liver metastasis went straight to surgery with no neoadjuvant treatment (Table 1).

3.1. Operative Management

Out of the five patients with rectal cancer, four underwent robotic low anterior resection (rLAR), one with a loop colostomy closure. Out of these, one underwent a synchronous robotic left hepatectomy, and the other four had minor hepatectomies with segmental, subsegmental, or wedge liver resections. All four rLAR patients also had a diverting loop ileostomy (DLI) created, and two female patients also had a bilateral salpingo-oophorectomy (BSO), one of them with a total abdominal hysterectomy (TAH) and a partial upper vaginectomy. One patient underwent a robotic abdominoperineal resection (APR) and an end colostomy creation, with a minor hepatectomy and segment 2 and 3 sub-segmentectomy. One patient had a left colectomy for a proximal sigmoid lesion, loop colostomy closure with a primary anastomosis, and a minor hepatectomy, segment 3 resection. Two patients with ascending colon cancer underwent right colectomies with primary anastomoses and minor hepatectomies (Table 2).

Table 1. Baseline Demographic, location of lesions, and neoadjuvant treatment.

Characteristic	n = 8
Age (years)—median (range)	59 (45–72)
Female sex—n (%)	4 (50%)
Body mass index (BMI) kg/m^2—median (range)	29 (20–33)
Location of CRC lesion	
Rectal cancer—n	5
Sigmoid colon cancer—n	1
Ascending colon cancer—n	2
Location of metastatic spread in the liver	
One metastasis—Right lobe	2
One metastasis—Left lobe	3
Two metastases—Bilobar	1
Three metastases—Left lobe	1
Three metastases—Bilobar	1
Prior loop colostomy creation for colonic obstruction—n	2
Neoadjuvant chemotherapy—n (%)	7 (87.5%)
Added neoadjuvant Bevacizumab—n (%)	3 (37.5%)
Neoadjuvant chemoradiotherapy for rectal cancer—n (%)	5 (100%)

Table 2. Operative management.

Characteristic	n = 8
Type of colorectal procedure	
Robotic low anterior resection (rLAR) with DLI—n	4
Robotic abdominoperineal resection (APR)—n	1
Robotic left colectomy—n	1
Robotic right colectomy—n	2
Type of liver resection	
Major hepatectomy	2
Minor Hepatectomy	6
Robotic ports array over the abdominal wall	
Horizontal line at the level of the umbilicus—n	6
Diagonal line from LUQ to RLQ—n	2
Liver resection performed first—n	5
Colorectal resection performed first—n	3
Colorectal anastomoses performed before the hepatic resection	2

Table 2. Cont.

Characteristic	n = 8
Specimens' extraction site	
Pfannenstiel incision—n	4
Colostomy incision—n	2
Perineal incision after APR—n	1
Limited supra-umbilical midline incision—n	1
Intraoperative complications—n	0
Conversion to an open approach—n	0
Estimated blood loss—ml-median (range)	200 (25–500)
Operative time—minutes-median (range)	448 (374–576)

DLI—Diverting loop ileostomy
LUQ—Left upper quadrant
RLQ—Right lower quadrant
ml—Milliliter

The six rectal and sigmoid cases required a two quadrants approach, repositioning the robotic boom once when transitioning between the rectal and liver resection. The two right colectomies did not require repositing the robotic boom and utilized a single abdominal quadrant approach. In the hepatectomy part, there were no hilar dissections or need for the Pringle maneuver. Parenchymal transection was performed with a combination of unipolar diathermy, bipolar diathermy, and a vessel sealer.

The liver resection was performed first, followed by the colorectal resection in five patients (63%). In two rectal resections and one colonic resection, the colorectal resection was performed first, followed by the liver resection, with the two colorectal anastomoses performed before the hepatic portion and the ileocolic anastomosis created after the hepatic portion was completed. Following the completion of both resections and reconstructions, the specimens were extracted through a Pfannenstiel incision in four patients, a colostomy site in two patients, a perineal incision in the APR case, and one through a limited supra-umbilical incision. There were no intraoperative complications, and none needed any conversion to an open approach. The median estimated blood loss was 200 mL (25–500), and the median operative time was 448 min (374–576) (Table 3).

Table 3. Patients list with the type of robotic colorectal and liver surgery and operative time.

Raw	Age/Gender	Colorectal Surgery	Liver Surgery	Operative Time (Hours)
1	56 M	Robotic abdominoperineal resection (APR)	Robotic left hepatectomy	6:18
2	45 M	Robotic low anterior resection (LAR)	Robotic partial hepatectomy (segments 3 + 4b)	9:36
3	72 F	Robotic right colectomy	Robotic partial hepatectomy (segments 4b + 5) & cholecystectomy	6:42
4	54 M	Robotic low anterior resection (LAR)	Robotic left hepatectomy	6:14
5	62 F	Robotic low anterior resection (LAR)	Robotic partial hepatectomy (segment 8) & cholecystectomy	8:24
6	63 M	Robotic sigmoid colectomy	Robotic partial hepatectomy (segment 3)	7:46
7	55 F	Robotic low anterior resection (LAR)	Robotic partial hepatectomy (segments 2 + 3 + 8) + ablation of liver lesion	8:34
8	62 F	Robotic right colectomy	Robotic partial hepatectomy (segments 2) + ablation of liver lesion	7:10

3.2. Post-Operative Period and Outcomes

The median length of stay of patients was 4 days, with a range of 3 to 14 days. Two of the eight patients (25%) had post-operative complications, with one patient having a post-operative ileus and one developing deep vein thrombosis (DVT), with a Clavien-Dindo post-operative complication grade of I and II. There were no cases of readmissions or reoperations.

Final pathology reports showed negative margins on all colorectal and liver resections, with six colorectal lesions having a penetration level of T3 and two of T4. Four patients were found to have positive lymph nodes in the mesentery, and four patients had no positive nodes found, the number of lymph nodes harvested ranged from 16 to 49. The average size of the hepatic lesions was 1.9 ± 1.3 cm, with lesions ranging from 0.5 cm to 4.5 cm. No post-operative mortality was reported through an average follow-up time of 29 ± 20 months (Table 4).

Table 4. Post-operative outcome and pathological characteristics.

Characteristic	n = 8
Length of post-operative hospital stay (LOS)—days-median (range)	4 (3–14)
Post-operative complications—n (%)	2 (25%)
Ileus	1
Deep vein thrombosis (DVT)	1
Clavien-Dindo postoperative complication grade I/II	2
Readmissions or reoperations—n	0
Positive resection margins—n	0
Level of colorectal tumor penetration	
T3—n	6
T4—n	2
Positive mesenteric lymph nodes—n	4
Size of the hepatic lesions—cm—mean $\pm$ SD (range)	1.9 ± 1.3 (0.5–4.5)
Post-operative mortality—n	0
Follow-up time—months—mean $\pm$ SD	29 ± 20

S.D.—Standard deviation
cm—Centimeter

4. Discussion

In this case series, we report our experience performing combined synchronous robotic colorectal and liver resections for mCRC. The surgical treatment of stage IV mCRC patients is still evolving, with no clear answer to the optimal strategy. The burden of systemic treatment with two major surgeries is challenging for some patients and can sometimes be mitigated by performing a combined minimally invasive surgical approach [6,10]. Presumably, the robotic approach allows for more flexibility in combining both CRC surgery and liver metastasis surgery compared to the laparoscopic approach, with improved visualization in a three-dimensional view, and wristed instruments that allow better reach and control in the pelvis for rectal lesions and over the liver for "hard to reach" liver lesions, so that a preferred outcome can be attained [11,12]. These assumptions are the results of small single-institution series, and the literature to support these assumptions is still lacking.

From a colorectal point of view, there is some difference between a right colon resection, a left or a sigmoid colon resection, and rectal resection. The difference is mainly in the added complexity of the rectal resection that requires a pelvic dissection, sometimes after neoadjuvant pelvic radiation that brings upon a protective diverting loop ileostomy. As an institutional practice, all patients with known metastatic rectal disease are generally referred to a short course of radiation in an effort to shorten treatment duration and minimize time off of systemic therapy prior to surgery. The duration of radiation is dictated by the morphology of the primary rectal cancer both at presentation and after neoadjuvant chemotherapy. For patients with threatened CRM, T4 tumors, and tumors with clinically positive extra-mesorectal lymph nodes, a long course of radiation is preferred. Another difference is the robotic ports array, which is more often a personal choice of the CRC and Liver surgeons. In this series, we used five trocars and positioned them over the abdominal wall in a horizontal line at the level of the umbilicus for the rectal and sigmoid cases and with a slight diagonal line from the left upper quadrant to the right lower quadrant for the cases with a right colon lesion as seen in Figure 1.

While robotic liver resection is gaining popularity, the vast majority of liver resections worldwide are still being done using an open approach. Given safety issues and the technical complexity of proper oncologic resections deep in the liver, or in the higher and posterior segments, most laparoscopic liver resections are being performed for peripheral lesions in favorable locations. With improved articulation, a robotic approach may offer better access to otherwise challenging locations such as segments 1, 7, and 8 [13]. Therefore, many patients with limited liver metastases could be potential candidates for robotic resections, as seen in the meta-analysis of Rocca et al. with a 131 robotic mCRC liver resection [14]. There are very few published series of synchronous robotic colorectal resection combined with liver resection for metastatic colorectal cancer. A recent meta-analysis by McGuirk et al. collected only 28 patients that underwent this simultaneous robotic approach. They showed a similar average operative time and a similar low rate of complications, but a hospital length of stay that was more than double in our cohort [15].

From a technical point of view, in a synchronous right colon and liver resection, the robotic platform is usually used in a single right upper quadrant orientation, which does not necessitate changes in the robotic arms array [16]. On the other hand, one of the challenges in a synchronous rectal and liver resection is the multi-quadrant approach and the need to "boom around" from a robotic pelvic dissection of the rectum to a right upper quadrant dissection for the liver and repositioning of the robotic tools. However, in a well-trained and dedicated robotic surgery team, this change in the robot position does not require more than a few minutes.

The optimal sequence of resection, colorectal first followed by liver resection or the other way around, is debatable, with advantages and disadvantages for each approach. The colorectal resection requires manipulation of the small bowel for exposure. It may be considered the "contaminated" part of the surgery with bowel resection. In contrast, the liver resection may necessitate portal vein occlusion (the Pringle maneuver) which can lead to bowel edema and low central venous pressure which can lead to hypotension and hypoperfusion. In our series, both sequences were employed based on the patient's disease specification, mainly the complexity of the liver resection part and the surgeon's preference. In addition, some thoughts were given to the timing of the bowel reconstruction by reserving the anastomosis creation to the final part of the surgery to avoid challenging the blood flow to the anastomosis while performing the liver resection.

In minimally invasive surgery and robotic surgery specifically, the specimens' extraction site can be chosen in a manner that will avoid a midline incision and a high risk for post-operative hernia and other wound complications. In this study, most specimens were taken out through a Pfannenstiel incision, a colostomy site incision, or through the perineal incision, with only one case needing a limited midline incision. With dedicated CRC and liver robotic surgeons and teams, the synchronous robotic approach can be performed with safety and relative ease, with limited intraoperative complications, no need for conversion to an open approach, and limited blood loss, as seen in this study. In the future, we believe that the robotic platform may be the platform of choice for more challenging cases like carcinomatosis management.

This study's limitations revolve around its small sample size, the heterogeneous mix of mCRC cases, and its retrospective nature. It might be challenging to extrapolate from this series for cases in other centers, yet, due to the limited number of cases published in the literature, no randomized control studies in the near future, and very few centers in the world that can perform a synchronous robotic colorectal and liver resection, this series can lay the groundwork for establishing these capabilities for future cases and show what is safe and feasible. Further studies should be planned and executed to prove its advantage to patients with mCRC. Further studies with larger cohorts and longer follow-ups are needed to assess the long-term outcomes of robotic combined resections.

5. Conclusions

Synchronous robotic colorectal and liver resection of colorectal cancer and liver metastases is a safe and feasible approach for select patients with liver mCRC. This approach can be performed effectively utilizing one port configuration with acceptable short-term outcomes and quality of oncologic resection. However, further studies are needed to assess the benefits of the robotic approach, especially compared to laparoscopy and open surgery.

Author Contributions: Conceptualization, Y.R.; methodology, Y.R., R.P. and K.T.B.; investigation, Y.R. and R.P.; data curation, Y.R. and R.P.; writing—original draft preparation, Y.R.; writing—review and editing, Y.R., R.P., S.S., S.W., S.P.C. and K.T.B.; supervision, K.T.B. All authors have read and agreed to the published version of the manuscript.

Funding: This study has received no funding or financial support.

Institutional Review Board Statement: This study was conducted in accordance with the ethical principles of the Declaration of Helsinki (Edinburgh 2000) and the approval of the Institutional Review Board. An exemption for informed consent was given by the IRB.

Informed Consent Statement: Patient consent was waived due to the retrospective nature of the study and the analysis used anonymous clinical data.

Data Availability Statement: Data will be available upon request from authors.

Conflicts of Interest: The authors declare no conflict of interest.

References

1. Araghi, M.; Soerjomataram, I.; Jenkins, M.; Brierley, J.; Morris, E.; Bray, F.; Arnold, M. Global trends in colorectal cancer mortality: Projections to the year 2035. *Int. J. Cancer* **2019**, *144*, 2992–3000. [CrossRef] [PubMed]
2. Kasi, P.M.; Shahjehan, F.; Cochuyt, J.J.; Li, Z.; Colibaseanu, D.T.; Merchea, A. Rising Proportion of Young Individuals with Rectal and Colon Cancer. *Clin. Color. Cancer* **2019**, *18*, e87–e95. [CrossRef] [PubMed]
3. Cardoso, R.; Guo, F.; Heisser, T.; Hackl, M.; Ihle, P.; De Schutter, H.; Van Damme, N.; Valerianova, Z.; Atanasov, T.; Majek, O.; et al. Colorectal cancer incidence, mortality, and stage distribution in European countries in the colorectal cancer screening era: An international population-based study. *Lancet Oncol.* **2021**, *22*, 1002–1013. [CrossRef] [PubMed]
4. Brouwer, N.P.M.; Bos, A.; Lemmens, V.; Tanis, P.J.; Hugen, N.; Nagtegaal, I.D.; de Wilt, J.H.W.; Verhoeven, R.H.A. An overview of 25 years of incidence, treatment and outcome of colorectal cancer patients. *Int. J. Cancer* **2018**, *143*, 2758–2766. [CrossRef] [PubMed]
5. Kanemitsu, Y.; Shitara, K.; Mizusawa, J.; Hamaguchi, T.; Shida, D.; Komori, K.; Ikeda, S.; Ojima, H.; Ike, H.; Shiomi, A.; et al. Primary Tumor Resection Plus Chemotherapy versus Chemotherapy Alone for Colorectal Cancer Patients with Asymptomatic, Synchronous Unresectable Metastases (JCOG1007; iPACS): A Randomized Clinical Trial. *J. Clin. Oncol.* **2021**, *39*, 1098–1107. [CrossRef] [PubMed]
6. Martin, J.; Petrillo, A.; Smyth, E.C.; Shaida, N.; Khwaja, S.; Cheow, H.K.; Duckworth, A.; Heister, P.; Praseedom, R.; Jah, A.; et al. Colorectal liver metastases: Current management and future perspectives. *World J. Clin. Oncol.* **2020**, *11*, 761–808. [CrossRef] [PubMed]
7. Wakabayashi, G.; Cherqui, D.; Geller, D.A.; Buell, J.F.; Kaneko, H.; Han, H.S.; Asbun, H.; O'Rourke, N.; Tanabe, M.; Koffron, A.J.; et al. Recommendations for laparoscopic liver resection: A report from the second international consensus conference held in Morioka. *Ann. Surg.* **2015**, *261*, 619–629. [CrossRef] [PubMed]
8. Sammarco, A.; de'Angelis, N.; Testini, M.; Memeo, R. Robotic synchronous treatment of colorectal cancer and liver metastasis: State of the art. *Mini-Invasive Surg.* **2019**, *3*, 31. [CrossRef]
9. Garritano, S.; Selvaggi, F.; Spampinato, M.G. Simultaneous minimally invasive treatment of colorectal neoplasm with synchronous liver metastasis. *BioMed Res. Int.* **2016**, *2016*, 9328250. [CrossRef] [PubMed]

10. Ceccarelli, G.; Rocca, A.; De Rosa, M.; Fontani, A.; Ermili, F.; Andolfi, E.; Bugiantella, W.; Levi Sandri, G.B. Minimally invasive robotic-assisted combined colorectal and liver excision surgery: Feasibility, safety and surgical technique in a pilot series. *Updates Surg.* **2021**, *73*, 1015–1022. [CrossRef] [PubMed]
11. Dwyer, R.H.; Scheidt, M.J.; Marshall, J.S.; Tsoraides, S.S. Safety and efficacy of synchronous robotic surgery for colorectal cancer with liver metastases. *J. Robot. Surg.* **2018**, *12*, 603–606. [CrossRef] [PubMed]
12. Shapera, E.; Ross, S.B.; Chudzinski, A.; Massarotti, H.; Syblis, C.C.; Crespo, K.; Rosemurgy, A.S.; Sucandy, I. Simultaneous Resection of Colorectal Carcinoma and Hepatic Metastases is Safe and Effective: Examining the Role of the Robotic Approach. *Am. Surg.* **2022**; *ahead of print*. [CrossRef]
13. Guerra, F.; Guadagni, S.; Pesi, B.; Furbetta, N.; Di Franco, G.; Palmeri, M.; Annecchiarico, M.; Eugeni, E.; Coratti, A.; Patriti, A.; et al. Outcomes of robotic liver resections for colorectal liver metastases. A multi-institutional analysis of minimally invasive ultrasound-guided robotic surgery. *Surg. Oncol.* **2019**, *28*, 14–18. [CrossRef] [PubMed]
14. Rocca, A.; Scacchi, A.; Cappuccio, M.; Avella, P.; Bugiantella, W.; De Rosa, M.; Costa, G.; Polistena, A.; Codacci-Pisanelli, M.; Amato, B. Robotic surgery for colorectal liver metastases resection: A systematic review. *Int. J. Med. Robot. Comput. Assist. Surg.* **2021**, *17*, e2330. [CrossRef] [PubMed]
15. McGuirk, M.; Gachabayov, M.; Rojas, A.; Kajmolli, A.; Gogna, S.; Gu, K.W.; Qiuye, Q.; Da Dong, X. Simultaneous robot assisted colon and liver resection for metastatic colon cancer. *JSLS J. Soc. Laparosc. Robot. Surg.* **2021**, *25*, e2020.00108. [CrossRef] [PubMed]
16. Murugan, S.; Grenn, E.E.; Earl, T.M.; Anderson, C.D.; Orr, W.S., III. Robot-Assisted Right Colectomy with Sequential Wedge Resection of Segments 4 and 5 of the Liver and Cholecystectomy for Colon Cancer with Metastasis to the Liver. *Am. Surg.* **2022**, *88*, 1566–1567. [CrossRef] [PubMed]

Disclaimer/Publisher's Note: The statements, opinions and data contained in all publications are solely those of the individual author(s) and contributor(s) and not of MDPI and/or the editor(s). MDPI and/or the editor(s) disclaim responsibility for any injury to people or property resulting from any ideas, methods, instructions or products referred to in the content.

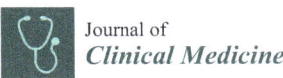

Review

Indocyanine Green Fluorescence Guided Surgery in Colorectal Surgery

Zoe Garoufalia and Steven D. Wexner *

Ellen Leifer Shulman and Steven Shulman Digestive Disease Center, Cleveland Clinic Florida, Weston, FL 33331, USA
* Correspondence: wexners@ccf.org; Tel.: +1-954-659-6020

Abstract: Background: Indocyanine green (ICG) imaging has been increasingly used for intraoperative guidance in colorectal surgery over the past decade. The aim of this study was to review and organize, according to different type of use, all available literature on ICG guided colorectal surgery and highlight areas in need of further research and discuss future perspectives. Methods: PubMed, Scopus, and Google Scholar databases were searched systematically through November 2022 for all available studies on fluorescence-guided surgery in colorectal surgery. Results: Available studies described ICG use in colorectal surgery for perfusion assessment, ureteral and urethral assessment, lymphatic mapping, and hepatic and peritoneal metastases assessment. Although the level of evidence is low, results are promising, especially in the role of ICG in reducing anastomotic leaks. Conclusions: ICG imaging is a safe and relatively cheap imaging modality in colorectal surgery, especially for perfusion assessment. Work is underway regarding its use in lymphatic mapping, ureter identification, and the assessment of intraperitoneal metastatic disease.

Keywords: colon; rectal; colorectal; indocyanine green (ICG); fluorescence; surgery

1. Introduction

Indocyanine green (ICG) is a fluorescent water-soluble dye that binds with plasma proteins, especially lipoproteins, and demonstrates fluorescent properties in the near-infrared (NIR) spectrum (750–950 nm). It was developed by Kodak Laboratories in 1955 for near-infrared photography and received FDA approval for human use in 1959 [1]. Since then, it has been used as an imaging method in several medical applications, including vascular, endocrine, hepatopancreaticobiliary, gynecologic, plastic, urologic, and colorectal surgery [2].

ICG is metabolized solely through the liver and excreted into the bile, and its half-life depends on liver function (typically 3–4 min) [2]. When it is not directly injected into the bloodstream, it is drained through the lymphatic network. The time required to reach the nearest lymph node is approximately 15 min [3]. ICG has been proven safe with dosages between 0.1–0.5 mg/mL/kg with only the relative contraindications of iodine or shellfish allergy. Depending on the target structure/organ that needs to be visualized, it can be administered through various routes, including intravenously, submucosally or into the ureteral system (Figure 1).

The different ICG applications in colorectal surgery are substantial and still evolving. ICG has been used in colorectal surgeries for perfusion assessment, intraoperative ureteral visualization, sentinel node identification, and lymphatic drainage visualization. Another described use is for the localization and intraoperative assessment of peritoneal and hepatic metastases. However, the evidence provided by published studies is poor. Therefore, the aim of this review was to review and organize, according to different type of use, the available published literature related to ICG-guided colorectal surgery, highlight areas in need of further research, and discuss future perspectives.

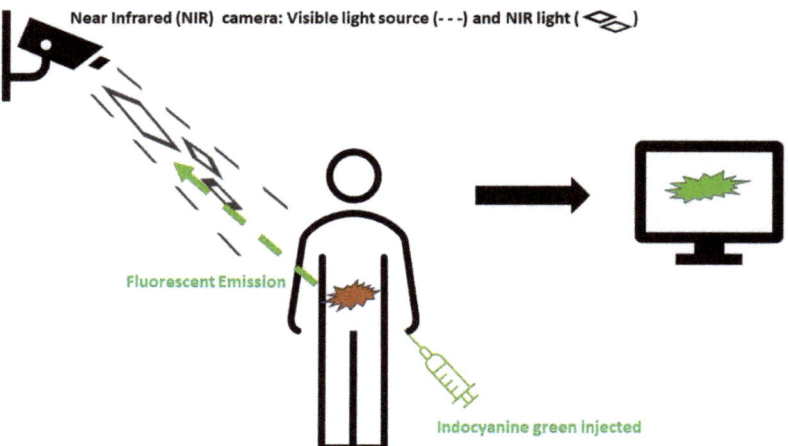

Figure 1. The basics of indocyanine green (ICG) imaging in colorectal surgery. ICG is injected (method of administration varies depending on the target). The ICG molecules are excited by the light source and demonstrate fluorescent properties in the near-infrared spectrum (750–950 nm). This signal is combined with real time image and transferred on the screen.

2. Methods

PubMed, Scopus, and Google Scholar databases were searched systematically through November 2022. The terms 'colorectal', 'colon', 'rectal', 'indocyanine green', 'ICG', and 'fluorescence' were used combined with the Boolean operators AND/OR in order to identify all available studies on fluorescence-guided surgery in colorectal surgery. The reference lists of retrieved articles were also screened for further eligible studies. After removal of duplicates, the abstract list generated by the above search was independently screened by the authors for potentially relevant studies. All English-text available studies involving humans (either cadaveric models or alive patients) on fluorescent guided colorectal surgery were retrieved and synthetized in a narrative manner to describe current applications of this technique as well as its future perspectives.

We did not seek ethics approval as this type of study, a literature review, does not require approval since no patient data were accessed or analyzed.

3. Current Uses of ICG in Colorectal Surgery

3.1. Perfusion Assessment

3.1.1. Anastomotic and Bowel Perfusion Assessment

Anastomotic leak (AL) remains a major dreaded colorectal surgery complication. AL rates vary by type of surgery with an incidence of up to 19% [4]. Multiple factors contribute to AL; nevertheless, a well perfused and tension-free anastomosis is necessary for an uneventful anastomotic healing process. ICG provides the ability to objectively intraoperatively assess anastomotic perfusion.

Several case series and cohort studies have demonstrated a reduced AL rate with the use of intraoperative ICG for the assessment of anastomotic perfusion, although not always statistically significant [5–9]. The first randomized trial (RCT) was published in 2020 by De Nardi et al. [10] and 252 patients. Although the authors concluded that ICG was safe and not time-consuming, it failed to show significantly lower AL rates (5% in the ICG group versus 9% in the control group). At the same time, another single center RCT was published by Alekseev et al. [11] that showed a significant reduction in AL rates of low (4–8 cm from the anal verge) stapled colorectal anastomoses (14.5% vs. 25.7%) and a change in resection margin in 20% of patients. Following these contradictory results, another randomized control trial was launched in the USA. Unfortunately, due to the low recruitment rate it was deemed underpowered and thus terminated early [12]. Two recent meta-analyses [13,14] concluded that the intraoperative use of ICG for perfusion assessment was associated with significantly lower odds for AL (OR 0.52, 95% CI 0.304–0.98, I2 = 0). One of these metanalyses [14] reported that the weighted mean rate of change in the surgical plan due to ICG imaging was 9.6% (95% CI 7.3–11.8). Currently, another phase III multicenter randomized controlled trial is being launched (NCT04712032; NL7502) [15] aiming to provide high quality evidence regarding the role of ICG in the reduction of clinically relevant ALs. The current literature reports that ICG assessment is a safe and rapid means of assessing anastomotic perfusion/bowel perfusion (Figure 2) and may result in reduction of AL. One of the main drawbacks of this method is the fact that assessment is subjective. Therefore, recent studies [16–19] have tried to address this issue with software assessing the ICG saturation. One study [16] reported the optimal distance of the camera from the colon to assess perfusion (5 cm) and the optimal time for assessment (1.5–3.5 min after intravenous infusion), indicating some progress in this area. Still, more research is required to identify the optimal software for validated, quantifiable, and reproducible perfusion assessment. Finally, a recent cost analysis [20] of the routine use of ICG for anastomotic perfusion assessment, using the assumption that the cost of AL is >USD 5616.29 and the cost of ICG-FA is <USD 634.44 [odds ratio (OR) for AL reduction with ICG use: 0.46], found that routine use of ICG imaging in colorectal surgery is cost-effective. Video S1 demonstrates the intraoperative use of ICG for bowel perfusion assessment.

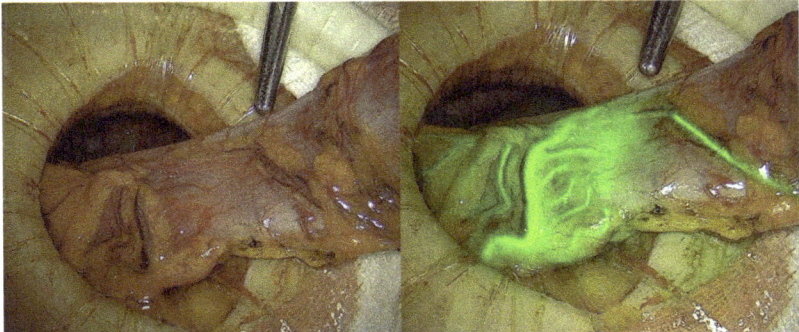

Figure 2. Bowel perfusion assessment using ICG. Courtesy of International Society for Fluorescence Guided Surgery (ISFGS).

3.1.2. Perfusion Assessment in Pedicled Omentoplasty

In 2019, Slooter et al. reported a pilot study for assessing omental perfusion during omentoplasty in salvage surgery for pelvic sepsis [21]. After establishing the feasibility of this technique, the same group went on to demonstrate the possible beneficial role in a subsequent cohort study [22]. They reported a much lower perineal non-healing rate in the group where ICG was utilized (22%) versus the controls (42%).

3.1.3. Perfusion Assessment in Gracilis Muscle Interposition

Graciloplasty is a technique that can be utilized to treat complex perianal fistulae [23]. Nevertheless, a well-perfused gracilis flap is of utmost importance for the success of this technique. A recent study by Lobbes et al. [24] reported a software-based approach for gracilis perfusion assessment, pointing to objective indicators for flap perfusion. This technique may be further developed and utilized in the future to optimize the outcome of gracilis muscle interposition.

3.1.4. Perfusion Assessment in Anal Advancement Flaps

Endorectal advancement flaps are used to treat complex perianal fistula repair; success depends on the viability of the anal flap to avoid flap dehiscence or recurrent fistula. Turner et al. [25] published a retrospective case series of six patients undergoing advancement flaps for perianal fistula. They reported a high rate (71.4%) of change in the surgical plan based on the results of intraoperative ICG perfusion assessment of the flap. This technology may be further developed in the future in terms of the quantification of the result to optimize the outcomes of this technique.

3.1.5. Perfusion Assessment in Ileal Pouch-Anal Anastomosis (IPAA)

Good perfusion is of utmost importance during construction of the anastomosis for IPAA. In 2021, Joosten et al. [26] published the first technical note on utilizing ICG technology to enable lengthening maneuvers. Following this, Freund et al. [27] confirmed the utility of ICG imaging in complex IPAA surgery requiring lengthening maneuvers in their patient series. Similarly, Slooter et al. [28] demonstrated the use of ICG in IPAA surgery, focusing on the time needed between ICG infusion and the assessment of pouch perfusion. They concluded that due to vascular ligation in lengthening maneuvers, a longer time interval might be needed between ICG infusion and the first signal. However, can this assessment be quantifiable? How can one assess the ICG signal with certainty and objectively? Lobbes et al. [29] sought to address this issue using novel software to assess the ICG signal for pouch perfusion in order to make this assessment quantifiable and comparable. Although the available literature supports the use of ICG in IPAA surgery, the level of evidence is still low.

3.2. Vital Structures Assessment

3.2.1. Intraoperative Ureteral Assessment

Ureteral injury is a devastating complication in colorectal surgery. The ureters are retroperitoneal structures that can be easily damaged during the dissection of the colon or rectum, especially in complicated surgeries, causing extensive inflammation and the need for re-operations. There are reports in the literature regarding ICG imaging utilization for intraoperative ureteral identification [30–36]. This method involves cystoscopic ureteral stenting and the injection of ICG dye through the stent into each ureter. Although the exact quantity of ICG instilled varies, the majority of studies report using 5 mL of 2.5 mg/mL ICG solution in each ureter. This dosage allows the ureters to glow green intraoperatively and are thus easier to identify throughout the surgery, especially in minimally invasive surgery where haptic feedback is unavailable. A recent systematic review of this technique [37] concluded that ICG ureter visualization (Figure 3) is safe and effective in minimally invasive colorectal surgery, with one caveat: this technique still entails ureteral stenting and its potential complications. The authors noted that current research is focusing on experimental dyes that could potentially combine imaging properties with renal excretion to minimize the adverse effects of ureteral stenting. In this scope, experimental novel fluorescent dyes are currently under development, similar to those reported by Dip et al. [38] and Mahalingam et al. [39], which could be systematically injected and excreted by the renal system, thus enabling intraoperative ureteral identification without the need for ureteral stenting. However, both reports concern in animal studies, and they have not yet been tested in humans.

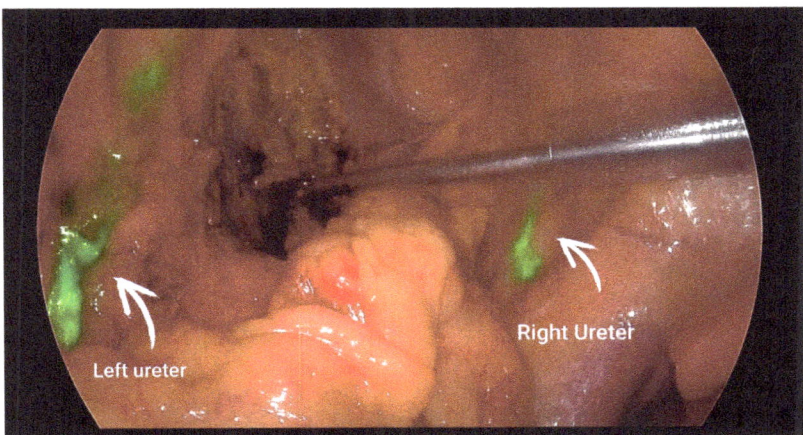

Figure 3. Ureter identification during pelvic dissection. Steven D. Wexner personal archive.

3.2.2. Intraoperative Urethral Assessment

With the progress made in transanal surgery and especially transanal total mesorectal (TaTME) excision, one of the main complications reported is urethral injury. The reported rates of urethral injury in TaTME range from 1% [40] to 6.7% [41]. First, Barnes et al. described the successful use of ICG mixed with Instillagel® (CliniMed, Buckinghamshire, UK) to visualize the male urethra in eight cadavers [42]. In another cadaver study, the same group demonstrated successful visualization of the male urethra with an ICG-silicone coated Foley catheter [43]. The authors also tested a new dye (IRDye800BK) in this same study, which has greater depth of penetration than ICG. Barberio et al. [44] demonstrated the efficacy of ICG/Instillagel® coated Foleys in cadaveric models [43]. Nitta et al. [45] successfully utilized the IRIS U kit (Stryker, Kalamazoo, MI, USA), an infrared lighted ureteral stent, for urethral visualization in a TaTME case report [45]. Although it seems reasonable that the ICG infusion used for ureteral visualization should also aid in visualizing the urethra, currently there are no available literature reports regarding the use of this technique for urethral visualization during transanal surgery.

3.2.3. Intraoperative Nerve Assessment

Intraoperative nerve identification is essential, especially in pelvic dissection, as it could potentially allow the surgeon to recognize and spare these anatomical structures from adverse urogenital and anorectal sequelae. Recently Jin et al. [46] reported a pilot trial in which ICG was used to guide intraoperative nerve identification in colorectal surgery. They injected 4.5 mg/kg ICG intravenously 24 h before surgery in seven patients. Using this technique, the authors confirmed the intraoperative identification of the inferior mesenteric artery plexus and sacral plexus. Their trial was the first to report ICG use for identifying pelvic nerves in colorectal surgery. However, further studies are needed to define the optimal dosage and administration time of ICG.

3.3. Tumor Assessment

Tumor visualization and localization can be beneficial in many scenarios of colorectal surgery. There can be discrepancies in tumor location between endoscopic assessment and intraoperative findings; this sometimes results in a different surgical strategy to the one originally planned. In addition, tumor visualization may sometimes allow the surgeon to better delineate the resection margins. The first report of intraoperative fluorescent tumor localization was published in 2016 by Handgraaf et al. [47], although the main focus was sentinel lymph node identification using ICG. There are several reports in the literature [48–52] regarding the feasibility of ICG imaging in primary tumor visualization and real-time navigation. Atallah et al. [53] reported a case wherein fluorescence-guided surgery along with a robotic-assisted stereotactic navigational system were successfully utilized for complex locally advanced rectal cancer surgery. More recently, Satoyoshi et al. [54] reported a case series wherein ICG was injected near the tumor in the submucosal layer of the bowel preoperatively using endoscopy. The tumor detection rate was 100% within six days of preoperative marking, and the ICG did not cause any inflammatory phenomena (compared to conventional preoperative tattooing) [54]. A similar later study by Ahn et al. [55] confirmed this finding but further focused on better lymph node visualization and retrieval using ICG. Another novel fluorescent adjunct for intraoperative tumor localization was presented by Narihiro et al. [56]. They reported the use of a novel fluorescent clip (ZEOCLIP FS, Zeon Medical Co, Tokyo, Japan), which was placed a few days prior to the surgery and was easily detected from the serosal side intraoperatively. Similar clips were more recently reported by Lee et al. [57] and Ryu et al. [58].

3.4. Lymphatic Mapping

Colorectal cancer spreads through the lumen to the submucosa, where it can start spreading through the lymph nodes. Thus, lymph node yield is critical, and the removal of all potential tumor involved lymph nodes is mandatory. Nishigori et al. [59] performed perioperative, peritumoral, and submucosal ICG injection in 21 patients. They noted that lymph flow was intraoperatively visible in 18/21 patients. Most importantly, they reported a change in the extent of mesenteric resection and vessel ligation in 23.5% of patients. Similar results are reported in later studies [54,60–62]. Along with the feasibility of the intraoperative ICG imaging of lymphovascular drainage in colorectal cancer, a later study by Chand et al. [63] also showed that the success of lymphatic imaging was affected by the quantity of ICG injected into the bowel wall and that India ink tattooing that could potentially block lymph drainage and cause inflammatory phenomena. Another study by Goo et al. [64] that included 1079 patients reported that the intraoperative ICG imaging of lymph drainage, although useful in adequate lymph node yield in early colorectal cancers, did not yield the same results for more advanced stages. This result may be explained by the later study of Kakizoe et al. [65]. The authors performed a histopathologic study on splenic flexure cancer specimens to compare the association of fluorescence and cancer spread. They reported that the lymph nodes with cancer did not show any fluorescence, while 80% of the non-occupied lymph nodes were visible with ICG imaging. This could be a downside to the surgery's lymphatic mapping and strategic planning since tumor metastasis might 'silence' the lymph nodes and lymphatic drainage that need to be included in the resected specimen. Similar results by Ushijima et al. [66] indicated that the ICG imaging of lymph flow was effective in early and not advanced colorectal cancer in their series of patients.

The idea of the better visualization of the lymphatic flow led to the utilization of intraoperative ICG imaging to perform CME and right hemicolectomies with D3 lymphadenectomy [67–70]. A recent matched control study by Park et al. involving patient with right-sided T3 and T4 colon cancer, showed that although ICG-guided lymphadenectomy resulted in a significantly higher lymph node yield (39 vs. 30, $p = 0.003$), the number of metastatic lymph nodes was not significantly different between the two groups [71].

More recently, the interim analysis of the GREENLIGHT trial, [72] a prospective non-randomized trial of ICG lymphatic mapping, showed that the extent of the lymphadenectomy was modified based on the results of imaging in 50% of the study population (35/70). What was more interesting is that they demonstrated that lymph node metastasis was not correlated with a paucity in ICG signal, as was shown in previous studies. In fact, one third of the fluorescent resected D3 lymph nodes were positive for malignancy.

3.5. Sentinel Lymph Node Assessment

An early systematic review and meta-analysis [73] that included 52 studies ($n = 3767$ patients) concluded that the sentinel node biopsy was sensitive regardless of tumor location and T stage The role of the sentinel node in lymph node metastasis detection was initiated by Gould et al. in 1960 [74]. Although it is well established in plastic, breast, and ENT surgery, there is no such consensus in colorectal surgery. Additional studies [75–83] have since been published on the matter, specifically related to techniques of detecting sentinel lymph nodes in colorectal cancer, such as ICG (Figure 4). Since then, even more systematic reviews and metanalyses on this subject have been published [84,85]. The most recent was published in 2021 [86] and the reported pooled detection and accuracy rates were 90% and 77%, respectively, for the T3–T34 and 91% and 98%, respectively, for the T1–T2 group using the ICG technique for sentinel lymph node assessment. Sensitivity and accuracy were 2.31 [CI: 1.15–4.67] and 1.25 [CI 1.05–1.47] times higher in the T1–T2 group than the T3–T4 group. A more recent study by Picchetto et al. [87] examined the use of ex vivo sentinel lymph node assessment, reporting promising and reliable results in 22 patients.

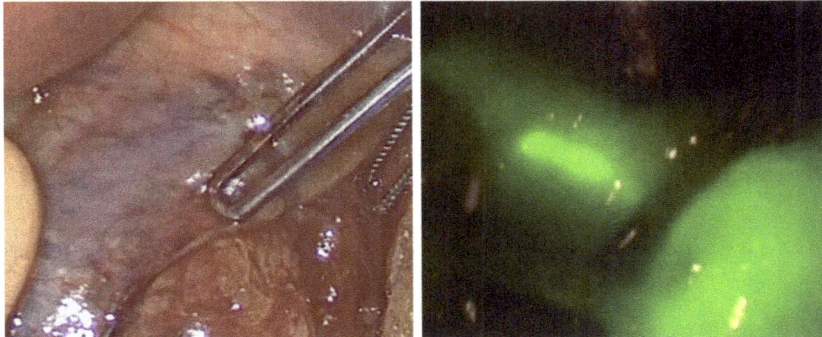

Figure 4. Sentinel lymph node identification using white light (**left**) and indocyanine green imaging (**right**). Courtesy of the International Society for Fluorescence Guided Surgery (ISFGS).

3.6. Lateral Pelvic Lymph Node Assessment

The role of lateral pelvic node dissection (LPND) in locally advanced rectal cancer is still controversial, with results from recent meta-analyses stating that it does not affect disease-free or overall survival but may reduce local recurrence risk [88,89]. Nevertheless, this procedure is associated with longer operative times, higher morbidity rates than TME [88,89], and poor visualization due to complex anatomy. In this context, there have been some recent reports [90–97] on the utilization of ICG for intraoperative visualization during lateral lymph node dissection for locally advanced rectal cancer. Zhou et al. [90] compared two patient cohorts undergoing LPND, one under ICG-guidance and a standard one and showed that using ICG led to significantly lower blood loss and higher lymph node yield. In a propensity score-matched analysis, Dai et al. [92] confirmed the previous results that ICG-guided LPND leads to significantly higher lymph node yield and lower intraoperative blood loss. This group also reported shorter hospital stays and lower rates of residual disease/recurrence in the ICG group. Another study by Yasui et al. [93] reported using ICG to identify the SNL in LPND. All 21 patients included in the study underwent SNL identification before laparoscopic LPND. All patients with negative SNL had no disease in the remaining lymph nodes retrieved [93]. The same concept had been previously supported by Noura et al. [82]. Another more recent propensity match analysis involving 172 patients showed that using ICG in LPND results in a significantly higher lymph node yield than the conventional method (14 vs. 9 lymph nodes), with no significant differences in short-term complications [94]. The use of ICG for LPND needs to be fully established, since there is still no solid evidence of the clear benefit of this procedure in terms of survival [95]. Finally, in 2020, Kim et al. [96] reported a new method combining ICG lateral pelvic lymph node identification with 3D reconstruction images using the results of preoperative CT scans. More research is needed to elucidate any potential value of LPDN for locally advanced rectal cancer. The results and perspectives of ICG-guidance, given the complexity and morbidity associated with LPDN, are promising.

3.7. Distant Disease Assessment

3.7.1. Peritoneal Metastases Assessment

The intraoperative detection of peritoneal metastases, even those not visible to the naked eye, is a great tool not only for diagnosis but also for treatment in select patients undergoing cytoreduction and intraperitoneal hyperthermic chemotherapy. First, Liberale et al. [97] reported the feasibility of ICG imaging in non-mucinous colorectal peritoneal metastases. They also reported a change in the surgery plan in 1/3 of the study population as ICG made visible peritoneal lesions that could not be seen with the naked eye [97]. A relevant metanalysis [98] published in 2020 included three studies and a total of 28 patients on the ICG imaging of colorectal cancer peritoneal metastases [97,99,100]. In all patients, ICG was intravenously administered between 0–24 h before surgery. The sensitivity of the method varied between 72.4% and 96.9%, while the specificity varied between 60% and 100%. Following this, in 2022, González-Abós et al. [101] reported preliminary results of the ICCP study, a prospective single center trial aiming to assess the diagnostic accuracy of the quantitative ICG imaging of non-mucinous colorectal peritoneal metastases. The authors reported that ICG uptake <100 units may suggest benign pathology while >181 units is suggestive of malignancy (sensitivity 89% and specificity 85%). The jury is still out as to whether this modality could be the standard of care in diagnosing/treating this specific category of patients with peritoneal metastases.

3.7.2. Liver Metastases Assessment

Colorectal liver metastases are treatable with resection. However, the indications for the hepatic metastasectomy of colorectal origin are still evolving. Nevertheless, up to 1/3 of patients undergoing the curative resection of colorectal hepatic metastases will have R1 resections (<1 mm resection margin) or residual disease due to the inability to properly detect intraoperatively [102]. This can severely impact disease-free survival and overall survival. The intraoperative imaging of the metastases is mostly performed using visual and haptic feedback and intraoperative ultrasound. There have been several reports on the use of ICG for intraoperatively localizing colorectal liver metastasis. The most recent review was by Picollo et al. [102] in 2022 and included 13 studies (literature search through April 2021). The authors reported a wide variation in the timing of ICG administration (1 to 14 days preoperatively) as well an average detection rate of metastases with ICG of 79.03% (range: 57.6–100) compared to 95.97% (range: 93.3–100%) with intraoperative ultrasound. Since then, four more studies have been published on this issue. In 2021, Picollo et al. [103] reported the advantage and the possible replacement of tactile feedback with ICG imaging, a potentially important feature, especially during minimally invasive surgery. Nevertheless, this study also included patients with hepatocellular carcinoma and cholangiocarcinoma, therefore, the results cannot be generalized. A prospective single-center UK study published in 2022 [104] included 15 patients undergoing ICG-assisted liver metastasectomy. The authors reported that ICG altered the operative plan in almost half of the patients (43%), despite the concurrent use of intraoperative ultrasound. Finally, a randomized control trial by He et al. [105] involving 64 patients undergoing hepatic metastasectomy for colorectal cancer showed that the mean number of intraoperatively identified colorectal metastases was significantly higher (3.03, SD:1.58) in the ICG imaging group compared to the non-ICG group (2.28 SD:1.35). The authors also noted that the 1-year recurrence rate was significantly lower in the ICG group, while postoperative complications were comparable between the two groups. Nevertheless, imaging with ICG, despite minimizing the need for tactile feedback, can be non-specific, especially regarding the resection margins. In this scope, Nishino et al. [106] recently published an animal study on the ICG-guided resection of colorectal metastases in mice previously injected with a carcinoembryonic antigen antibody conjugated with a fluorophore. At three weeks after surgery, tumor weight was significantly lower in the ICG imaging group compared to the control group. The authors concluded that this technique might potentially improve hepatic metastasectomy [106].

4. Discussions and Future Perspectives

ICG in colorectal surgery can be beneficial in multiple ways (Table 1). Although it has been FDA-approved since 1959, [1] the use of ICG has become more prominent in colorectal surgery over the past ten years. Still, it is still not routinely adopted by colorectal surgeons as some question its real benefit due to the lack of high-level evidence. In addition, some have also raised the issue of additional costs of ICG without a scientifically proven benefit. Nevertheless, a recent cost analysis [20] on the routine use of ICG imaging for anastomotic perfusion assessment reported that it is cost effective. Based on the assumption that the cost of AL is more than USD 5616.29 and the cost of ICG-FA is <USD 634.44, and that the given odds ratio for AL reduction with ICG-use (based on a literature review) is 0.46, the authors showed that routine use of ICG for anastomotic assessment can reduce the financial burden of AL.

Table 1. Reported applications of indocyanine green (ICG) imaging in colorectal surgery in literature.

ICG Applications in Colorectal Surgery
Perfusion Assessment
• Bowel Perfusion [5–20]
• Anastomotic Perfusion [5–20,26–29]
• Gracilis Muscle Perfusion [24]
• Anal Advancement Flap Perfusion [25]
• Pedicled Omentoplasty [21,22]
Anatomic Visualization
• Ureteral Visualization [31–36,38,39]
• Urethral Visualization [42–45]
• Nerve assessment [46]
Tumor Localization [47–58]
Lymphatic Mapping [59–72]
Sentinel Lymph Node Identification [75–85]
Lateral pelvic node dissection [88–95]
Distant Metastases Assessment
• Peritoneal Metastases [96–101]
• Liver Metastases [101–107]

ICG is a safe and relatively inexpensive method of perfusion assessment; current data show its beneficial role in reducing AL. Nevertheless, this is yet to be proven in well-conducted and powered randomized control trials. Hopefully, the results of the AVOID study will provide the evidence needed to dissolve any ensuing skepticism on this modality [15]. A recently published Delphi consensus of international experts on the use of ICG further supported the use of ICG for anastomotic perfusion assessment (100% consensus reached), as well as issues such as timing and dosage of ICG for perfusion assessment during colorectal surgery [108,109]. The other ICG applications for perfusion assessment, including for gracilis and advancement flaps, although promising, require further research in order to be routinely implemented into daily practice.

The available studies show promising results with potential practice-changing applications of this technique including lymph node evaluation. The prematurity and contradictive nature of the available data is also reflected in the recent Delphi survey: while experts agreed that ICG lymphangiography might increase the lymph node yield, they debated whether the routine use of ICG is needed in cancer surgery for lymph node evaluation or whether it will impact the resection plan [108,109]. Furthermore, the use of ICG for the intraoperative visualization of colorectal peritoneal and liver metastases seems revolutionary, yet more research is needed for the quantification of ICG signal as well as safely defining the boundary where fluorescence ceases and healthy tissue ensues. Finally, intraoperative ICG ureteral visualization, although helpful especially in complicated cases, still lacks the necessary evidence for routinely implementing this technique in everyday practice. The parameters listed in Table 2 need to be considered when ICG is utilized for bowel perfusion assessment and lymph node evaluation.

Table 2. Important parameters during evaluation of blood flow and lymphatic mapping using ICG.

Important Parameters during Evaluation of Blood Flow and Lymphatic Mapping Using ICG
Dosage of ICG
Concentration of ICG
Route of administration
Assessment time (time from ICG injection until assessment)
Quantification of the result

The future may be a combination of ICG applications optimized by artificial intelligence (AI) programs. In 2020, Park et al. [110] reported on an AI/ICG based real-time micro perfusion application that was more accurate and consistent than conventional ICG imaging. A similar hybrid model was reported by Seeliger et al. [111] The authors performed a quantitative mucosal and serosal perfusion analysis in porcine ischemic colons using ICG and computer assisted FLER analysis. They suggested that serosal ICG assessment might be less indicative of the actual extent of ischemia than the mucosal ICG assessment. These are only some examples of the evolving AI technology in ICG imaging studies with potential applications in better quantifying ICG signal and delineating tumor location and resection margins for colorectal metastases.

5. Conclusions

ICG imaging is undoubtedly a helpful adjunct. ICG perfusion assessment seems to reduce AL. Its use in ureteric identification, lymphatic mapping and assessing liver and peritoneal metastases remain developmental. To date, these are the reported applications of ICG in colorectal surgery. Evidence is low for the majority of these applications.

Supplementary Materials: The following supporting information can be downloaded at: https://www.mdpi.com/article/10.3390/jcm12020494/s1, Video S1: demonstrates the intraoperative use of ICG for bowel perfusion assessment.

Author Contributions: Conceptualization, S.D.W. writing—original draft preparation, Z.G.; writing—review and editing, S.D.W.; visualization, S.D.W.; supervision, S.D.W. All authors have read and agreed to the published version of the manuscript.

Funding: This research received no external funding.

Informed Consent Statement: Not applicable.

Data Availability Statement: Not applicable.

Conflicts of Interest: Wexner reports receiving consulting fees from ARC/Corvus, Astellas, Baxter, Becton Dickinson, GI Supply, ICON Language Services, Intuitive Surgical, Leading BioSciences, Livsmed, Medtronic, Olympus Surgical, Stryker, Takeda and receiving royalties from Intuitive Surgical, Karl Storz Endoscopy America Inc, Medtronic, Unique Surgical Innovations, LLC.

References

1. Alander, J.T.; Kaartinen, I.; Laakso, A.; Pätilä, T.; Spillmann, T.; Tuchin, V.V.; Venermo, M.; Välisuo, P. A Review of Indocyanine Green Fluorescent Imaging in Surgery. *Int. J. Biomed. Imaging* **2012**, *2012*, 940585. [CrossRef] [PubMed]
2. Available online: https://www.cancer.gov/publications/dictionaries/cancer-drug/def/indocyanine-green-solution?redirect=true (accessed on 25 November 2022).
3. Tajima, Y.; Murakami, M.; Yamazaki, K.; Masuda, Y.; Kato, M.; Sato, A.; Goto, S.; Otsuka, K.; Kato, T.; Kusano, M. Sentinel node mapping guided by indocyanine green fluorescence imaging during laparoscopic surgery in gastric cancer. *Ann. Surg. Oncol.* **2010**, *17*, 1787–1793. [CrossRef]
4. Ellis, C.T.; Maykel, J.A. Defining Anastomotic Leak and the Clinical Relevance of Leaks. *Clin. Colon Rectal Surg.* **2021**, *34*, 359–365. [CrossRef] [PubMed]
5. Benčurik, V.; Škrovina, M.; Martínek, L.; Bartoš, J.; Macháčková, M.; Dosoudil, M.; Štěpánová, E.; Přibylová, L.; Briš, R.; Vomáčková, K. Intraoperative fluorescence angiography and risk factors of anastomotic leakage in mini-invasive low rectal resections. *Surg. Endosc.* **2021**, *35*, 5015–5023. [CrossRef]
6. Bonadio, L.; Iacuzzo, C.; Cosola, D.; Cipolat Mis, T.; Giudici, F.; Casagranda, B.; Biloslavo, A.; de Manzini, N. Indocyanine green-enhanced fluorangiography (ICGf) in laparoscopic extraperitoneal rectal cancer resection. *Updates Surg.* **2020**, *72*, 477–482. [CrossRef] [PubMed]
7. Dinallo, A.M.; Kolarsick, P.; Boyan, W.P.; Protyniak, B.; James, A.; Dressner, R.M.; Arvanitis, M.L. Does routine use of indocyanine green fluorescence angiography prevent anastomotic leaks? A retrospective cohort analysis. *Am. J. Surg.* **2019**, *218*, 136–139. [CrossRef] [PubMed]
8. Kin, C.; Vo, H.; Welton, L.; Welton, M. Equivocal effect of intraoperative fluorescence angiography on colorectal anastomotic leaks. *Dis. Colon Rectum* **2015**, *58*, 582–587. [CrossRef] [PubMed]
9. Jafari, M.D.; Wexner, S.D.; Martz, J.E.; McLemore, E.C.; Margolin, D.A.; Sherwinter, D.A.; Lee, S.W.; Senagore, A.J.; Phelan, M.J.; Stamos, M.J. Perfusion assessment in laparoscopic left-sided/anterior resection (PILLAR II): A multi-institutional study. *J. Am. Coll. Surg.* **2015**, *220*, 82–92.e1. [CrossRef]
10. De Nardi, P.; Elmore, U.; Maggi, G.; Maggiore, R.; Boni, L.; Cassinotti, E.; Fumagalli, U.; Gardani, M.; De Pascale, S.; Parise, P.; et al. Intraoperative angiography with indocyanine green to assess anastomosis perfusion in patients undergoing laparoscopic colorectal resection: Results of a multicenter randomized controlled trial. *Surg. Endosc.* **2020**, *34*, 53–60. [CrossRef]
11. Alekseev, M.; Rybakov, E.; Shelygin, Y.; Chernyshov, S.; Zarodnyuk, I. A study investigating the perfusion of colorectal anastomoses using fluorescence angiography: Results of the FLAG randomized trial. *Color. Dis.* **2020**, *22*, 1147–1153. [CrossRef]
12. Jafari, M.D.; Pigazzi, A.; McLemore, E.C.; Mutch, M.G.; Haas, E.; Rasheid, S.H.; Wait, A.D.; Paquette, I.M.; Bardakcioglu, O.; Safar, B.; et al. Perfusion Assessment in Left-Sided/Low Anterior Resection (PILLAR III): A Randomized, Controlled, Parallel, Multicenter Study Assessing Perfusion Outcomes with PINPOINT Near-Infrared Fluorescence Imaging in Low Anterior Resection. *Dis. Colon Rectum* **2021**, *64*, 995–1002. [CrossRef] [PubMed]
13. Safiejko, K.; Tarkowski, R.; Kozlowski, T.P.; Koselak, M.; Jachimiuk, M.; Tarasik, A.; Pruc, M.; Smereka, J.; Szarpak, L. Safety and Efficacy of Indocyanine Green in Colorectal Cancer Surgery: A Systematic Review and Meta-Analysis of 11,047 Patients. *Cancers* **2022**, *14*, 1036. [CrossRef] [PubMed]
14. Emile, S.H.; Khan, S.M.; Wexner, S.D. Impact of change in the surgical plan based on indocyanine green fluorescence angiography on the rates of colorectal anastomotic leak: A systematic review and meta-analysis. *Surg. Endosc.* **2022**, *36*, 2245–2257. [CrossRef] [PubMed]
15. Meijer, R.P.J.; Faber, R.A.; Bijlstra, O.D.; Braak, J.P.B.M.; Meershoek-Klein Kranenbarg, E.; Putter, H.; Mieog, J.S.D.; Burggraaf, K.; Vahrmeijer, A.L.; Hilling, D.E.; et al. AVOID; a phase III, randomised controlled trial using indocyanine green for the prevention of anastomotic leakage in colorectal surgery. *BMJ Open* **2022**, *12*, e051144. [CrossRef] [PubMed]
16. Serra-Aracil, X.; Lucas-Guerrero, V.; Garcia-Nalda, A.; Mora-López, L.; Pallisera-Lloveras, A.; Serracant, A.; Navarro-Soto, S. When should indocyanine green be assessed in colorectal surgery, and at what distance from the tissue? Quantitative measurement using the SERGREEN program. *Surg. Endosc.* **2022**, *36*, 8943–8949. [CrossRef]
17. Gomez-Rosado, J.C.; Valdes-Hernandez, J.; Cintas-Catena, J.; Cano-Matias, A.; Perez-Sanchez, A.; Del Rio-Lafuente, F.J.; Torres-Arcos, C.; Lara-Fernandez, Y.; Capitan-Morales, L.C.; Oliva-Mompean, F. Feasibility of quantitative analysis of colonic perfusion using indocyanine green to prevent anastomotic leak in colorectal surgery. *Surg. Endosc.* **2022**, *36*, 1688–1695. [CrossRef]
18. D'Urso, A.; Agnus, V.; Barberio, M.; Seeliger, B.; Marchegiani, F.; Charles, A.L.; Geny, B.; Marescaux, J.; Mutter, D.; Diana, M. Computer-assisted quantification and visualization of bowel perfusion using fluorescence-based enhanced reality in left-sided colonic resections. *Surg. Endosc.* **2021**, *35*, 4321–4331. [CrossRef]
19. Hayami, S.; Matsuda, K.; Iwamoto, H.; Ueno, M.; Kawai, M.; Hirono, S.; Okada, K.; Miyazawa, M.; Tamura, K.; Mitani, Y.; et al. Visualization and quantification of anastomotic perfusion in colorectal surgery using near-infrared fluorescence. *Tech. Coloproctol.* **2019**, *23*, 973–980. [CrossRef]
20. Liu, R.Q.; Elnahas, A.; Tang, E.; Alkhamesi, N.A.; Hawel, J.; Alnumay, A.; Schlachta, C.M. Cost analysis of indocyanine green fluorescence angiography for prevention of anastomotic leakage in colorectal surgery. *Surg. Endosc.* **2022**, *36*, 9281–9287. [CrossRef]

21. Slooter, M.D.; Blok, R.D.; Wisselink, D.D.; Buskens, C.J.; Bemelman, W.A.; Tanis, P.J.; Hompes, R. Near-infrared fluorescence angiography for intra-operative assessment of pedicled omentoplasty for filling of a pelvic cavity: A pilot study. *Tech. Coloproctol.* **2019**, *23*, 723–728. [CrossRef]
22. Slooter, M.D.; Blok, R.D.; de Krom, M.A.; Buskens, C.J.; Bemelman, W.A.; Tanis, P.J.; Hompes, R. Optimizing omentoplasty for management of chronic pelvic sepsis by intra-operative fluorescence angiography: A comparative cohort study. *Color. Dis.* **2020**, *22*, 2252–2259. [CrossRef] [PubMed]
23. Garoufalia, Z.; Gefen, R.; Emile, S.H.; Silva-Alvarenga, E.; Horesh, N.; Freund, M.R.; Wexner, S.D. Gracilis Muscle Interposition for Complex Perineal Fistulae: A Systematic Review and Meta-Analysis of the Literature. *Color. Dis.* **2022**; *ahead of print*. [CrossRef] [PubMed]
24. Lobbes, L.A.; Hoveling, R.J.M.; Schmidt, L.R.; Berns, S.; Weixler, B. Objective Perfusion Assessment in Gracilis Muscle Interposition—A Novel Software-Based Approach to Indocyanine Green Derived Near-Infrared Fluorescence in Reconstructive Surgery. *Life* **2022**, *12*, 278. [CrossRef] [PubMed]
25. Turner, J.S.; Okonkwo, A.; Chase, A.; Clark, C.E. Early outcomes of fluorescence angiography in the setting of endorectal mucosa advancement flaps. *Tech. Coloproctol.* **2018**, *22*, 25–30. [CrossRef] [PubMed]
26. Joosten, J.J.; Reijntjes, M.A.; Slooter, M.D.; Duijvestein, M.; Buskens, C.J.; Bemelman, W.A.; Hompes, R. Fluorescence angiography after vascular ligation to make the ileo-anal pouch reach. *Tech. Coloproctol.* **2021**, *25*, 875–878. [CrossRef] [PubMed]
27. Freund, M.R.; Kent, I.; Agarwal, S.; Wexner, S.D. Use of indocyanine green fluorescence angiography during ileal J-pouch surgery requiring lengthening maneuvers. *Tech. Coloproctol.* **2022**, *26*, 181–186. [CrossRef]
28. Slooter, M.D.; van der Does de Willebois, E.M.L.; Joosten, J.J.; Reijntjes, M.A.; Buskens, C.J.; Tanis, P.J.; Bemelman, W.A.; Hompes, R. Fluorescence Perfusion Assessment of Vascular Ligation during Ileal Pouch-Anal Anastomosis. *Tech. Coloproctol.* **2022**; *ahead of print*. [CrossRef]
29. Lobbes, L.A.; Hoveling, R.J.M.; Berns, S.; Schmidt, L.R.; Strobel, R.M.; Schineis, C.; Lauscher, J.C.; Beyer, K.; Weixler, B. Feasibility of Novel Software-Based Perfusion Indicators for the Ileal J-Pouch-On the Path towards Objective and Quantifiable Intraoperative Perfusion Assessment with Indocyanine Green Near-Infrared Fluorescence. *Life* **2022**, *12*, 1144. [CrossRef]
30. Kanabur, P.; Chai, C.; Taylor, J. Use of indocyanine green for intraoperative ureteral identification in nonurologic surgery. *JAMA Surg.* **2020**, *155*, 520–521. [CrossRef]
31. White, L.A.; Joseph, J.P.; Yang, D.Y.; Kelley, S.R.; Mathis, K.L.; Behm, K.; Viers, B.R. Intraureteral indocyanine green augments ureteral identification and avoidance during complex robotic-assisted colorectal surgery. *Color. Dis.* **2021**, *23*, 718–723. [CrossRef]
32. Hamada, M.; Matsumi, Y.; Sekimoto, M.; Kurokawa, H.; Kita, M.; Kinoshita, H. Image navigation surgery with the fluorescent ureteral catheter of recurrent tumors in the pelvic cavity. *Dis. Colon Rectum* **2022**, *65*, e72–e76. [CrossRef] [PubMed]
33. Mandovra, P.; Kalikar, V.; Patankar, R.V. Real-time visualization of ureters using indocyanine green during laparoscopic surgeries: Can we make surgery safer? *Surg. Innov.* **2019**, *26*, 464–468. [CrossRef] [PubMed]
34. Ryu, S.; Hara, K.; Kitagawa, T.; Okamoto, A.; Marukuchi, R.; Ito, R.; Nakabayashi, Y. Fluorescence vessel and ureter navigation during laparoscopic lateral lymph node dissection. *Langenbeck's Arch. Surg.* **2022**, *407*, 305–312. [CrossRef] [PubMed]
35. Satish, V.N.V.R.; Acharya, A.; Ramachandran, S.; Narasimhan, M.; Ardhanari, R. Fluorescent ureterography with indocyanine green in laparoscopic colorectal surgery: A safe method to prevent intraoperative ureteric injury. *J. Minim. Access Surg.* **2022**, *18*, 320–323.
36. Soriano, C.R.; Cheng, R.R.; Corman, J.M.; Moonka, R.; Simianu, V.V.; Kaplan, J.A. Feasibility of injected indocyanine green for ureteral identification during robotic left-sided colorectal resections. *Am. J. Surg.* **2022**, *223*, 14–20. [CrossRef]
37. Garoufalia, Z.; Wexner, S.D. Ureter identification utilizing indocyanine green (ICG) imaging in colorectal surgery: A systematic review of the literature. *Mini-Invasive Surg.* **2022**, *6*, 51. [CrossRef]
38. Dip, F.D.; Nahmod, M.; Anzorena, F.S.; Moreira, A.; Sarotto, L.; Ampudia, C.; Kalaskar, S.N.; Ferraina, P.; Rosenthal, R.J.; Wexner, S.D. Novel technique for identification of ureters using sodium fluorescein. *Surg. Endosc.* **2014**, *28*, 2730–2733. [CrossRef]
39. Mahalingam, S.M.; Dip, F.; Castillo, M.; Roy, M.; Wexner, S.D.; Rosenthal, R.J.; Low, P.S. Intraoperative Ureter Visualization Using a Novel Near-Infrared Fluorescent Dye. *Mol. Pharm.* **2018**, *15*, 3442–3447. [CrossRef]
40. Penna, M.; Hompes, R.; Arnold, S.; Wynn, G.; Austin, R.; Warusavitarne, J.; Moran, B.; Hanna, G.B.; Mortensen, N.J.; Tekkis, P.P. Transanal total mesorectal excision: International registry results of the first 720 cases. *Ann. Surg.* **2017**, *266*, 111–117. [CrossRef]
41. Rouanet, P.; Mourregot, A.; Azar, C.C.; Carrere, S.; Gutowski, M.; Quenet, F.; Saint-Aubert, B.; Colombo, P.E. Transanal endoscopic proctectomy: An innovative procedure for difficult resection of rectal tumors in men with narrow pelvis. *Dis. Colon Rectum* **2013**, *56*, 408–415. [CrossRef]
42. Barnes, T.G.; Penna, M.; Hompes, R.; Cunningham, C. Fluorescence to highlight the urethra: A human cadaveric study. *Tech. Coloproctol.* **2017**, *21*, 439–444. [CrossRef] [PubMed]
43. Barnes, T.G.; Volpi, D.; Cunningham, C.; Vojnovic, B.; Hompes, R. Improved urethral fluorescence during low rectal surgery: A new dye and a new method. *Tech. Coloproctol.* **2018**, *22*, 115–119. [CrossRef] [PubMed]
44. Barberio, M.; Al-Taher, M.; Forgione, A.; Hoskere Ashoka, A.; Felli, E.; Agnus, V.; Marescaux, J.; Klymchenko, A.; Diana, M. A novel method for near-infrared fluorescence imaging of the urethra during perineal and transanal surgery: Demonstration in a cadaveric model. *Color. Dis.* **2020**, *22*, 1749–1753. [CrossRef] [PubMed]
45. Nitta, T.; Tanaka, K.; Kataoka, J.; Ohta, M.; Ishii, M.; Ishibashi, T.; Okuda, J. Novel technique with the IRIS U kit to prevent urethral injury in patients undergoing transanal total mesorectal excision. *Ann. Med. Surg.* **2019**, *46*, 1–3. [CrossRef] [PubMed]

46. Jin, H.; Zheng, L.; Lu, L.; Cui, M. Near-infrared intraoperative imaging of pelvic autonomic nerves: A pilot study. *Surg. Endosc.* **2022**, *36*, 2349–2356. [CrossRef] [PubMed]
47. Handgraaf, H.J.; Boogerd, L.S.; Verbeek, F.P.; Tummers, Q.R.; Hardwick, J.C.; Baeten, C.I.; Frangioni, J.V.; van de Velde, C.J.; Vahrmeijer, A.L. Intraoperative fluorescence imaging to localize tumors and sentinel lymph nodes in rectal cancer. *Minim. Invasive Ther. Allied Technol.* **2016**, *25*, 48–53. [CrossRef]
48. Watanabe, M.; Tsunoda, A.; Narita, K.; Kusano, M.; Miwa, M. Colonic tattooing using fluorescence imaging with light-emitting diode-activated indocyanine green: A feasibility study. *Surg. Today* **2009**, *39*, 214–218. [CrossRef]
49. Poris, S.P.; Tanishima, H.; Albert, M.R. Use of intraoperative submucosal tattooing with indocyanine green immunofluorescence angiography for tumor localization during colectomy. *Tech. Coloproctol.* **2017**, *21*, 165–166. [CrossRef]
50. Kim, Y.J.; Park, J.W.; Lim, H.K.; Kwon, Y.H.; Kim, M.J.; Choe, E.K.; Moon, S.H.; Ryoo, S.B.; Jeong, S.Y.; Park, K.J. Preoperative Colonoscopic Tattooing Using a Direct Injection Method with Indocyanine Green for Localization of Colorectal Tumors: An Efficacy and Safety Comparison Study. *J. Minim. Invasive Surg.* **2020**, *23*, 186–190. [CrossRef]
51. Kim, J.H. Small Efforts Can Prevent Big Mistakes: Preoperative Colonoscopic Tattooing Using Indocyanine Green. *J. Minim. Invasive Surg.* **2020**, *23*, 159–160. [CrossRef]
52. Lee, S.J.; Sohn, D.K.; Han, K.S.; Kim, B.C.; Hong, C.W.; Park, S.C.; Kim, M.J.; Park, B.K.; Oh, J.H. Preoperative tattooing using indocyanine green in laparoscopic colorectal surgery. *Ann. Coloproctol.* **2018**, *34*, 206–211. [CrossRef] [PubMed]
53. Atallah, S.; Parra-Davila, E.; Melani, A.G.F.; Romagnolo, L.G.; Larach, S.W.; Marescaux, J. Robotic-assisted stereotactic real-time navigation: Initial clinical experience and feasibility for rectal cancer surgery. *Tech. Coloproctol.* **2019**, *23*, 53–63. [CrossRef] [PubMed]
54. Satoyoshi, T.; Okita, K.; Ishii, M.; Hamabe, A.; Usui, A.; Akizuki, E.; Okuya, K.; Nishidate, T.; Yamano, H.; Nakase, H.; et al. Timing of indocyanine green injection prior to laparoscopic colorectal surgery for tumor localization: A prospective case series. *Surg. Endosc.* **2021**, *35*, 763–769. [CrossRef] [PubMed]
55. Ahn, H.M.; Son, G.M.; Lee, I.Y.; Shin, D.H.; Kim, T.K.; Park, S.B.; Kim, H.W. Optimal ICG dosage of preoperative colonoscopic tattooing for fluorescence-guided laparoscopic colorectal surgery. *Surg. Endosc.* **2022**, *36*, 1152–1163. [CrossRef]
56. Narihiro, S.; Yoshida, M.; Ohdaira, H.; Sato, T.; Suto, D.; Hoshimoto, S.; Suzuki, N.; Marukuchi, R.; Kamada, T.; Takeuchi, H.; et al. Effectiveness and safety of tumor site marking with near-infrared fluorescent clips in colorectal laparoscopic surgery: A case series study. *Int. J. Surg.* **2020**, *80*, 74–78. [CrossRef]
57. Lee, D.W.; Sohn, D.K.; Han, K.S.; Hong, C.W.; Park, H.C.; Oh, J.H. Promising Novel Technique for Tumor Localization in Laparoscopic Colorectal Surgery Using Indocyanine Green-Coated Endoscopic Clips. *Dis. Colon Rectum* **2021**, *64*, e9–e13. [CrossRef]
58. Ryu, S.; Okamoto, A.; Nakashima, K.; Hara, K.; Ishida, K.; Ito, R.; Nakabayashi, Y.; Eto, K.; Ikegami, T. Usefulness of Preoperative Endoscopic Fluorescent Clip Marking in Laparoscopic Gastrointestinal Surgery. *Anticancer Res.* **2020**, *40*, 6517–6523. [CrossRef]
59. Nishigori, N.; Koyama, F.; Nakagawa, T.; Nakamura, S.; Ueda, T.; Inoue, T.; Kawasaki, K.; Obara, S.; Nakamoto, T.; Fujii, H.; et al. Visualization of Lymph/Blood Flow in Laparoscopic Colorectal Cancer Surgery by ICG Fluorescence Imaging (Lap-IGFI). *Ann. Surg. Oncol.* **2016**, *23* (Suppl. S2), 266–274. [CrossRef]
60. Ho, M.F.; Futaba, K.; Mak, T.W.C.; Ng, S.S.M. Personalized laparoscopic resection of colon cancer with the use of indocyanine green lymph node mapping: Technical and clinical outcomes. *Asian J. Endosc. Surg.* **2022**, *15*, 563–568. [CrossRef]
61. Caprioli, M.; Garosio, I.; Botteri, E.; Vettoretto, N.; Molteni, B.; Molfino, S.; Yiu, D.; Portolani, N.; Baiocchi, G.L. Fluorescence-guided nodal navigation during colectomy for colorectal cancer. *Minim. Invasive Ther. Allied Technol.* **2022**, *31*, 879–886. [CrossRef]
62. Soares, A.S.; Lovat, L.B.; Chand, M. Intracorporeal lymph node mapping in colon cancer surgery. *Eur. J. Surg. Oncol.* **2019**, *45*, 2316–2318. [CrossRef] [PubMed]
63. Chand, M.; Keller, D.S.; Joshi, H.M.; Devoto, L.; Rodriguez-Justo, M.; Cohen, R. Feasibility of fluorescence lymph node imaging in colon cancer: FLICC. *Tech. Coloproctol.* **2018**, *22*, 271–277. [CrossRef] [PubMed]
64. Goo, J.J.; Ryu, D.G.; Kim, H.W.; Park, S.B.; Kang, D.H.; Choi, C.W.; Kim, S.J.; Nam, H.S.; Kim, H.S.; Son, G.M.; et al. Efficacy of preoperative colonoscopic tattooing with indocyanine green on lymph node harvest and factors associated with inadequate lymph node harvest in colorectal cancer. *Scand. J. Gastroenterol.* **2019**, *54*, 666–672. [CrossRef] [PubMed]
65. Kakizoe, M.; Watanabe, J.; Suwa, Y.; Nakagawa, K.; Suwa, H.; Ozawa, M.; Ishibe, A.; Masui, H.; Nagahori, K. The histopathological evaluation based on the indocyanine green fluorescence imaging of regional lymph node metastasis of splenic flexural colon cancer by near-infrared observation. *Int. J. Colorectal Dis.* **2021**, *36*, 717–723. [CrossRef]
66. Ushijima, H.; Kawamura, J.; Ueda, K.; Yane, Y.; Yoshioka, Y.; Daito, K.; Tokoro, T.; Hida, J.I.; Okuno, K. Visualization of lymphatic flow in laparoscopic colon cancer surgery using indocyanine green fluorescence imaging. *Sci. Rep.* **2020**, *10*, 14274. [CrossRef]
67. Young, R.; Rajkomar, A.K.S.; Smart, P.; Warrier, S.K. Robotic complete mesocolic excision using indocyanine fluorescence imaging in colorectal cancer: A case study and technical approach. *Int. J. Surg. Case Rep.* **2020**, *69*, 32–34. [CrossRef]
68. Petz, W.; Bertani, E.; Borin, S.; Fiori, G.; Ribero, D.; Spinoglio, G. Fluorescence-guided D3 lymphadenectomy in robotic right colectomy with complete mesocolic excision. *Int. J. Med. Robot.* **2021**, *17*, e2217. [CrossRef]
69. Spinoglio, G.; Petz, W.; Borin, S.; Piccioli, A.N.; Bertani, E. Robotic right colectomy with complete mesocolic excision and indocyanine green guidance. *Minerva Chir.* **2019**, *74*, 165–169. [CrossRef]
70. Trujillo-Díaz, J.J.; Pérez-Corbal, L.; Alarcón Del Agua, I.; Licardie Bolaños, E.; Senent Boza, A.; Morales-Conde, S. Complete mesocolon excision guided by indocyanine green for right colonic cancer. *Color. Dis.* **2021**, *23*, 2779–2780. [CrossRef]

71. Park, S.Y.; Park, J.S.; Kim, H.J.; Woo, I.T.; Park, I.K.; Choi, G.S. Indocyanine Green Fluorescence Imaging-Guided Laparoscopic Surgery Could Achieve Radical D3 Dissection in Patients with Advanced Right-Sided Colon Cancer. *Dis. Colon Rectum* **2020**, *63*, 441–449. [CrossRef]
72. Ribero, D.; Mento, F.; Sega, V.; Lo Conte, D.; Mellano, A.; Spinoglio, G. ICG-Guided Lymphadenectomy during Surgery for Colon and Rectal Cancer-Interim Analysis of the GREENLIGHT Trial. *Biomedicines* **2022**, *10*, 541. [CrossRef]
73. van der Pas, M.H.; Meijer, S.; Hoekstra, O.S.; Riphagen, I.I.; de Vet, H.C.; Knol, D.L.; van Grieken, N.C.; Meijerink, W.J. Sentinel-lymph-node procedure in colon and rectal cancer: A systematic review and meta-analysis. *Lancet Oncol.* **2011**, *12*, 540–550. [CrossRef]
74. Gould, E.A.; Winship, T.; Philbin, P.H.; Kerr, H.H. Observations on a "sentinel node" in cancer of the parotid. *Cancer* **1960**, *13*, 77–78. [CrossRef] [PubMed]
75. Andersen, H.S.; Bennedsen, A.L.B.; Burgdorf, S.K.; Eriksen, J.R.; Eiholm, S.; Toxværd, A.; Riis, L.B.; Rosenberg, J.; Gögenur, I. In vivo and ex vivo sentinel node mapping does not identify the same lymph nodes in colon cancer. *Int. J. Colorectal Dis.* **2017**, *32*, 983–990. [CrossRef] [PubMed]
76. Cahill, R.A.; Anderson, M.; Wang, L.M.; Lindsey, I.; Cunningham, C.; Mortensen, N.J. Near-infrared (NIR) laparoscopy for intraoperative lymphatic road-mapping and sentinel node identification during definitive surgical resection of early-stage colorectal neoplasia. *Surg. Endosc.* **2012**, *26*, 197–204. [CrossRef] [PubMed]
77. Currie, A.C.; Brigic, A.; Thomas-Gibson, S.; Suzuki, N.; Moorghen, M.; Jenkins, J.T.; Faiz, O.D.; Kennedy, R.H. A pilot study to assess near infrared laparoscopy with indocyanine green (ICG) for intraoperative sentinel lymph node mapping in early colon cancer. *Eur. J. Surg. Oncol.* **2017**, *43*, 2044–2051. [CrossRef]
78. Hirche, C.; Mohr, Z.; Kneif, S.; Doniga, S.; Murawa, D.; Strik, M.; Hünerbein, M. Ultrastaging of colon cancer by sentinel node biopsy using fluorescence navigation with indocyanine green. *Int. J. Colorectal Dis.* **2012**, *27*, 319–324. [CrossRef]
79. Kusano, M.; Tajima, Y.; Yamazaki, K.; Kato, M.; Watanabe, M.; Miwa, M. Sentinel node mapping guided by indocyanine green fluorescence imaging: A new method for sentinel node navigation surgery in gastrointestinal cancer. *Dig. Surg.* **2008**, *25*, 103–108. [CrossRef]
80. Liberale, G.; Galdon, M.G.; Moreau, M.; Vankerckhove, S.; El Nakadi, I.; Larsimont, D.; Donckier, V.; Bourgeois, P. Ex vivo detection of tumoral lymph nodes of colorectal origin with fluorescence imaging after intraoperative intravenous injection of indocyanine green. *J. Surg. Oncol.* **2016**, *114*, 348–353. [CrossRef]
81. Liberale, G.; Vankerckhove, S.; Galdon, M.G.; Larsimont, D.; Ahmed, B.; Bouazza, F.; Moreau, M.; El Nakadi, I.; Donckier, V.; Bourgeois, P.; et al. Sentinel Lymph Node Detection by Blue Dye versus Indocyanine Green Fluorescence Imaging in Colon Cancer. *Anticancer Res.* **2016**, *36*, 4853–4858. [CrossRef]
82. Noura, S.; Ohue, M.; Seki, Y.; Tanaka, K.; Motoori, M.; Kishi, K.; Miyashiro, I.; Ohigashi, H.; Yano, M.; Ishikawa, O.; et al. Feasibility of a lateral region sentinel node biopsy of lower rectal cancer guided by indocyanine green using a near-infrared camera system. *Ann. Surg. Oncol.* **2010**, *17*, 144–151. [CrossRef] [PubMed]
83. Weixler, B.; Rickenbacher, A.; Raptis, D.A.; Viehl, C.T.; Guller, U.; Rueff, J.; Zettl, A.; Zuber, M. Sentinel Lymph Node Mapping with Isosulfan Blue or Indocyanine Green in Colon Cancer Shows Comparable Results and Identifies Patients with Decreased Survival: A Prospective Single-Center Trial. *World J. Surg.* **2017**, *41*, 2378–2386. [CrossRef] [PubMed]
84. Emile, S.H.; Elfeki, H.; Shalaby, M.; Sakr, A.; Sileri, P.; Laurberg, S.; Wexner, S.D. Sensitivity and specificity of indocyanine green near-infrared fluorescence imaging in detection of metastatic lymph nodes in colorectal cancer: Systematic review and meta-analysis. *J. Surg. Oncol.* **2017**, *116*, 730–740. [CrossRef] [PubMed]
85. Villegas-Tovar, E.; Jimenez-Lillo, J.; Jimenez-Valerio, V.; Diaz-Giron-Gidi, A.; Faes-Petersen, R.; Otero-Piñeiro, A.; De Lacy, F.B.; Martinez-Portilla, R.J.; Lacy, A.M. Performance of Indocyanine green for sentinel lymph node mapping and lymph node metastasis in colorectal cancer: A diagnostic test accuracy meta-analysis. *Surg. Endosc.* **2020**, *34*, 1035–1047. [CrossRef]
86. Burghgraef, T.A.; Zweep, A.L.; Sikkenk, D.J.; van der Pas, M.H.G.M.; Verheijen, P.M.; Consten, E.C.J. In vivo sentinel lymph node identification using fluorescent tracer imaging in colon cancer: A systematic review and meta-analysis. *Crit. Rev. Oncol. Hematol.* **2021**, *158*, 103149. [CrossRef]
87. Picchetto, A.; Diana, M.; Swanström, L.L.; Magliocca, F.M.; Pronio, A.; Choppin, E.; Rocca, S.; Marescaux, J.; D'Ambrosio, G. Upstaging nodal status in colorectal cancer using ex vivo fluorescence sentinel lymph node mapping: Preliminary results. *Minim. Invasive Ther. Allied Technol.* **2022**, *31*, 223–229. [CrossRef]
88. Kroon, H.M.; Hoogervorst, L.A.; Hanna-Rivero, N.; Traeger, L.; Dudi-Venkata, N.N.; Bedrikovetski, S.; Kusters, M.; Chang, G.J.; Thomas, M.L.; Sammour, T. Systematic review and meta-analysis of long-term oncological outcomes of lateral lymph node dissection for metastatic nodes after neoadjuvant chemoradiotherapy in rectal cancer. *Eur. J. Surg. Oncol.* **2022**, *48*, 1475–1482. [CrossRef]
89. Emile, S.H.; Elfeki, H.; Shalaby, M.; Sakr, A.; Kim, N.K. Outcome of lateral pelvic lymph node dissection with total mesorectal excision in treatment of rectal cancer: A systematic review and meta-analysis. *Surgery* **2021**, *169*, 1005–1015. [CrossRef]
90. Zhou, S.C.; Tian, Y.T.; Wang, X.W.; Zhao, C.D.; Ma, S.; Jiang, J.; Li, E.N.; Zhou, H.T.; Liu, Q.; Liang, J.W.; et al. Application of indocyanine green-enhanced near-infrared fluorescence-guided imaging in laparoscopic lateral pelvic lymph node dissection for middle-low rectal cancer. *World J. Gastroenterol.* **2019**, *25*, 4502–4511. [CrossRef]

91. Dai, J.Y.; Han, Z.J.; Wang, J.D.; Liu, B.S.; Liu, J.Y.; Wang, Y.C. Short-term outcomes of near-infrared imaging using indocyanine green in laparoscopic lateral pelvic lymph node dissection for middle-lower rectal cancer: A propensity score-matched cohort analysis. *Front. Med.* **2022**, *9*, 1039928. [CrossRef]
92. Kawada, K.; Yoshitomi, M.; Inamoto, S.; Sakai, Y. Indocyanine Green Fluorescence-Guided Laparoscopic Lateral Lymph Node Dissection for Rectal Cancer. *Dis. Colon Rectum* **2019**, *62*, 1401. [CrossRef] [PubMed]
93. Yasui, M.; Ohue, M.; Noura, S.; Miyoshi, N.; Takahashi, Y.; Matsuda, C.; Nishimura, J.; Haraguchi, N.; Ushigome, H.; Nakai, N.; et al. Exploratory analysis of lateral pelvic sentinel lymph node status for optimal management of laparoscopic lateral lymph node dissection in advanced lower rectal cancer without suspected lateral lymph node metastasis. *BMC Cancer* **2021**, *21*, 911. [CrossRef] [PubMed]
94. Ohya, H.; Watanabe, J.; Suwa, H.; Suwa, Y.; Ozawa, M.; Ishibe, A.; Kunisaki, C.; Endo, I. Near-Infrared Imaging Using Indocyanine Green for Laparoscopic Lateral Pelvic Lymph Node Dissection for Clinical Stage II/III Middle-Lower Rectal Cancer: A Propensity Score-Matched Cohort Study. *Dis. Colon Rectum* **2022**, *65*, 885–893. [CrossRef]
95. Kazanowski, M.; Al Furajii, H.; Cahill, R.A. Near-infrared laparoscopic fluorescence for pelvic side wall delta mapping in patients with rectal cancer—'PINPOINT' nodal assessment. *Colorectal Dis.* **2015**, *17* (Suppl. S3), 32–35. [CrossRef] [PubMed]
96. Kim, H.J.; Choi, G.S.; Park, J.S.; Park, S.Y.; Cho, S.H.; Seo, A.N.; Yoon, G.S. S122: Impact of fluorescence and 3D images to completeness of lateral pelvic node dissection. *Surg. Endosc.* **2020**, *34*, 469–476. [CrossRef] [PubMed]
97. Liberale, G.; Vankerckhove, S.; Caldon, M.G.; Ahmed, B.; Moreau, M.; Nakadi, I.E.; Larsimont, D.; Donckier, V.; Bourgeois, P.; Group R & D for the Clinical Application of Fluorescence Imaging of the Jules Bordet's Institute. Fluorescence Imaging after Indocyanine Green Injection for Detection of Peritoneal Metastases in Patients Undergoing Cytoreductive Surgery for Peritoneal Carcinomatosis from Colorectal Cancer: A Pilot Study. *Ann. Surg.* **2016**, *264*, 1110–1115. [CrossRef]
98. Baiocchi, G.L.; Gheza, F.; Molfino, S.; Arru, L.; Vaira, M.; Giacopuzzi, S. Indocyanine green fluorescence-guided intraoperative detection of peritoneal carcinomatosis: Systematic review. *BMC Surg.* **2020**, *20*, 158. [CrossRef]
99. Barabino, G.; Klein, J.P.; Porcheron, J.; Grichine, A.; Coll, J.L.; Cottier, M. Intraoperative near-infrared fluorescence imaging using indocyanine green in colorectal carcinomatosis surgery: Proof of concept. *Eur. J. Surg. Oncol.* **2016**, *42*, 1931–1937. [CrossRef]
100. Lieto, E.; Auricchio, A.; Cardella, F.; Mabilia, A.; Basile, N.; Castellano, P.; Orditura, M.; Galizia, G. Fluorescence-guided surgery in the combined treatment of peritoneal Carcinomatosis from colorectal Cancer: Preliminary results and considerations. *World J. Surg.* **2018**, *42*, 1154–1160. [CrossRef]
101. González-Abós, C.; Selva, A.B.; de Lacy, F.B.; Valverde, S.; Almenara, R.; Lacy, A.M. Quantitative Indocyanine Green Fluorescence Imaging Assessment for Nonmucinous Peritoneal Metastases: Preliminary Results of the ICCP Study. *Dis. Colon Rectum* **2022**, *65*, 314–321. [CrossRef]
102. Piccolo, G.; Barabino, M.; Pesce, A.; Diana, M.; Lecchi, F.; Santambrogio, R.; Opocher, E.; Bianchi, P.P.; Piozzi, G.N. Role of Indocyanine Green Fluorescence Imaging in Minimally Invasive Resection of Colorectal Liver Metastases. *Surg. Laparosc. Endosc. Percutan Tech.* **2022**, *32*, 259–265. [CrossRef] [PubMed]
103. Piccolo, G.; Barabino, M.; Diana, M.; Lo Menzo, E.; Epifani, A.G.; Lecchi, F.; Santambrogio, R.; Opocher, E. Application of Indocyanine Green Fluorescence as an Adjuvant to Laparoscopic Ultrasound in Minimally Invasive Liver Resection. *J. Laparoendosc. Adv. Surg. Tech. A* **2021**, *31*, 517–523. [CrossRef] [PubMed]
104. Patel, I.; Bartlett, D.; Dasari, B.V.; Chatzizacharias, N.; Isaac, J.; Marudanayagam, R.; Mirza, D.F.; Roberts, J.K.; Sutcliffe, R.P. Detection of Colorectal Liver Metastases Using Near-Infrared Fluorescence Imaging during Hepatectomy: Prospective Single Centre UK Study. *J. Gastrointest. Cancer*, 2022; ahead of print. [CrossRef] [PubMed]
105. He, K.; Hong, X.; Chi, C.; Cai, C.; An, Y.; Li, P.; Liu, X.; Shan, H.; Tian, J.; Li, J. Efficacy of Near-Infrared Fluorescence-Guided Hepatectomy for the Detection of Colorectal Liver Metastases: A Randomized Controlled Trial. *J. Am. Coll. Surg.* **2022**, *234*, 130–137. [CrossRef] [PubMed]
106. Nishino, H.; Turner, M.A.; Amirfakhri, S.; Hollandsworth, H.M.; Lwin, T.M.; Hosseini, M.; Framery, B.; Cailler, F.; Pèlegrin, A.; Hoffman, R.M.; et al. Proof of concept of improved fluorescence-guided surgery of colon cancer liver metastasis using color-coded imaging of a tumor-labeling fluorescent antibody and indocyanine green restricted to the adjacent liver segment. *Surgery* **2022**, *172*, 1156–1163. [CrossRef]
107. Fretland, A.A.; Dagenborg, V.J.; Bjornelv, G.M.W.; Kazaryan, A.M.; Kristiansen, R.; Fagerland, M.W.; Hausken, J.; Tønnessen, T.I.; Abildgaard, A.; Barkhatov, L.; et al. Laparoscopic versus Open Resection for Colorectal Liver Metastases: The OSLO-COMET Randomized Controlled Trial. *Ann. Surg.* **2018**, *267*, 199–207. [CrossRef]
108. Wexner, S.; Abu-Gazala, M.; Boni, L.; Buxey, K.; Cahill, R.; Carus, T.; Chadi, S.; Chand, M.; Cunningham, C.; Emile, S.H.; et al. Use of fluorescence imaging and indocyanine green during colorectal surgery: Results of an intercontinental Delphi survey. *Surgery* **2022**, *172*, S38–S45. [CrossRef] [PubMed]
109. Dip, F.; Menzo, E.L.; Bouvet, M.; Schols, R.M.; Sherwinter, D.; Wexner, S.D.; White, K.P.; Rosenthal, R.J. Intraoperative fluorescence imaging in different surgical fields: Consensus among 140 intercontinental experts. *Surgery* **2022**, *172*, S54–S59. [CrossRef]

110. Park, S.H.; Park, H.M.; Baek, K.R.; Ahn, H.M.; Lee, I.Y.; Son, G.M. Artificial intelligence based real-time microcirculation analysis system for laparoscopic colorectal surgery. *World J. Gastroenterol.* **2020**, *26*, 6945–6962. [CrossRef] [PubMed]
111. Seeliger, B.; Agnus, V.; Mascagni, P.; Barberio, M.; Longo, F.; Lapergola, A.; Mutter, D.; Klymchenko, A.S.; Chand, M.; Marescaux, J.; et al. Simultaneous computer-assisted assessment of mucosal and serosal perfusion in a model of segmental colonic ischemia. *Surg. Endosc.* **2020**, *34*, 4818–4827. [CrossRef]

Disclaimer/Publisher's Note: The statements, opinions and data contained in all publications are solely those of the individual author(s) and contributor(s) and not of MDPI and/or the editor(s). MDPI and/or the editor(s) disclaim responsibility for any injury to people or property resulting from any ideas, methods, instructions or products referred to in the content.

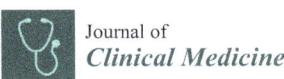 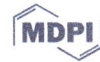

Article

New Perianal Sepsis Risk Score Predicts Outcome of Elderly Patients with Perianal Abscesses

Martin Reichert [1,2,*], Lukas Eckerth [1], Moritz Fritzenwanker [2,3], Can Imirzalioglu [2,3], Anca-Laura Amati [1,2], Ingolf Askevold [1], Winfried Padberg [1], Andreas Hecker [1,2], Juliane Liese [1,†] and Fabienne Bender [1,†]

1 Department of General, Visceral, Thoracic, Transplant and Pediatric Surgery, University Hospital of Giessen, Rudolf-Buchheim Strasse 7, 35390 Giessen, Germany; l.eckerth@web.de (L.E.); anca-laura.amati@chiru.med.uni-giessen.de (A.-L.A.); ingolf.askevold@chiru.med.uni-giessen.de (I.A.); winfried.padberg@chiru.med.uni-giessen.de (W.P.); andreas.hecker@chiru.med.uni-giessen.de (A.H.); juliane.liese@chiru.med.uni-giessen.de (J.L.); fabienne.bender@chiru.med.uni-giessen.de (F.B.)
2 German Center for Infection Research (DZIF), Site Giessen-Marburg-Langen, Justus-Liebig-University of Giessen, Schubertstrasse 81, 35392 Giessen, Germany; moritz.fritzenwanker@uk-gm.de (M.F.); can.imirzalioglu@mikrobio.med.uni-giessen.de (C.I.)
3 Institute of Medical Microbiology, Justus-Liebig-University of Giessen, Schubertstrasse 81, 35392 Giessen, Germany
* Correspondence: martin.reichert@chiru.med.uni-giessen.de; Tel.: +49-641-985-44701; Fax: +49-641-985-44709
† These authors contributed equally to this work.

Abstract: Antibiotic therapy following surgical perianal abscess drainage is debated, but may be necessary for high-risk patients. Frailty has been shown to increase the risk of unfavorable outcomes in elderly surgical patients. This study aims to identify high-risk patients by retrospectively analyzing a single-center cohort and using a pretherapeutic score to predict the need for postoperative antibiotics and extended nursing care following perianal abscess drainage surgery. The perianal sepsis risk score was developed through univariable and multivariable analysis. Internal validation was assessed using the area under receiver-operating characteristic curve. Elderly, especially frail patients exhibited more severe perianal disease, higher frequency of antibiotic therapy, longer hospitalization, poorer clinical outcomes. Multivariable analysis revealed that scores in the 5-item modified frailty index, severity of local infection, and preoperative laboratory markers of infection independently predicted the need for prolonged hospitalization and anti-infective therapy after abscess drainage surgery. These factors were combined into the perianal sepsis risk score, which demonstrated better predictive accuracy for prolonged hospitalization and antibiotic therapy compared with chronological age or frailty status alone. Geriatric assessments are becoming increasingly important in clinical practice. The perianal sepsis risk score identifies high-risk patients before surgery, enabling early initiation of antibiotic therapy and allocation of additional nursing resources.

Keywords: perianal abscess; sepsis; microbiome; elderly; frailty; fistula; emergency surgery; hospital resources

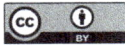

1. Introduction

Perianal abscesses are common diseases in general surgery that require urgent therapy [1]. While simple skin abscesses are usually caused by Staphylococci or Streptococci [2–4], the bacteriology, etiology and treatment principles of perianal abscesses are more complex [1]. Perianal abscesses are frequently complicated by fistula-in-ano due to their cryptoglandular origin, which depends on their location [5–9]. Hence, the treatment principles of perianal abscesses are drainage of purulence followed by exploration of potential fistula-in-ano with the consecutive drainage of the fistula, if present, in the emergency setting [6–9]. The microbiome present in purulence from perianal abscesses is diverse, but specific types of microbiota may indicate certain conditions. For example, the enteric microbiome is predominantly found in abscesses accompanied by fistula-in-ano [1]. Furthermore, certain pre-existing conditions in patients like chronic inflammatory bowel diseases or diabetes can be expected to result in distinct bacteriology [1,10–12]. As we have recently shown, the complexity and severity of perianal abscesses including the severity of perineal sepsis are mainly determined by two important factors: the microbial pattern and their acquired drug resistances [1]. While it is still a matter of debate, if antibiotic therapy should be necessary routinely after surgical abscess drainage, it is generally considered appropriate for patients at high risk of extensive perianal infection and consequently poor outcomes [1,13–16]. Nevertheless, the criteria for postoperative antimicrobial therapy have not been adequately defined.

It is known from other formally trivial diseases in general surgery, that elderly patients are at higher risk for experiencing a more severe and complicated course [17]. However, it is less the chronologic age than the multidimensional frailty syndrome, which dramatically increases the risk for poor outcome and consecutively for additional resource utilization after various elective and urgent surgical interventions [17–22]. This is currently unknown for patients with perianal abscesses, thus further research is needed to investigate this relevant issue in more detail. Frailty can simply be measured by the multidimensional modified frailty index (mFi), which shows high predictive values for poor outcome after emergency surgery in elderly patients [17].

The aim of this study was to identify high-risk patients with perianal abscesses who urgently required prolonged nursing resources and additional anti-infective therapy following surgical drainage. Therefore, the study analyzed the relevant risk factors for worse patient outcome and focused on the impact of either older age or frailty on the outcomes of patients with perianal abscesses. This enabled the development of a scoring system which can identify these high-risk patients on admission to the emergency department. With a reliable assessment, the score predicts the need for perioperative antibiotic therapy and additional nursing resources after surgery.

2. Materials and Methods

This exploratory, retrospective single-center cohort study was performed in accordance with the latest version of the Declaration of Helsinki and was approved by the local ethics committee of the medical faculty of the University of Giessen (approval No. 66/19). All patients were treated according to the institutional standard-of-care.

From January 2008 to December 2019, all patients (≥ 12 y of age), who underwent surgical treatment at the University Hospital of Giessen for perianal abscess (i.e., surgical abscess drainage or local abscess excision both with exploration for an accompanying perianal fistula-in-ano and, if present, primary excision or drainage of the fistula) as well as for extended surgical tissue excision for advanced perianal/perineal soft tissue infection originated from perianal abscesses were included in this study.

Patient data were obtained from the prospectively maintained institutional database. Retrospective availability of presented data was >97%. The present work focused on the preoperative frailty status of patients who underwent surgery for perianal abscess. Frailty was assessed independently by two authors of the study in patients ≥ 60 y of age by using the 5-item and 11-item modified frailty index (mFi-5, mFi-11) [23,24]. Discrepancies were resolved by a third party. Two or more points in mFi-5 and/or ≥ 3 points in mFi-11 indicated frailty.

C-reactive protein (CRP) values and white blood cell counts (WBC) in peripheral blood were obtained from clinical routine data to assess the extent of systemic inflammation due to perineal infection or sepsis in patients with perianal abscesses. The rates of antibiotic therapy and re-do surgery after the index operation were used to assess the complexity of the disease. Length of hospital stay after index abscess drainage surgery as well as duration until definitive fistula repair or lost in follow-up rate were used as the surrogate parameters for short- as well as long-term outcome, respectively.

Two experienced microbiologists independently reviewed the results of the bacterial cultures and susceptibility tests of swabs obtained from the purulence of perianal abscesses during surgery. The review included assessment of drug resistance of the identified microorganisms based on EUCAST (The European Committee on Antimicrobial Susceptibility Testing) breakpoint tables for interpretation of minimum inhibitory concentrations and zone diameters, v11.0, 2021, as well as intrinsic resistance and unusual phenotypes, v3.2, 2020 (http://www.eucast.org), with focus on acquired drug resistances as described previously [1]. Furthermore, detected isolates were classified according to the ESKAPE definition, which includes highly virulent and frequently drug-resistant pathogens [25].

2.1. Surgery and Perioperative Care

The institutional treatment strategies adhere to the German guidelines for anal abscess and cryptoglandular fistula [9]. The standard treatments include emergency surgical drainage or excision of the abscess, followed by careful exploration of the fistula during the index surgery. Primary fistulectomy is typically performed during index surgery for superficial fistulas. In cases of unclear findings or complex fistulas, a temporary loose seton is placed during the index surgery for drainage of the fistula. Fistula repair is then performed after 4–6 weeks, once the infectious situation has been resolved. Surgeons have the discretion to obtain swabs from purulence during abscess-drainage surgery. Thus, swabs are routinely taken from purulence and infected tissue in cases of more severe and complicated perianal disease with extended soft tissue involvement. However, in cases of milder and uncomplicated disease, swabs are not routinely obtained.

Antibiotic therapy is not routinely administered after surgery. Indications for postoperative antibiotic therapy include complicated perianal infection and situations with perianal as well as perineal sepsis with locally advanced phlegmonous or gangrenous soft tissue infection. Postoperatively, patients self-rinse the perianal wounds and are discharged as soon as possible on postoperative day one or two.

2.2. Statistical Analyses

The patient cohort was divided into two groups according to age at time of surgery: <60 y and ≥60 y. Subsequently, patients with an age of ≥60 y were subdivided regarding their frailty status to assess the impact of frailty on perioperative patient outcome.

Statistical analyses were performed using GraphPad Prism (Version 9 for Windows, GraphPad Software, San Diego, CA, USA; www.graphpad.com). Two-group comparisons were performed using Fisher's exact test for categorical data and unpaired, two-tailed Student's t-test for continuous variables. Data are given in n (%) or mean ± standard deviation, respectively. If applicable, odds ratios (OR) were calculated using the Baptista–Pike method.

In cases of fistula-in-ano found during index surgery, the duration until definitive fistula repair was calculated by Kaplan–Meier estimation. Patients with an initial drainage of the fistula during index surgery, but were lost in follow-up were censored from this analysis upon the last contact. This is indicated in the Kaplan–Meier curves by vertical ticks. Log rank test was used for Kaplan–Meier curve comparisons.

Spearman's rho rank correlation was used to determine statistical dependencies between age, frailty, bacteriology and outcome. Results are given as the Spearman's rank correlation coefficient (r^{SP}) and respective significances. Heatmaps display correlation coefficients between the variables.

p-Values ≤ 0.05 indicate statistical significance. Because of the exploratory character of the study, no adjustments of p-values were performed.

Simple linear regression and multiple linear regression were used for univariable and multivariable analyses, respectively, to evaluate relevant parameters that impact on the outcomes "postoperative antibiotic therapy" and "prolonged length of postoperative hospital stay". Variables with p-values ≤ 0.01 in univariable regression were included in the multivariable analysis. Variables with significance in multiple regression analysis, were included in the perianal sepsis risk score. Areas under the receiver-operating characteristic (ROC) curves were used to estimate the ability of the score, age or frailty alone in predicting the need for postoperative antibiotic therapy or prolonged postoperative hospitalization.

To define prolonged hospitalization, we used a threshold of ≥4 d, which exceeded the mean postoperative length of stay of the entire patient cohort (i.e., 3.2 d). To obtain comparability of the ROC curves, areas under the curves (AUC) were directly compared by the method described by Hanley and McNeil [26].

3. Results

3.1. Patient Characteristics

Overall, 817 patients underwent surgical drainage procedure for perianal abscess during the study period and were included in the data analysis. Of the patients, 693 were younger than 60 y and 124 patients were ≥60 y of age. Older patients suffered more frequently from chronic cardio-pulmonary and metabolic diseases. However, perianal abscesses were rarely associated with chronic inflammatory bowel diseases in the elderly. Although no differences were seen in the rate of fistula-in-ano, perianal disease was more complex in elderly patients, reflected by higher preoperative CRP values, longer operation times as well as higher odds for local severe (gangrenous) tissue infection (OR: 4.281, 95%CI: 1.455–12.680), need for postoperative antibiotic therapy (OR: 1.832, 95%CI: 1.217–2.731) and re-do surgery during short-term follow-up (OR: 2.629, 95%CI: 1.374–4.915). More individuals from the elderly cohort were transferred to the intensive care unit postoperatively and, accordingly, postoperative hospitalization was much longer (Table 1). In this regard, regression analyses reveal discrete linear correlations between patient age, CRP elevation and duration of postoperative hospitalization (Supplementary Figure S1). Nevertheless, no differences were seen in duration until fistula repair nor in overall recurrence rates between younger and older patients (Table 1, Figure 1).

Table 1. Characteristics of patients stratified by age.

Variable	Age < 60 Years n = 693	Age ≥ 60 Years n = 124	p-Value
Female sex, n (%)	190 (27.4%)	20 (16.1%)	0.0074
Age, years ± SD	38.9 ± 11.7	67.8 ± 6.1	-
Body mass index, kg/m^2 ± SD	27.7 ± 7.0	29.2 ± 6.4	0.0246
Diabetes mellitus, n (%)	32 (4.6%)	31 (25.0%)	<0.0001
Active smoking, n (%)	261 (37.7%)	20 (16.2%)	<0.0001
Chronic pulmonary disease, n (%)	43 (6.2%)	19 (15.3%)	0.0013
Coronary artery disease, n (%)	12 (1.7%)	18 (14.5%)	<0.0001
CIBD, n (%)	73 (10.5%)	5 (4.0%)	0.0201
Systemic immunosuppression #, n (%)	32 (4.6%)	10 (8.1%)	0.1211
Duration of surgery, min ± SD	17.33 ± 13.80	22.17 ± 17.81	0.0006
Preoperative laboratory parameters White blood cell count, giga/L ± SD C-reactive protein, mg/L ± SD	11.4 ± 6.1 45.0 ± 61.2	12.1 ± 7.5 77.5 ± 84.4	0.2929 <0.0001
Supralevatoric or pararectal abscess, n (%)	25 (3.6%)	4 (3.2%)	1
Gangrenous infection of surrounding tissue, n (%)	8 (1.2%)	6 (4.8%)	0.0123
Detection of fistula during index surgery, n (%)	426 (61.5%)	80 (64.5%)	0.5481
Primary fistula drainage, n (%) Primary fistulectomy, n (%)	323 (75.8%) 103 (24.2%)	55 (68.8%) 25 (31.3%)	0.2069
Failure to fistula repair in long-term follow-up, n (%)	75 (17.6%)	15 (18.8%)	0.8734
Stool deviation/stoma rate, n (%)	9 (1.3%)	8 (6.5%)	0.0017

Table 1. Cont.

Variable	Age < 60 Years n = 693	Age ≥ 60 Years n = 124	p-Value
Postoperative antibiotic therapy, n (%)	160 (23.1%)	44 (35.5%)	0.0047
Change in antibiotic therapies, n (%)	10 (1.4%)	2 (1.6%)	1
Re-do surgery (short-term follow-up), n (%)	32 (4.6%)	14 (11.3%)	0.0057
Overall recurrency [§], n (%)	138 (19.9%)	19 (15.3%)	0.2661
Postoperative stay at intensive or intermediate care unit, n (%)	12 (1.7%)	9 (7.2%)	0.0019
Duration of postoperative in-hospital stay, d ± SD	2.9 ± 6.6	5.4 ± 10.0	0.0003
30 day mortality, n (%)	1 (0.001%)	1 (0.01%)	0.5889
n patients without intraoperative abscess swab	389 (56.1%)	67 (54.0%)	0.6950
n patients with intraoperative abscess swab	304 (43.9%)	57 (46.0%)	
n patients without germ detection	24 (7.9%)	2 (3.5%)	0.3996
n patients with germ detection	280 (92.1%)	55 (96.5%)	
n patients with polybacterial culture [&]	112 (36.8%)	34 (59.6%)	0.0018
n patients with ESKAPE [$] bacteria	202 (66.4%)	42 (73.7%)	0.3550
n patients with > 1 ESKAPE bacteria	31 (10.2%)	8 (14.0%)	0.3608
n patients with (acquired) drug-resistant germ(s)	177 (58.2%)	43 (75.4%)	0.0175

[#] Including chemotherapy within eight weeks before abscess surgery. [§] Including patients with recurrent perianal abscess in long-term follow-up after index surgery or perianal abscess in the patient's history. [&] Excluding fungi. [$] Although not intended to classify community-acquired infections, the ESKAPE (Enterococcus faecium, Staphylococcus aureus, Klebsiella pneumoniae, Acinetobacter baumanii, Pseudomonas aeruginosa, Enterobacter sp.) definition was used. SD = standard deviation. CIBD = chronic inflammatory bowel disease. CRP = C-reactive protein.

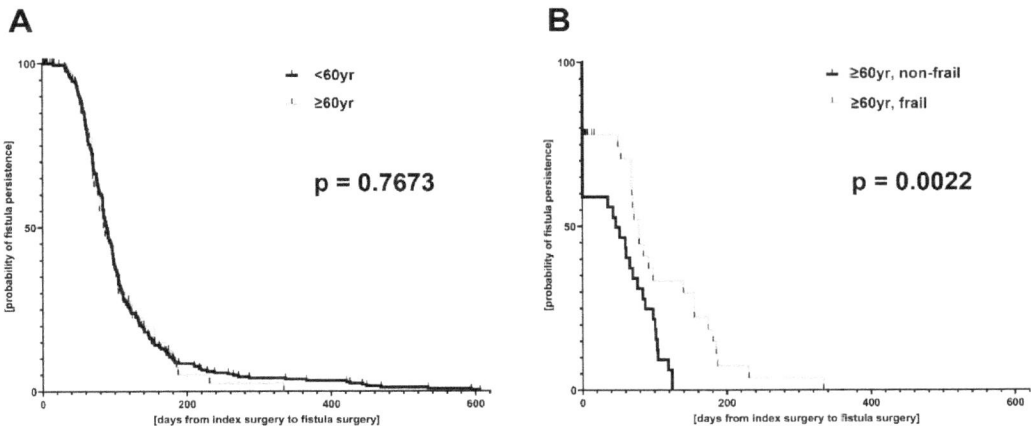

Figure 1. Kaplan–Meier estimation of duration from index surgery to definitive fistula repair. The total patient cohort (A) was stratified by age (<60 y versus ≥60 y of age); (B) the elderly patient cohort (i.e., patients with an age ≥ 60 y) was subdivided regarding their frailty status (frail versus non-frail).

3.2. Impact of Frailty on Patient Outcome

From the older patient cohort, 63 patients were classified as being non-frail and 61 as frail. Group comparisons demonstrated that not chronological age alone but rather frailty impacted perioperative outcome. Frail patients suffered from more complex and severe diseases, indicated by higher preoperative CRP and—by tendency—WBC, longer operation times, higher rates of postoperative antibiotic therapy (OR: 4.690, 95%CI: 2.139–10.19), re-do surgery (OR: 7.469, 95%CI: 1.702–34.33) and stool deviation (OR: 8.037, 95%CI: 1.352–91.80) compared with elderly but non-frail patients. Frailty was accompanied with higher odds for postoperative intensive care (OR: 9.358; 95%CI: 1.327–105.4) and prolonged postoperative hospitalization (Table 2). In this regard, especially, the indices from mFi-5 correlated with preoperative markers of systemic inflammation and length of postoperative hospitalization in linear regression analyses (Supplementary Figure S1).

Table 2. Characteristics of aged patients stratified by frailty status.

Variable	Age ≥ 60 Years Non-Frail n = 63	Age ≥ 60 Years Frail n = 61	p-Value
Female sex, n (%)	13 (20.6%)	7 (11.5%)	0.2230
mFi-5, score ± SD	0.5 ± 0.5	2.4 ± 0.8	-
mFi-11, score ± SD	0.7 ± 0.7	3.1 ± 1.2	-
Duration of surgery, min ± SD	18.4 ± 12.0	26.6 ± 21.8	0.0123
Preoperative laboratory parameters			
White blood cell count, giga/L ± SD	10.9 ± 3.9	13.4 ± 9.9	0.0625
C-reactive protein, mg/L ± SD	58.3 ± 69.6	97.9 ± 94.1	0.0090
Supralevatoric or pararectal abscess, n (%)	2 (3.2%)	2 (3.3%)	1
Gangrenous infection of surrounding tissue, n (%)	0	6 (9.8%)	0.0124
Detection of fistula during index surgery, n (%)	39 (61.9%)	41 (67.2%)	0.5770
Primary fistula drainage, n (%)	23 (59.0%)	32 (78.0%)	0.0915
Primary fistulectomy, n (%)	16 (41.0%)	9 (22.0%)	
Failure to fistula repair in long-term follow-up, n (%)	4 (6.3%)	11 (18.0%)	0.0852
Stool deviation/stoma rate, n (%)	1 (1.6%)	7 (11.5%)	0.0312
Postoperative antibiotic therapy, n (%)	12 (19.0%)	32 (52.5%)	0.0001
Change in antibiotic therapies, n (%)	0	2 (3.3%)	0.2400
Re-do surgery (short-term follow-up), n (%)	2 (3.2%)	12 (19.7%)	0.0042
Overall recurrency [§], n (%)	7 (11.1%)	12 (19.7%)	0.2185
Postoperative stay at intensive or intermediate care unit, n (%)	1 (1.6%)	8 (13.1%)	0.0160
Duration of postoperative in-hospital stay, d ± SD	2.6 ± 2.9	8.4 ± 13.3	0.0009
30 day mortality, n (%)	1 (1.6%)	0	1
n patients without intraoperative abscess swab	41 (65.1%)	26 (42.6%)	0.0188
n patients with intraoperative abscess swab	22 (34.9%)	35 (57.4%)	
n patients without germ detection	0	2 (5.7%)	0.5175
n patients with germ detection	22 (100%)	33 (94.3%)	
n patients with polybacterial culture [&]	14 (63.6%)	20 (57.1%)	0.2287
n patients with ESKAPE [$] bacteria	19 (86.4%)	23 (65.7%)	0.1242
n patients with >1 ESKAPE bacteria	4 (6.3%)	4 (6.6%)	0.6975
n patients with (acquired) drug-resistant germ(s)	16 (72.7%)	27 (77.1%)	0.7584

Two points or more in mFi-5 and/or ≥3 points in mFi-11 indicate frailty. [§] Including patients with recurrent perianal abscess in long-term follow-up after index surgery or perianal abscess in the patient's history. [&] Excluding fungi. [$] Although not intended to classify community-acquired infections, the ESKAPE (*Enterococcus faecium*, *Staphylococcus aureus*, *Klebsiella pneumoniae*, *Acinetobacter baumanii*, *Pseudomonas aeruginosa*, *Enterobacter* sp.) definition was used. CIBD = chronic inflammatory bowel disease. CRP = C-reactive protein.

Although advanced age was not, frailty was a potential risk factor for patients to be lost in follow-up for fistula repair by tendency (OR: 3.208, 95%CI: 0.9410–9.808). Furthermore, the duration until fistula repair was significantly longer in frail patients (Table 2, Figure 1).

3.3. Bacteriology and Correlation Analyses

Correlation analyses basically confirmed the results of the two-group comparisons. Especially the scores in mFi-5 correlated with relevant outcome data including elevation of preoperative CRP (mFi-5: r^{SP} = 0.211, p = 0.020; frailty: r^{SP} = 0.247, p = 0.006, age: r^{SP} = 0.110, p = 0.002), rates of gangrenous tissue infection (mFi-5 r^{SP} = 0.315, p = 0.002; frailty: r^{SP} = 0.232, p = 0.010; age: r^{SP} = 0.100, p = 0.004), postoperative antibiotic therapy (mFi-5: r^{SP} = 0.355, p < 0.0001; frailty: r^{SP} = 0.354, p < 0.0001; age: r^{SP} = 0.122, p = 0.001), stool deviation (mFi-5: r^{SP} = 0.276, p = 0.002; frailty: r^{SP} = 0.205, p = 0.019; age: r^{SP} = 0.126, p < 0.0001.), re-do surgery (mFi-5: r^{SP} = 0.266, p = 0.003; frailty: r^{SP} = 0.265, p = 0.003; age: r^{SP} = 0.065, p = 0.063), intensive care (mFi-5: r^{SP} = 0.254, p = 0.004; frailty: r^{SP} = 0.222, p = 0.013; age: r^{SP} = 0.150, p < 0.0001), duration of postoperative hospital stay (mFi-5: r^{SP} = 0.442, p < 0.0001; frailty: r^{SP} = 0.431, p < 0.0001; age: r^{SP} = 0.174, p < 0.0001) and the rate of patients who were lost in follow-up for fistula repair (mFi-5: r^{SP} = 0.225, p = 0.045; frailty: r^{SP} = 0.212, p = 0.059; age: r^{SP} = −0.080, p = 0.071).

According to the clinical standard [1], overall, 44.2% of the patients received intraoperative swabs from abscesses with a consequent detection of germs in 41.0%. Older age alone but not frailty was associated with higher risk for polybacterial culture. Furthermore, the rate of acquired drug resistances of the detected germs according to EUCAST guidelines was higher in the elderly population. Correlation analyses revealed the detection rate of Streptococcus sp. was higher in elderly patients (mFi-5: r^{SP} = 0.083, p = 0.540; frailty: r^{SP} = −0.004, p = 0.976; age: r^{SP} = 0.117, p = 0.027). The detection rate of E. coli was markedly lower in frail patients; however, age itself did not play a role in that finding (mFi-5: r^{SP} = -0.315, p = 0.017; frailty: r^{SP} = −0.285, p = 0.032; age: r^{SP} = −0.030, p = 0.566). Furthermore, mFi scores but not chronological age correlated by tendency with the finding of Prevotella in perianal abscess swabs (mFi-5: r^{SP} = 0.246, p = 0 068; mFi-11: r^{SP} = 0.237, p = 0.069; age: r^{SP} = 0.002, p = 0.977). No other significant and clinically relevant influences of age or frailty on the specific bacteriology to be expected in perianal abscesses were found in the correlation analyses (Tables 1 and 2, Figure 2).

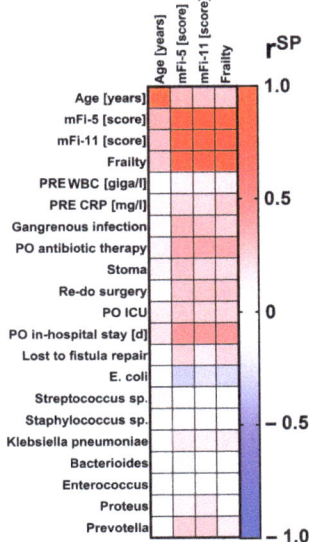

Figure 2. Correlation analysis of chronological age, scores in modified frailty indices or frailty status with relevant perianal disease characteristics. As shown in the legend, the colors code for the Spearman's rank correlation coefficient (r^{SP}). Redder colors indicate the more positive correlation, bluer colors the more negative correlation. mFi-5 = 5-item modified frailty index. mFi-11 = 11-item modified frailty index. PRE = preoperative. WBC = white blood cell count. CRP = C-reactive protein. PO = postoperative. ICU = Intensive Care Unit (including the stay at the intermediate care unit). E. = Escherichia. Sp. = species.

3.4. Score Development and Validation

Data analysis shows that preoperative scores in mFi-5, CRP, WBC and signs of severe local tissue infection are important factors to consider for postoperative antibiotic therapy and longer hospital stay, i.e., a prolonged need for professional nursing resources (Tables 3 and 4).

Table 3. Perioperative determinants for the need for postoperative antibiotic therapy.

Variable	Univariable Analysis		Multivariable Analysis						Included in Score
			Coefficients						
	r^2	p Value	B	Std. Error	95% CI		t	p Value	
Postoperative antibiotic therapy									
Age [years]	0.016	**0.0003**	0.003	0.007	−0.010–0.017		0.489	0.6260	
mFi-5 [score]	0.125	**<0.0001**	0.094	0.038	0.018–0.170		2.461	**0.0154**	Yes
BMI [kg/m^2]	0.000	0.5257	-	-	-		-	-	
WBC [giga/L]	0.015	**0.0005**	0.001	0.006	-0.010–0.012		0.142	0.8872	
CRP [mg/L]	0.176	**<0.0001**	0.002	0.001	0.001–0.004		4.216	**<0.0001**	Yes
Complex abscess [#]	0.000	0.7036	-	-	-		-	-	
Fistula-in-ano	−0.000	0.8681	-	-	-		-	-	
Fistual seton inserted	0.001	0.3714	-	-	-		-	-	
Gangrenous infection [§]	0.043	**<0.0001**	0.065	0.205	−0.340–0.471		0.318	0.7507	
CIBD	0.003	0.1308	-	-	-		-	-	
Immunosuppression	0.016	**0.0004**	−0.095	0.138	−0.368–0.177		0.6926	0.4900	
Acquired drug resistances	0.005	0.1845	-	-	-		-	-	
ESKAPE [&]	0.002	0.4234	-	-	-		-	-	

Perioperative variables that have a significant influence on the need for additional anti-infective therapy in univariable analysis were included in the multivariable regression model. Variables that pass significance in multivariable analysis were included in the new perianal sepsis risk score. [#] i.e., Pararectal or supralevatoric abscess. [§] Gangrenous infection of surrounding tissue. [&] Although not intended to classify community-acquired infections, the ESKAPE (*Enterococcus faecium*, *Staphylococcus aureus*, *Klebsiella pneumoniae*, *Acinetobacter baumanii*, *Pseudomonas aeruginosa*, *Enterobacter* sp.) definition was used. mFi-5 = (preoperative) 5-item modified frailty index. BMI = body mass index. WBC = (preoperative) white blood cell count in peripheral blood. CRP = (preoperative) C-reactive protein value. CIBD = chronic inflammatory bowel disease.

Table 4. Perioperative determinants for prolonged hospital stay, i.e., need for prolonged professional nursing resources.

Variable	Univariable Analysis		Multivariable Analysis						Included in Score
			Coefficients						
	r^2	p Value	B	Std. Error	95% CI		t	p Value	
Length of postoperative in-hospital stay									
Age [years]	0.014	**0.0008**	−0.292	0.191	−0.675–0.091		1.534	0.1317	
mFi-5 [score]	0.144	**<0.0001**	2.714	1.244	0.213–5.216		2.182	**0.0341**	Yes
BMI [kg/m^2]	0.006	0.0238	-	-	-		-	-	
WBC [giga/L]	0.022	**<0.0001**	0.780	0.267	0.243–1.316		2.923	**0.0053**	Yes
CRP [mg/L]	0.123	**<0.0001**	0.032	0.016	−0.001–0.064		1.944	0.0577	Yes
Complex abscess [#]	−0.001	0.5172	-	-	-		-	-	

Table 4. Cont.

Variable	Univariable Analysis		Multivariable Analysis					Included in Score
	r^2	p Value	Coefficients			t	p Value	
			B	Std. Error	95% CI			
Fistula-in-ano	−0.015	**0.0005**	0.151	2.566	−5.008–5.310	0.059	0.9533	
Fistual seton inserted	−0.005	0.0424	-	-	-	-	-	
Gangrenous infection §	0.318	**<0.0001**	17.460	5.281	6.839–28.080	3.306	**0.0018**	Yes
CIBD	0.000	0.9412	-	-	-	-	-	
Immunosuppression	0.003	0.1411	-	-	-	-	-	
Acquired drug resistances	0.023	**0.0037**	3.594	2.860	−2.157–9.345	1.256	0.2150	
ESKAPE &	−0.007	0.1277	-	-	-	-	-	

Perioperative variables that have a significant influence on the length of postoperative in-hospital stay in univariable analysis were included in the multivariable regression model. Variables that pass significance in multivariable analysis were included in the new perianal sepsis risk score. # i.e., Pararectal or supralevatoric abscess. § Gangrenous infection of surrounding tissue. & Although not intended to classify community-acquired infections, the ESKAPE (Enterococcus faecium, Staphylococcus aureus, Klebsiella pneumoniae, Acinetobacter baumanii, Pseudomonas aeruginosa, Enterobacter sp.) definition was used. mFi-5 = (preoperative) 5-item modified frailty index. BMI = body mass index. WBC = (preoperative) white blood cell count in peripheral blood. CRP = (preoperative) C-reactive protein value. CIBD = chronic inflammatory bowel disease.

As a result, mFi-5 score, elevated CRP, abnormal WBC and signs of severe local tissue infection were included in the proposed perianal sepsis risk score (Table 5) for perianal abscesses.

Table 5. Perianal sepsis risk score.

Perianal Sepsis Risk Score [0–9 points]		
Variable	Value	Score
Preoperative **mFi-5** [score]	0	0
	1–5	1–5
Preoperative **C-reactive protein** [mg/L]	0–49	0
	≥50	1
	≥100	2
Preoperative **white blood cell count** [giga/L]	≤4	1
	4–10.9	0
	≥11	1
Local severe surrounding **tissue reaction** *	No	0
	Yes	1

* phlegmonous or gangrenous, surrounding the perianal abscess, assessed preoperatively or intraoperatively.

The preoperative CRP mean value of the entire patient cohort (49.97 mg/l) was used as the cutoff for a positive score, and each doubling of the value was given an extra point. The sepsis guidelines recommended a preoperative WBC threshold of <4 giga/l and ≥11 giga/L [27].

The score was internally validated using ROC analysis in the retrospective patient cohort, demonstrating a significant predictive power for the need for postoperative antibiotic therapy and prolonged in-hospital stay for perianal sepsis following surgical abscess drainage. This was observed in both the total patient cohort and the elderly patient subgroup (all: $p < 0.0001$).

In the direct comparison of AUC by the Hanley and McNeil method [26], the score demonstrated significantly higher predictive values in elderly patients with perianal abscesses compared to the overall patient cohort for both postoperative antibiotic therapy (all patients: AUC = 0.7149 ± 0.0221; 95%CI: 0.6717–0.7582 versus elderly patients: AUC = 0.8518 ± 0.0334; 95%CI: 0.7864–0.9173; $p < 0.0001$) as well as prolonged in-hospital stay (all patients: AUC = 0.7845 ± 0.0246; 95%CI: 0.7364–0.8327 versus elderly patients: AUC = 0.8220 ± 0.0399; 95%CI: 0.7438–0.9001; p = 0.0095). Specifically, the predictive value of the score was superior to either age or frailty assessment alone (Figure 3).

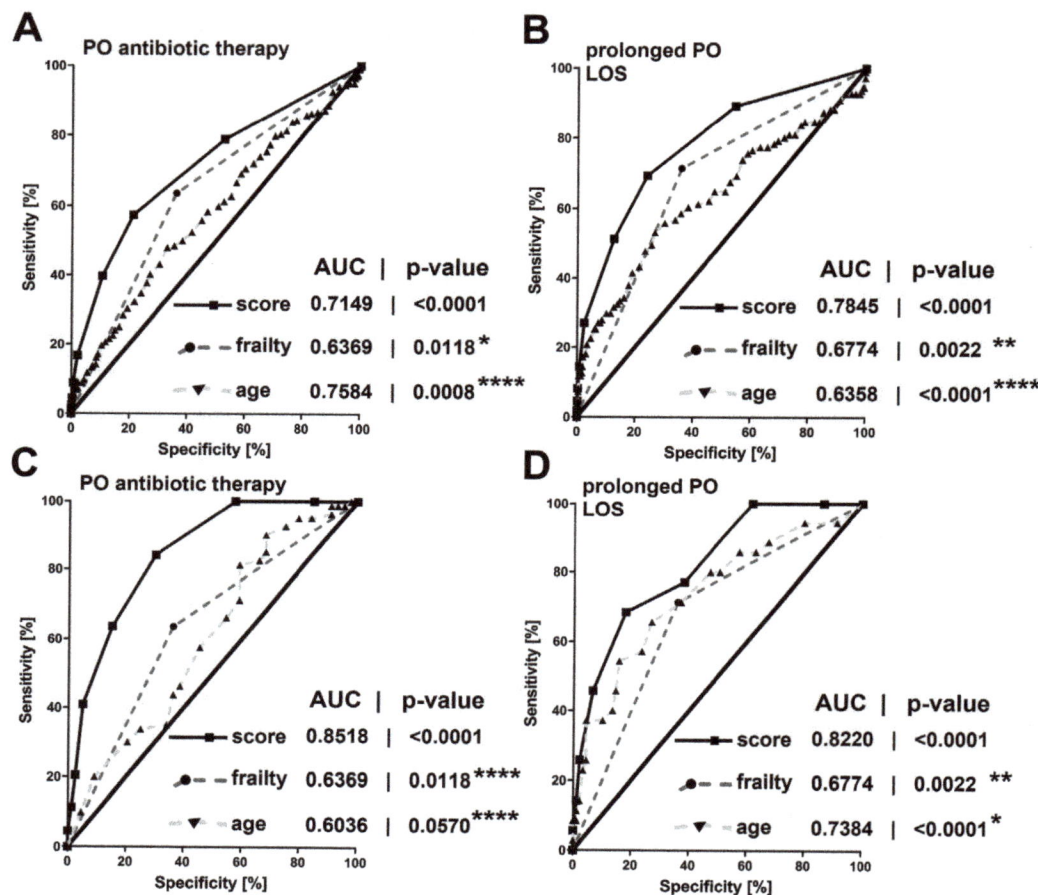

Figure 3. Areas under the receiver-operating characteristic curves of the new perianal sepsis risk score or chronological age and native frailty status alone in predicting the need for postoperative antibiotic therapy (**A,C**) or prolonged postoperative hospitalization (**B,D**): either in the total patient cohort (**A,B**) or in the elderly patient cohort (≥60 y of age; **C,D**). Areas under the receiver-operating characteristic curve are given with their respective p-values. Asterisks indicate p-values obtained from direct comparisons of the areas under the receiver-operating characteristic curves between the new perianal sepsis risk score with native frailty and chronological age alone: * ≤0.1; ** ≤0.05; *** <0.01; **** <0.0001. Four days or more was defined as a prolonged postoperative hospitalization. PO = postoperative. LOS = length of (postoperative) hospital stay. AUC = area under the receiver-operating characteristic curve. Score = new perianal sepsis risk score.

In patients with a score of two or higher, there was a higher occurrence of antibiotic therapy and longer hospital stays after surgery. The score was especially effective in elderly patients, with excellent sensitivity at a score of two or higher. The specificity improved either by increasing the score or by adding points from different domains of the score (Table 6).

Table 6. Perioperative determinants for prolonged hospital stay, i.e., need for prolonged stay.

	Score	All Patients (n = 817)				Elderly Patients (n = 124)			
	Value	≥2	≥2 #	≥3	≥3 #	≥2	≥2 #	≥3	≥3 #
Need for PO antibiotic therapy	Sensitivity	0.57	0.52	0.40	0.38	1	0.91	0.84	0.77
	Specificity	0.79	0.82	0.89	0.89	0.43	0.59	0.70	0.70
	Positive PV	0.47	0.48	0.56	0.55	0.49	0.55	0.61	0.59
	Negative PV	0.85	0.84	0.82	0.81	1	0.92	0.89	0.85
	Likelihood ratio	2.70	2.82	3.75	3.61	1.74	2.20	2.80	2.58
	Rate of PO antibiotic therapy [n]								
	Score <	15.3%	16.4%	18.3%	18.7%	0	7.8%	11.1%	15.2%
	Score ≥	47.4% ***	48.4% ***	55.5% ***	54.5% ***	48.9% ***	54.8% ***	60.7% ***	58.6% ***
Prolonged PO hospital stay	Sensitivity	0.69	0.62	0.51	0.51	1	0.89	0.77	0.74
	Specificity	0.76	0.79	0.87	0.88	0.38	0.53	0.62	0.64
	Positive PV	0.31	0.32	0.39	0.39	0.39	0.43	0.44	0.45
	Negative PV	0.94	0.93	0.92	0.92	1	0.92	0.87	0.86
	Likelihood ratio	2.88	2.93	4.07	4.09	1.62	1.88	2.02	2.07
	Length of PO hospital stay [d]								
	Score <	2.3 ± 5.1	2.3 ± 5.1	2.4 ± 4.8	2.4 ± 4.8	1.9 ± 0.6	2.4 ± 2.3	2.5 ± 1.8	2.7 ± 2.5
	Score ≥	5.4 ± 10.3 ***	5.7 ± 10.8 ***	7.2 ± 13.0 ***	7.2 ± 13.1 ***	6.7 ± 11.4 *	7.5 ± 12.4 **	8.5 ± 13.5 **	8.5 ± 13.7 **
	Rate of prolonged PO hospital stay [n]								
	Score <	6.0%	7.0%	8.1%	8.2%	0	7.8%	12.7%	13.6%
	Score ≥	31.2% ***	31.5% ***	39.0% ***	39.2% ***	38.9% ***	42.5% ***	44.3% ***	44.8% **

Characteristics of the score in predicting the need for antibiotic therapy in addition to surgical abscess drainage as well as prolonged postoperative length of hospitalization already at first presentation in the emergency department obtained either from the whole patient cohort or exclusively in the subcohort of elderly patients, i.e., ≥60 years of age. # Points from at least two different domains of the perianal sepsis risk score; *** $p < 0.0001$; ** $p < 0.01$; * $p < 0.05$. PO = postoperative. PV = predictive value.

4. Discussion

Our data suggest that the etiology and bacteriology of perianal abscesses in elderly patients differ from the disease in younger patients. However, as is known from other surgical interventions [17–22], our data also reveal that the frailty status of aged people—and not their chronological age—mainly determines the outcome in both the short as well as longer term after surgery for perianal abscesses. These findings are the expression of the multidimensional frailty syndrome, which involves physiological and psychological aspects and results in loss of functional reserve and increased vulnerability upon surgery, as stated recently by Cappe et al. [18]. However, not only is the postsurgical situation precarious, because frail patients in our study suffered from more severe and complex diseases (higher rates of severe surrounding tissue infection, higher preoperative CRP values), they also, as a consequence, needed stool deviation, re-do surgery and postoperative antibiotic therapy more frequently.

Routine antibiotic treatment for controlling perianal infection initiated primarily either perioperatively or immediately after surgical abscess drainage with or without approaching fistula-in-ano is disputed in the current literature and certainly not generally necessary for every patient [13–16,28]. However, our data show that there are patients in whom the well-known principles of abscess therapy "ubi pus, ibi evacua" do not seem to be sufficient alone. Thus, antibiotic therapy in addition to abscess drainage would be beneficial. In this regard, the univariable and multivariable analyses presented here reveal that not only the clinical signs of severe local tissue infection and the laboratory signs of severe systemic inflammatory response but also the frailty status of (aged) patients increase the odds for anti-infective treatment in addition to surgical drainage of perianal abscesses. Furthermore, the sum of these parameters additionally predicts the need for prolonged hospitalization in terms of more intensive treatment and nursing, as well, in these patients. For the sake of simplicity, these parameters either derive preoperatively from clinical routine or can be easily and time-sparingly determined at initial presentation in the emergency room, as is the case for mFi-5 [17]. The parameters were included in the novel perianal sepsis risk score. Thereby, ≥ 2 points in elderly patients (i.e., ≥ 60 years of age), best obtained from different domains of the score, were investigated as being highly predictive of the need for both antibiotic therapy and prolonged hospitalization already at the time of first presentation in the emergency room. Hence, the score provides important new insights into treatment modalities of a putative old disease whose therapy is currently debated in an outpatient setting. The score identifies sensitively those patients with high risk for perianal sepsis, poor outcome and situations in which surgery alone is not sufficient for the treatment of perianal abscesses. The perianal sepsis risk score consequently indicates with high sensitivity the need for additional antibiotic therapy and the prolonged need for professional (nursing) care. This correlation analysis presented here as well as the bacteriology and resistance heatmap from the former work by Bender et al. [1] may guide the most effective antibiotic therapy. However, local differences in the resistances profile should be carefully considered.

Our study has impressively shown that frailty status is associated with more complex and severe disease, poorer short-term and long-term outcomes. Despite the high predictive power of the scoring system developed here for the need for antibiotic therapy and prolonged professional (nursing) care in elderly patients with perianal abscesses and perianal sepsis, our study has relevant limitations. The perianal sepsis risk score has been developed and internally validated based on clinical signs of local severe soft tissue infection, laboratory signs of systemic inflammatory response and the frailty status of our cohort of over 800 patients. However, the external validation of the score and thus the evidence to introduce the perianal sepsis risk score into clinical routine is currently pending. This must now be carried out in a future prospective study, so that the score can prove its clinical applicability with its time-efficient calculation as well as diagnostic accuracy. In this prospective setting, it is essential to assess the clinical effectiveness of perioperative antibiotic therapy following abscess drainage, particularly concerning its impact on the outcomes especially of older and frail patients.

5. Conclusions

In summary, outpatient care is not favorable for the patients concerned, and the perianal sepsis risk score allows the appropriate measures to be initiated—antibiotic therapy, additional resource calculation and organized ambulatory nursing care—already at the time of initial presentation in the emergency department. The score identifies these high-risk patients, who should be given further optimal access to ambulatory long-term follow-up after acute care.

Supplementary Materials: The following supporting information can be downloaded at: https://www.mdpi.com/article/10.3390/jcm12165219/s1, Figure S1: Linear relationships between chronological age and modified frailty indices with preoperative markers of systemic inflammation and length of postoperative hospitalization as surrogate parameters for disease severity and short-term outcome, respectively.

Author Contributions: Conceptualization, M.R., L.E. and F.B.; methodology, M.R. and I.A.; software, M.R. and A.H.; validation, M.F., C.I., A.-L.A. and W.P.; formal analysis, M.R. and J.L.; investigation, L.E. and F.B.; resources, C.I. and W.P.; data curation, M.R., L.E. and F.E.; writing—original draft preparation, M.R. and F.B.; writing—review and editing, M.F., C.I., A.H. and J.L.; visualization, I.A. and A.-L.A.; supervision, M.R.; project administration, F.B. All authors have read and agreed to the published version of the manuscript.

Funding: This research received no external funding. M.R. was supported by the Justus-Liebig University Giessen Clinician Scientist Program in Biomedical Research (JLU-CAREER) funded by the German Research Foundation (DFG No. GU405/14-1).

Institutional Review Board Statement: This exploratory, retrospective single-center cohort study was performed in accordance with the latest version of the Declaration of Helsinki and was approved by the local ethics committee of the medical faculty of the University of Giessen (approval No. 66/19, approved on 24 April 2019). All patients were treated according to the institutional standard-of-care.

Informed Consent Statement: Patient consent was waived due to the retrospective nature of data analysis.

Data Availability Statement: The data presented in this study are available on request from the corresponding author.

Conflicts of Interest: The authors declare no conflict of interest.

References

1. Bender, F.; Eckerth, L.; Fritzenwanker, M.; Liese, J.; Askevold, I.; Imirzalioglu, C.; Padberg, W.; Hecker, A.; Reichert, M. Drug resistant bacteria in perianal abscesses are frequent and relevant. *Sci. Rep.* **2022**, *12*, 14866. [CrossRef] [PubMed]
2. Daum, R.S.; Miller, L.G.; Immergluck, L.; Fritz, S.; Creech, C.B.; Young, D.; Kumar, N.; Downing, M.; Pettibone, S.; Hoagland, R.; et al. A placebo-controlled trial of antibiotics for smaller skin abscesses. *N. Engl. J. Med.* **2017**, *376*, 2545–2555. [CrossRef] [PubMed]
3. Talan, D.A.; Mower, W.R.; Krishnadasan, A.; Abrahamian, F.M.; Lovecchio, F.; Karras, D.J.; Steele, M.T.; Rothman, R.E.; Hoagland, R.; Moran, G.J. Trimethoprim-sulfamethoxazole versus placebo for uncomplicated skin abscess. *N. Engl. J. Med.* **2016**, *374*, 823–832. [CrossRef]
4. Miller, L.G.; Daum, R.S.; Creech, C.B.; Young, D.; Downing, M.D.; Eells, S.J.; Pettibone, S.; Hoagland, R.J.; Chambers, H.F. Clindamycin versus trimethoprim-sulfamethoxazole for uncomplicated skin infections. *N. Engl. J. Med.* **2015**, *372*, 1093–1103. [CrossRef] [PubMed]
5. Wright, W.F. Infectious diseases perspective of anorectal abscess and fistula-in-ano disease. *Am. J. Med. Sci.* **2016**, *351*, 427–434. [CrossRef] [PubMed]
6. Malik, A.I.; Nelson, R.L.; Tou, S. Incision and drainage of perianal abscess with or without treatment of anal fistula. *Cochrane Database Syst. Rev.* **2010**, CD006827. [CrossRef]
7. Ramanujam, P.S.; Prasad, M.L.; Abcarian, H.; Tan, A.B. Perianal abscesses and fistulas. A study of 1023 patients. *Dis. Colon Rectum* **1984**, *27*, 593–597. [CrossRef]
8. Ommer, A.; Herold, A.; Berg, E.; Farke, S.; Fürst, A.; Hetzer, F.; Köhler, A.; Post, S.; Ruppert, R.; Sailer, M.; et al. S3-Leitlinie: Analabszess. *Coloproctology* **2016**, *38*, 378–398. [CrossRef]

9. Ommer, A.; Herold, A.; Berg, E.; Fürst, A.; Post, S.; Ruppert, R.; Schiedeck, T.; Schwandner, O.; Strittmatter, B. German S3 guidelines: Anal abscess and fistula (second revised version). *Langenbeck's Arch. Surg.* **2017**, *402*, 191–201. [CrossRef]
10. Liu, C.-K.; Liu, C.-P.; Leung, C.-H.; Sun, F.-J. Clinical and microbiological analysis of adult perianal abscess. *J. Microbiol. Immunol. Infect.* **2011**, *44*, 204–208. [CrossRef]
11. Kelm, M.; Kusan, S.; Surat, G.; Anger, F.; Reibetanz, J.; Germer, C.-T.; Schlegel, N.; Flemming, S. Disease- and medication-specific differences of the microbial spectrum in perianal fistulizing Crohn's disease–Relevant aspects for antibiotic therapy. *Biomedicines* **2022**, *10*, 2682. [CrossRef] [PubMed]
12. Albright, J.B.; Pidala, M.J.; Cali, J.R.; Snyder, M.J.; Voloyiannis, T.; Bailey, H.R. MRSA-related perianal abscesses: An underrecognized disease entity. *Dis. Colon Rectum* **2007**, *50*, 996–1003. [CrossRef] [PubMed]
13. Leung, E.; McArdle, K.; Yazbek-Hanna, M. Pus swabs in incision and drainage of perianal abscesses: What is the point? *World J. Surg.* **2009**, *33*, 2448–2451. [CrossRef] [PubMed]
14. Xu, R.W.; Tan, K.-K.; Chong, C.-S. Bacteriological study in perianal abscess is not useful and not cost-effective. *ANZ J. Surg.* **2016**, *86*, 782–784. [CrossRef]
15. Seow-En, I.; Ngu, J. Routine operative swab cultures and post-operative antibiotic use for uncomplicated perianal abscesses are unnecessary. *ANZ J. Surg.* **2017**, *87*, 356–359. [CrossRef]
16. Lalou, L.; Archer, L.; Lim, P.; Kretzmer, L.; Elhassan, A.M.; Awodiya, A.; Seretis, C. Auditing the routine microbiological examination of pus swabs from uncomplicated perianal abscesses: Clinical necessity or old habit? *Gastroenterol. Res.* **2020**, *13*, 114–116. [CrossRef]
17. Reinisch, A.; Reichert, M.; Ondo Meva, C.C.; Padberg, W.; Ulrich, F.; Liese, J. Frailty in elderly patients with acute appendicitis. *Eur. J. Trauma Emerg. Surg.* **2022**, *48*, 3033–3042. [CrossRef]
18. Cappe, M.; Laterre, P.-F.; Dechamps, M. Preoperative frailty screening, assessment and management. *Curr. Opin. Anaesthesiol.* **2023**, *36*, 83–88. [CrossRef]
19. Daddimani, R.M.; Madhava Murthy, S.K.; Sharan, P.M.; Patil, A.D. A prospective study correlating preoperative modified frailty index with one-year mortality in the elderly with hip fractures. *Cureus* **2022**, *14*, e30951. [CrossRef]
20. Bludevich, B.M.; Emmerick, I.; Uy, K.; Maxfield, M.; Ash, A.S.; Baima, J.; Lou, F. Association between the modified frailty index and outcomes following lobectomy. *J. Surg. Res.* **2022**, *283*, 559–571. [CrossRef]
21. Lin, Z.-Q.; Chen, X.-J.; Dai, X.-F.; Chen, L.-W.; Lin, F. Impact of frailty status on clinical and functional outcomes after concomitant valve replacement and bipolar radiofrequency ablation in patients aged 65 years and older. *J. Cardiothorac. Surg.* **2022**, *17*, 295. [CrossRef] [PubMed]
22. Balasundaram, N.; Chandra, I.; Sunilkumar, V.T.; Kanake, S.; Bath, J.; Vogel, T.R. Frailty index (mFI-5) predicts resource utilization after nonruptured endovascular aneurysm repair. *J. Surg. Res.* **2022**, *283*, 507–513. [CrossRef]
23. Velanovich, V.; Antoine, H.; Swartz, A.; Peters, D.; Rubinfeld, I. Accumulating deficits model of frailty and postoperative mortality and morbidity: Its application to a national database. *J. Surg. Res.* **2013**, *183*, 104–110. [CrossRef] [PubMed]
24. Subramaniam, S.; Aalberg, J.J.; Soriano, R.P.; Divino, C.M. New 5-factor modified frailty index using American College of Surgeons NSQIP data. *J. Am. Coll. Surg.* **2018**, *226*, 173–181.e8. [CrossRef] [PubMed]
25. Mulani, M.S.; Kamble, E.E.; Kumkar, S.N.; Tawre, M.S.; Pardesi, K.R. Emerging strategies to combat ESKAPE pathogens in the era of antimicrobial resistance: A review. *Front. Microbiol.* **2019**, *10*, 539. [CrossRef]
26. Hanley, J.A.; McNeil, B.J. A method of comparing the areas under receiver operating characteristic curves derived from the same cases. *Radiology* **1983**, *148*, 839–843. [CrossRef]
27. Hecker, A.; Reichert, M.; Reuss, C.J.; Schmoch, T.; Riedel, J.G.; Schneck, E.; Padberg, W.; Weigand, M.A.; Hecker, M. Intra-abdominal sepsis: New definitions and current clinical standards. *Langenbeck's Arch. Surg.* **2019**, *404*, 257–271. [CrossRef]
28. Alabbad, J.; Abdul Raheem, F.; Alkhalifa, F.; Hassan, Y.; Al-Banoun, A.; Alfouzan, W. Retrospective clinical and microbiologic analysis of patients with anorectal abscess. *Surg. Infect.* **2019**, *20*, 31–34. [CrossRef]

Disclaimer/Publisher's Note: The statements, opinions and data contained in all publications are solely those of the individual author(s) and contributor(s) and not of MDPI and/or the editor(s). MDPI and/or the editor(s) disclaim responsibility for any injury to people or property resulting from any ideas, methods, instructions or products referred to in the content.

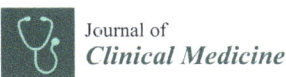 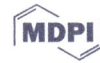

Article

Evaluation of Clinical Manifestations of Hemorrhoidal Disease, Carried Out Surgeries and Prolapsed Anorectal Tissues: Associations with ABO Blood Groups of Patients

Inese Fišere [1,2,*], Valērija Groma [3,*], Šimons Svirskis [4], Estere Strautmane [5] and Andris Gardovskis [2]

1. Department of Doctoral Studies, Rīga Stradiņš University, Dzirciema Street 16, LV-1007 Riga, Latvia
2. Surgery Clinic, Pauls Stradins Clinical University Hospital, Pilsonu Street 13, LV-1002 Riga, Latvia; andris.gardovskis@rsu.lv
3. Institute of Anatomy and Anthropology, Rīga Stradiņš University, Dzirciema Street 16, LV-1007 Riga, Latvia
4. Institute of Microbiology and Virology, Rīga Stradiņš University, Ratsupītes Street 5, LV-1067 Riga, Latvia; ssvirskis@latnet.lv
5. Medical Faculty, Rīga Stradiņš University, Dzirciema Street 16, LV-1007 Riga, Latvia; esterestrautmene99@gmail.com
* Correspondence: inese_fisere@inbox.lv (I.F.); valerija.groma@rsu.lv (V.G.); Tel.: +371-26419636 (I.F.)

Abstract: Hemorrhoidal disease (HD) is a chronic multifactorial disease. Increased abdominal pressure, along with hyperperfusion, neovascularization, overexpression of inflammatory mediators, and dysbiosis, contributes to the development of HD. The deterioration of the anchoring connective tissue with reduced collagen content and altered collagen ratios, dilatation of blood vessels and thrombosis, muscle injury, and inflammation gradually lead to clinically manifesting prolapse and bleeding from hemorrhoids. The associations of the ABO blood types with a disease have been investigated for the upper gastrointestinal tract only. This study aimed to evaluate HD clinical manifestations, surgeries carried out, and the status of prolapsed anorectal tissues by exploring the associations with the patients' ABO blood groups. Clinical and various morphological methods, combined with extensive bioinformatics, were used. The blood type 0, grade III and IV HD individuals constituted the largest group in a moderately-sized cohort of equally represented males and females studied and submitted to surgical treatment of hemorrhoids. There were significantly more complaints reported by HD females compared to males ($p = 0.0094$). The Longo technique appeared mostly used, and there were proportionally more surgeries performed below the dentate line for HD individuals with blood type 0 compared to other blood type patients (24% vs. 11%). HD males were found to present with significantly more often inflamed rectal mucosa ($p < 0.05$). Loosening and weakening of collagenous components of the rectal wall combined with vascular dilation and hemorrhage was found to differ in 0 blood type HD individuals compared to other types. HD males were demonstrated to develop the ruptures of vascular beds significantly more often when compared to HD females ($p = 0.0165$). Furthermore, 0 blood type HD males were significantly more often affected by a disease manifested with tissue hemorrhage compared to the 0 blood type HD females ($p = 0.0081$). Collectively, the local status of chronically injured anorectal tissue should be considered when applying surgical techniques. Future studies could include patients with HD grades I and II to gain a comprehensive understanding of the disease progression, allowing for a comparison of tissue changes at different disease stages.

Keywords: hemorrhoidal disease; clinical manifestations; surgery; prolapsed anorectal tissue; ABO blood groups; morphology

Citation: Fišere, I.; Groma, V.; Svirskis, Š.; Strautmane, E.; Gardovskis, A. Evaluation of Clinical Manifestations of Hemorrhoidal Disease, Carried Out Surgeries and Prolapsed Anorectal Tissues: Associations with ABO Blood Groups of Patients. *J. Clin. Med.* **2023**, *12*, 5119. https://doi.org/10.3390/jcm12155119

Academic Editor: Shmuel Avital

Received: 19 June 2023
Revised: 25 July 2023
Accepted: 28 July 2023
Published: 4 August 2023

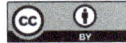

Copyright: © 2023 by the authors. Licensee MDPI, Basel, Switzerland. This article is an open access article distributed under the terms and conditions of the Creative Commons Attribution (CC BY) license (https://creativecommons.org/licenses/by/4.0/).

1. Introduction

Hemorrhoidal disease (HD) is one of the most common anorectal diseases, affecting 13–36% of the general population [1–8]. The prevalence of HD is estimated as high as 88%, depending on the definition used [9,10]. About 50% of people over the age of 50 years have complaints due to HD [1,4,11,12]. Identical in both genders, the disease commonly affects individuals aged 45 to 65 [1,4,11–18], while external thrombosed hemorrhoids are reported at a younger age (<45) and are more pronounced in women [12,19].

The most studied and generally accepted risk factors for HD are chronic constipation and slow bowel movements [4,11,12,15,20,21]. However, several additional risk factors—aging, obesity, straining, pregnancy, lifestyle, spicy food, alcohol, sedentary lifestyle, and physical activity are mentioned [7,15,20,22,23]. Low fiber intake (<12 g/day) and insufficient hydration (<2 L/day) are reported to increase the risk of HD development [22]. Reversely, sufficient use of a fiber-rich diet is demonstrated to reduce HD symptoms and bleeding by 50% [24]. Advancing age and strenuous lifting, straining with defecation, and prolonged sitting are believed to contribute sufficiently to the abnormal downward displacement of the anal cushions causing venous dilatation in HD [1,3,4,25]. Pathophysiological studies highlight increased abdominal pressure as a significant factor [2,11,25,26], along with hyperperfusion, neovascularization [7,27], overexpression of inflammatory mediators [21], and dysbiosis [28]. Histopathological changes include the deterioration of anchoring connective tissue with reduced collagen content and altered collagen ratios [24,29–31]. All these factors collectively weaken the perivascular connective tissue and lead to the dilation of blood vessels, resulting in the formation of hemorrhoids.

HD has very different symptoms and manifestations—itching, swelling, anal discharge, hygienic problems, bleeding, and pain [2]. A total of 40% of individuals with HD are asymptomatic [1,3,4,14,32]. For internal hemorrhoids, the most commonly reported symptom is bleeding and the sensation of tissue prolapse [1,6], whereas the most frequently reported patient complaints are dyschezia, constipation, and diarrhea [2,6,13–15,21].

Surgery is recommended for high-graded internal hemorrhoids, failed non-operative approaches, or HD complications [1,2,4,11–14,26,33]. Commonly, only 5 to 10% of patients require surgical hemorrhoidectomy [2–4,11–13,34]. Minimally invasive procedures, such as LigaSure hemorrhoidectomy, Doppler-guided hemorrhoidal artery ligation, and stapled hemorrhoidopexy have been introduced as alternatives to excisional hemorrhoidectomy. However, it is still used for patients presented with complications [1,4,11,21,25,26,35]. Both the conventional Milligan–Morgan (MM) and closed Ferguson and Parks hemorrhoidectomy techniques have similar complications: tissue trauma, pain, bleeding, mucosal discharge, prolonged local care, and anal stricture [13,25,26]. The Ferguson technique shows better results in terms of wound healing, postoperative pain, and bleeding [8,16,19,36]. The Longo technique preserves hemorrhoidal tissue by relocating and anchoring prolapsed internal hemorrhoids and anoderm [1,4,11,13,14,25]. Therefore, the use of stapled hemorrhoidopexy has some rationale behind it [9,37]. Stapled hemorrhoidopexy addresses mucosal prolapse, but traditional stapled hemorrhoidopexy may cause unnecessary tissue damage [6,38]. A higher hemorrhoidopexy staple line is shown to demonstrate better functional results, with a lower risk of incorporating part of the internal sphincter and the anal transitional zone [39–41].

A link between the ABO blood group system and disease has been demonstrated [32,42–45]. The ABO blood group system, consisting of three main alleles, is controlled by a single gene located on chromosome 9. The association between ABO blood type and bleeding risk and thromboembolic diseases is influenced primarily by the plasma levels and biologic activity of the Von Willebrand factor (VWF) and glycosyltransferase activity [8,23,24,46–48]. In the case of VWF, glycosylation is essential for its proper folding, multimerization, and stability in circulation. In turn, alterations in glycosylation can lead to structural and functional changes in VWF, affecting its ability to mediate platelet adhesion and clot formation. On the other hand, the ABO blood group system is reported to affect some specific aspects of platelet function as well [12] found that blood group 0 is a potential genetic risk factor for bleeding, while [29] found that blood group 0 is associated with increased bleeding severity in patients with bleeding of unknown cause. Moreover, blood group 0 has been associated with an increased risk of severe hemorrhages and lower hemostatic potency observed in upper gastrointestinal bleeding [23,28–30]. For the upper gastrointestinal tract, oral mucosal bleeding, peptic ulcer disease, erosive disease, and cirrhosis-associated gastroesophageal variceal bleeding are recognized as the most common causes of bleeding [31]. Although some evidence suggests an association between ABO blood type and bleeding from hemorrhoids, most often confirmed in patients with blood group 0 and the least common in B and AB blood group individuals [44,49], current understanding of the relationship between the development of hemorrhoids and different ABO blood groups is incomplete. Therefore, several research questions appeared to be addressed in the given study, as follows: (i) what are the clinical manifestations of HD in patients of different ABO blood groups? (ii) How does the local status of chronically injured anorectal tissue influence the choice and success of surgical techniques for HD? (iii) Are there significant differences in reported complaints between male and female HD patients, particularly related to ABO blood types? (iv) How do the composition and condition of collagenous components of the rectal wall and anal canal differ in HD patients with blood type 0 compared to other blood types? (v) Are there any gender differences among HD patients with blood type 0 experiencing hemorrhage? (vi) Are there differences in the presence of chronically injured anorectal tissue and inflamed rectal mucosa between male and female HD patients? To address the aforementioned issues, we conducted this study to evaluate HD clinical manifestations, surgeries carried out, and the status of prolapsed anorectal tissues by exploring the associations with patients' ABO blood groups. In pursuit of this goal, we also attempted the assessment of possible differences between HD in younger and older male and female patients.

2. Materials and Methods

2.1. Patients' Characteristics

In this observational study, the study population was chosen from the database of 316 patients who were treated surgically from September 2020 to June 2021 at Pauls Stradins Clinical University Hospital, Riga, Latvia. The database used for patient selection was comprehensive and included HD patients from regional medical centers, thus enhancing the representativeness of the study population. Sixty adult, equally distributed male and female patients clinically presented with HD grades III and IV were found eligible for inclusion in the study. The recruited participants were representative of the target population, ensuring external validity. Inclusion criteria were defined as follows: age over 18 years, HD grades III and IV, refractory to conservative measures, and persistent clinical manifestation for the last year. Exclusion criteria were concomitant anorectal inflammatory disease (fistula, abscess, inflammatory bowel disease), colon or anal cancer, history of colon or anorectal operation, additional or multiple surgeries required, and active use of immunosuppressants. Patients underwent a thorough anamnesis and physical examination, including inspection, digital-rectal examination, and ano/rectoscopy. The hemorrhoidal disease was defined as symptomatic according to the Goligher classification. All patients underwent hemorrhoidectomy or hemorrhoidopexy surgery. Post-interventional follow-up included clinical examination and ano/rectoscopy after four weeks. Medical records and anorectal tissues of these patients were used in this retrospective study. The certified proctologist collected the data, thus ensuring accuracy and consistency. The information on gender, age, blood group, complaints, type of operation, complications, and data from the histopathological examination was extracted from the record and assessed for each patient. Only standardized data collection protocols and measurement tools were used to minimize observer bias and ensure objectivity and consistency in data gathering. The sum of reported complaints was scored as follows: 1—one complaint recorded; 2—two complaints recorded; 3—three complaints recorded; and 4—four different complaints recorded. The study was approved by the Ethical Committee of Riga Stradins University (Decision No. 22-2/264/2021) and conducted according to the Declaration of Helsinki. Any sensitive information was excluded, and the necessity for informed consent was waived due to the retrospective design of the study.

2.2. Histopathological and Histochemical Investigation of Anorectal Tissues

Sixty surgically obtained formalin-fixed and paraffin-embedded (FFPE) anorectal tissue samples were sectioned and mounted on SuperFrost Plus slides (Gerhard Menzel GmbH, Braunschweig, Germany). Routine histopathological staining with hematoxylin and eosin was performed to confirm the diagnosis of HD and accurately detect the site either above or below the dentate (pectinate) line and surfaced by simple columnar or stratified squamous epithelium, accordingly. Van Gieson's and Picro Sirius red staining were used for the assessment of collagen. The sections stained in Picro Sirius red were further observed under interference and polarized light that improves the visualization and assessment of collagen fibers using a Biolar microscope (BIOLAR, Warsaw, Poland) [30,31,49]. The density of connective tissue fibers appearing in Van Gieson's and Picro Sirius red staining was graded semiquantitatively from 0 to 4, where: 0—loose, 1—minimally dense, 2—moderately dense, 3—markedly dense, and 4—very dense. Furthermore, in each of the slides, the presence of inflammatory cells, various blood vessels, and hemorrhage was assessed. The structures were estimated in 5 properly oriented microscopic fields for each region of interest. The sections were examined by a Leitz light microscope (LEICA, LEITZ DMRB, Wetzlar, Germany) using a digital camera DC 300F, whereas the images of interest were captured using a Glissando Slide Scanner (Objective Imaging Ltd., Cambridge, UK).

2.3. Immunohistochemical Investigation of Anorectal Tissues

The expression of vascular type V collagen and CD34 was assessed immunohistochemically. For this purpose, 4–5 μm-thick FFPE sections mounted on SuperFrost Plus slides (Gerhard Menzel GmbH, Braunschweig, Germany) were used. The IHC protocol recommended by the manufacturer was applied. Briefly, deparaffinized sections were incubated overnight with the primary mouse monoclonal anti-collagen type V antibody (Abcam, Cambridge, UK, 1:300 dilution, ab201980) and mouse monoclonal anti-CD34 antibody (Invitrogen, Camarillo, CA, USA, 1:200 dilution, BI-3C5) at 4 °C. A HiDef Detection HRP Polymer system and a diaminobenzidine tetrahydrochloride substrate kit (Cell Marque, Rocklin, CA, USA) were used to visualize the products of IHC reactions. Cell nuclei were counterstained with Mayer's hematoxylin. Primary antibodies were omitted in the negative controls of IHC reactions. The reaction results were assessed by two independent observers blind to the clinical data.

2.4. Statistical Data Analysis

Statistical data analysis, as well as graphing, were performed using Prism 9 software for macOS (GraphPad Software, LLC, San Diego, CA, USA) and JMP 16 (SAS, Cary, NC, USA). To improve the comparability of patient groups and increase the reliability of associations between ABO blood groups and clinical manifestations, a propensity score matching (PSM) test was performed using the XLSTAT 2023.1.6 (1410) package for Mac as a preliminary analysis. Clinical parameters were presented as medians with an interquartile range (IQR). The histopathology and histochemistry data and immunostaining values within the group were analyzed using the Wilcoxon signed ranks. The Chi-squared test was applied to compare the distribution of variables used to characterize the extent of inflammation in HD tissue samples of males and females. Spearman's rank correlation analysis was applied to detect the possible correlation between patients' complaints and histopathology data, as well as the relation between sex, age, type of surgery, and ABO blood type. A hierarchical clustering method was used to explore the similarities and differences of data, and to see a pattern of data obtained, whereas alluvial plots were constructed to show how associations across categorical dimensions of variables are allocated. The difference between variables was considered significant at $p < 0.05$.

3. Results

3.1. General Clinical Information

During the study time span, 60 subjects were diagnosed with HD stage III and IV and further submitted to hemorrhoidectomy surgery and anorectal tissue retrieval. The patients' age, sex, HD staging, complaints, comorbidities, and stratification into four blood groups are summarized in Figures 1–3. Among all recruited patients, 13 (21.67%) female patients and 14 (23.33%) male patients were diagnosed with HD stage III, whereas 17 (28.33%) female patients and 16 (26.67%) male patients were diagnosed with HD stage IV (Figure 2). In the present study, a major portion of patients presented by blood group 0. There were 55.56, 22.22, 14.81, and 7.41% of HD grade III patients presented by blood groups 0, A, B, and AB, respectively. Simultaneously, there were 57.58, 21.21, and 21.21% of HD grade IV patients presented by blood groups 0, A, and B, respectively. Among HD grade IV patients, no one presented by blood group AB. Two HD grade III males presented by blood group AB (Figure 2). There were no significant differences found between males and females presented by different blood groups. Equal numbers of females were presented in a group of patients aged from 28 to 50 years and in a group of patients aged from 51 to 82 years. In turn, 19 (31.67%) males constituted a group of patients aged under 50 years, whereas 11 (18.33%) males constituted a group of patients aged above 51 years (Figure 1). There were no significant differences found between males and females under and above 50 years, as well as males and females diagnosed with HD stage III and stage IV (Figure 2).

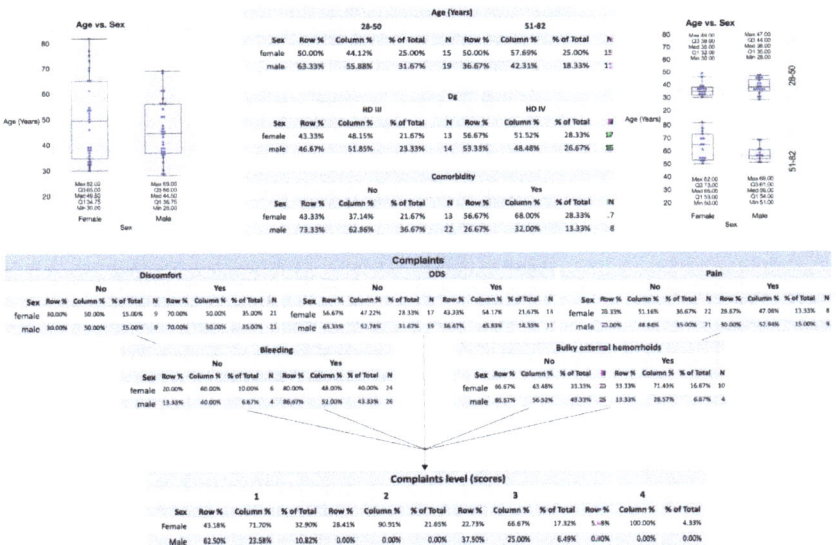

Figure 1. A summary of patients' characteristics related to age, sex, HD staging, complaints, and comorbidities.

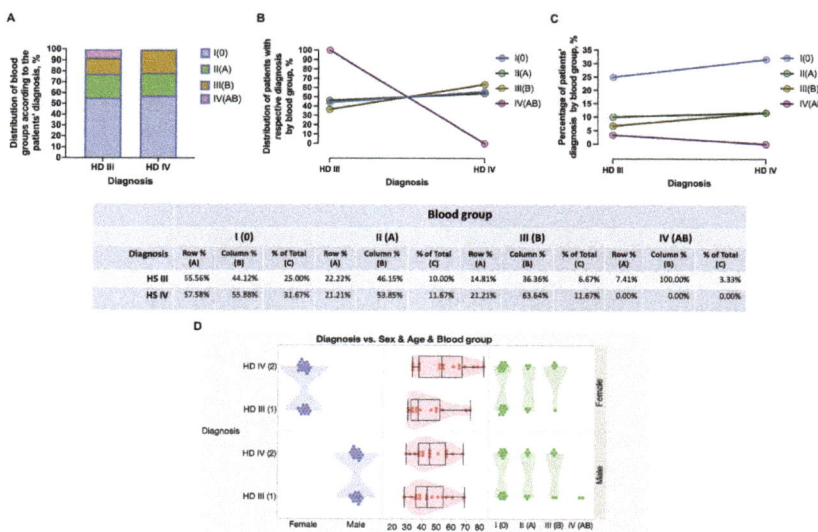

Figure 2. Distribution of female and male patients of different ages presented with HD grade III and IV according to their blood group data. The distribution of blood groups according to diagnosis (**A**). Distribution of patients with respective diagnosis by blood group (**B**). Percentage of patient diagnosis by blood group (**C**). Diagnosis vs. sex and age and blood groups (**D**).

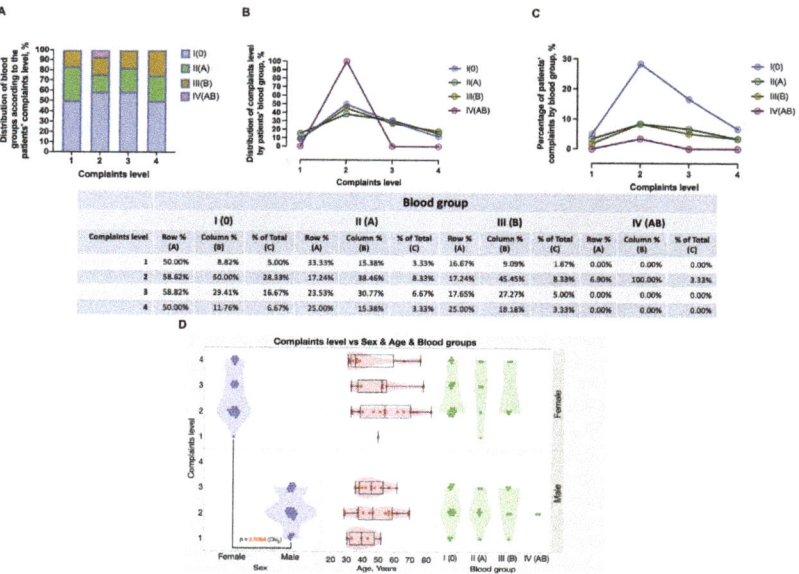

Figure 3. A spectrum and distribution of complaints reported in HD patients with different blood groups. Distribution of blood groups according to the complaints level (**A**–**C**). Distribution of complaints level vs. sex and age and blood groups (**D**).

3.2. Comorbidities, HD Patients' Complaints, and Types of Surgery Used

There were seventeen females and seven males presented with comorbidities, whereas 13 (21.67%) females and 22 (36.67%) males did not reveal any comorbidity. Nearly the same number of female and male subjects reported patient complaints. Hemorrhoidal bleeding, anal and perianal discomfort, and ODS were the most common complaints reported. In this study, nine males and eight females reported pain, whereas four males and ten females reported the presence of bulky external hemorrhoids (Figure 1). Specifically, all individuals with blood group A reported only one complaint. In this study, blood group 0 individuals reported several complaints most often. Males had two or three complaints, whereas females had two, three, or more complaints. There were significantly more complaints reported by HD females compared to males ($p = 0.0094$). Simultaneously, no differences were found between males and females in different age groups (Figure 3D). The Longo technique appeared mostly used for HD individuals with blood type 0 compared to other blood type patients (24% vs. 11%) (Figure 4).

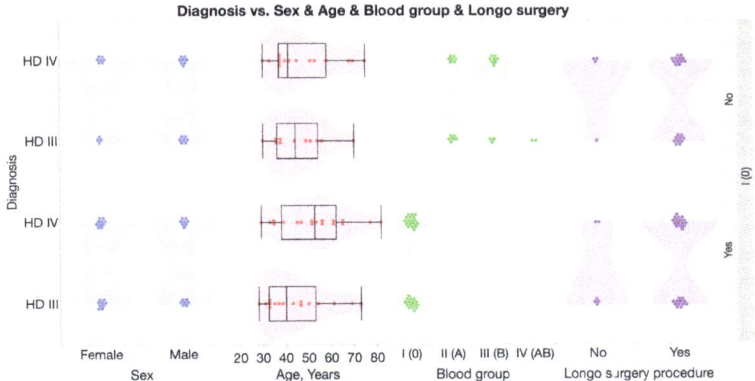

Figure 4. Type of surgery carried out on patients of grade III and IV HD with different blood groups.

3.3. Histopathological Stratification and Assessment of Tissue Samples Localized above and below the Dentate Line

Sixty surgically obtained tissue samples of grade III and IV HD cases were used in this study. Histopathologically, the tissues were stratified into those showing either a simple columnar or stratified squamous epithelium as a lining of a mucous membrane and those that included both types joined by the transition zone, and, therefore, reflecting the tissues of internal and external hemorrhoids, respectively (Figure 5). Differently shaped crypts were embedded in the loose connective tissue of the lamina propria mucosae (Figure 5E,F), whereas a stratified squamous epithelium was found to be resting on more tightly packed connective tissue bundles that supported the basement membrane (Figure 5G,H). The HD 0 blood group individuals constituted a larger group of patients whose surgical samples were obtained above the dentate line, followed by A, B, and AB blood group individuals—55.32, 25.53. 14.89, and 4.26%, respectively. In turn, the presence of stratified squamous epithelium was confirmed in 72.73, 0.00, 27.27, and 0.00% of 0, A, B, and AB blood group individuals, respectively (Figure 5A). Finally, the surgical samples across the transition zone with both types of epithelia accounted for 50% of A and B blood group individuals only (Figure 5A–C). Females presented with surgical samples below the dentate line more often than males. In turn, two males only presented with tissue samples across the transitional zone (Figure 5D).

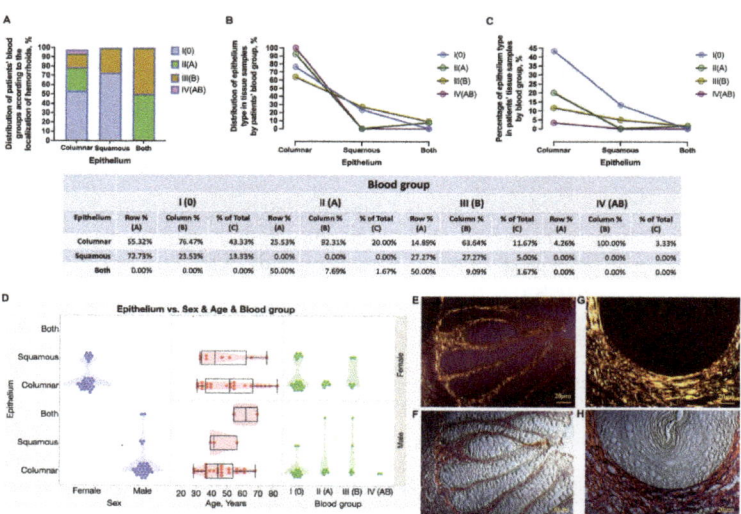

Figure 5. This figure demonstrates a pattern of the histopathological stratification of tissue samples localized above and below the dentate line in HD males and females presented with different blood types (**A–D**). Elongated and paralleled crypts that are embedded in the loose connective tissue can be viewed in a polarized light (**E**) and a differential interference mode (**F**). A stratified squamous epithelium that rests on the basement membrane is followed by tightly packed collagenous bundles supporting the basement membrane and is assessed using a polarized light (**G**) and a differential interference mode (**H**). When observed under polarized light, the lamina propria mucosae reveals type I and type III collagen fibers stained in yellow-red and green, respectively. Picro Sirius red staining (**E–H**). Scale bars: 20 μm.

3.4. Assessment of Chronic Anorectal Tissue Injury in Hemorrhoidal Disease Patients

Chronic mucosal injury of the rectum, including the presence of inflammatory cells, follicular lymphoid hyperplasia, crypt distortion, and crypt shortfall, was evidenced in the tissue samples obtained from HD patients (Figure 6A,B). In this study, anorectal tissues obtained in males were significantly more often inflamed (96.7% vs. 3.3%) than those in HD females (Figure 6C). In addition, for a better exploration of chronic mucosal lesions in HD, immunostaining was performed to specify the involvement of vascular and immune cells. Specifically, CD34 immunohistochemistry was applied to track the mucosa coat vascularity and the presence and distribution of immune cells contributing to crypt distortion. Endothelial cells of small mucosal blood vessels were positively stained with the anti-CD34 antibody and, therefore, easily tracked and analyzed. As a surface molecule, CD34 was found decorating immunocompetent cells infiltrating mucosa (Figure 7E,F). The mucosa crypt status was assessed extensively, and a degree of crypt damage was scored (Figure 7A–D). Severely lesioned and inflamed mucosa was found in 47.62, 28.57, 14.29, and 9.52% of 0, A, B, and AB blood group individuals, respectively (Figure 7D). Both females and males of 0, A, and B blood groups and males of AB blood type presented with severely lesioned rectal mucosa. The significant differences between females and males and different age groups of HD patients when estimating chronic mucosal lesions were not found. The estimation of anorectal tissues was extended to the submucosa, and the integrity and density of collagen fibers, including perivascular fibers, were explored by the use of special stainings—Van Gieson's and Picro Sirius's red stainings (Figure 8E–J) and scored (Figure 8A–C). Loosening of connective tissue collagen was confirmed in HD tissue samples. The presence of loosened collagen arrangement in the tissue samples was confirmed and further assessed proportionally to the representative number of HD subjects studied. It was determined in a large proportion of HD individuals of 0 blood type—42.86%, followed by HD individuals of A and B blood types—28.57 and 28.57%, respectively. No significant differences were found when assessing collagen density in HD males' and females' samples and different age groups (Figure 8D). Immunohistochemistry was applied to target the expression and distribution of vascular type V collagen and explore its contribution to the integrity of the vascular wall. The results were assessed using Picro Sirius red staining and type V collagen immunohistochemistry in all anorectal tissue samples (Figure 9E–H). The presence of dilated and ruptured submucosal veins was confirmed in 72.73, 13.64, 13.64, and 0%, and 51.35, 27.03, 18.92, and 2.70% of HD individuals of 0, A, B, and AB blood types, respectively (Figure 9A–C). There were significant differences found when assessing the vascular integrity in HD males' and females' samples but not the age groups (Figure 9D). In this study, HD males were demonstrated to develop the ruptures of vascular beds significantly more often when compared to HD females ($p = 0.0165$). Furthermore, 0 blood type HD males were significantly more often affected by a disease manifested with tissue hemorrhage compared to the 0 blood type HD females ($p = 0.0081$).

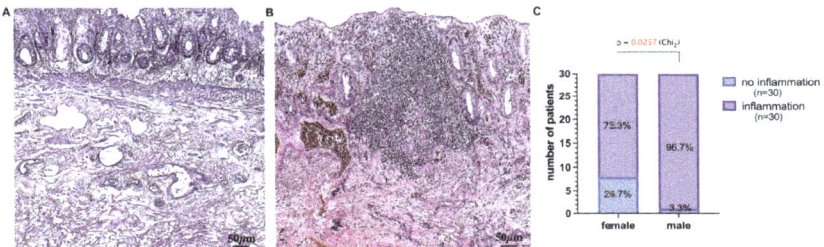

Figure 6. A representative image that depicts the histopathological features of mucosa and submucosa in HD in the absence (**A**) and presence (**B**) of inflammation. (**C**) The extent of inflammation in the anorectal samples obtained from males is significantly higher than that in females. (**A**) The rectal mucosa reveals paralleled crypts; however, the glands do not rest on the muscular mucosae; the submucosa houses thin- and thick-walled vessels. (**B**) The culprit bleeding vessels are visualized in the rectal mucosa. Inflammatory infiltrate brings to the reduction and distortion of crypts and produces insertions toward the haphazardly patterned muscular mucosae. Van Gieson's staining (**A**,**B**). Scale bars: 50 μm.

3.5. Hierarchical Clustering Used for the Exploration of Data Similarities and Visualization Using Alluvial Plotting

A hierarchical clustering method was used to assess the similarity and differences in the levels of studied factors. Data for patients in the HD 0 blood group were analyzed separately from data of HD subjects of A, B, and AB blood types (Figure 10). There were four different clusters recognized for patients in the group HD 0. A small, orange-colored cluster was distinguished in the HD 0 blood group only. However, some similarities have emerged regarding patient complaints and comorbidities, but not the site of surgery, with a blue cluster representing HD subjects with blood type A, B, and AB. Green cluster consisting only of HD 0 blood group males undergoing Longo surgery presented with an inflamed mucosa, heavily deformed crypts, and ruptured blood vessels revealing hemorrhage. In a red-colored cluster consisting of HD patients of A, B, and AB blood types submitted to Longo surgery, the levels of certain studied factors, specifically, the presence of inflammation, deformation of crypts, and damage of blood vessels, were recognized to resemble those determined for HD 0 blood type individuals. Additionally, alluvial diagrams were plotted to show how associations across categorical dimensions of variables are allocated. This type of data representation was used to better visualize an individual spectrum of the variables studied (HD patients of 0 blood type vs. HD patients of A, B, and AB blood types, and HD patients submitted to Longo surgery vs. HD patients submitted to other types of surgical treatments) and the relationship between variables such as sex, age, HD grade, comorbidity, complaints, submission to Longo surgery, and anorectal tissue-related characteristics (Figure 11).

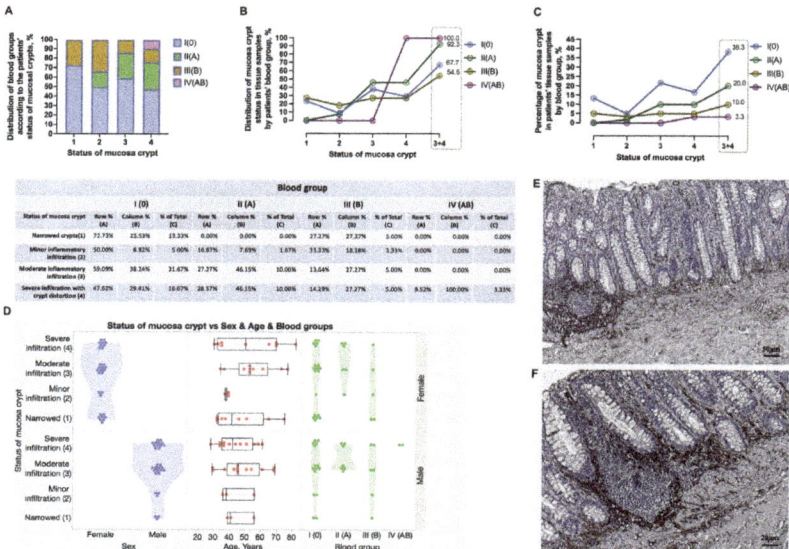

Figure 7. The histopathological assessment of chronic mucosal lesions in HD males and females presented with different blood groups. The schematic presentation of the structural appearance of crypts in HD patients of 0, A, B, and AB blood types (**A–C**). The status of mucosal glands is graded and estimated in HD males and females of different age groups (**D**). A representative image that depicts the histopathological features of inflamed mucosa HD (**E,F**). CD34 immunohistochemistry (**A,B**). Scale bars: 50 μm (**A**), 20 μm (**B**).

3.6. Multivariate Analysis of Hemorrhoidal Disease Contributing Factors

Multivariate analysis was used to better recognize a pattern of data obtained and to investigate the dependence between multiple variables at the same time. A correlation matrix, as plotted and demonstrated in Figure 12, indicates that in this study, females reported complaints slightly more often than males ($r = -0.30$). Elderly persons with HD were more likely to develop inflammation than younger patients with HD ($r = 0.24$). As predicted, one patient's complaints were positively associated with comorbidities ($r = 0.35$). The application of the Longo technique appeared to be more beneficial for patients presented with a simple columnar epithelium in their tissue samples when compared to those presented with a stratified squamous epithelium or the transitional zone ($r = -0.52$). This technique was applied to patients who presented with crypt distortion ($r = 0.46$), hemorrhage ($r = 0.45$), and inflammation ($r = 0.39$). Inflammatory infiltrate that surrounded a crypt was determined more frequently when compared to the stratified squamous epithelium ($r = -0.63$), and hemorrhage was confirmed more often in the mucosa coat covered by a simple columnar epithelium ($r = -0.62$). A decrease in the density of connective tissue was associated with hemorrhage ($r = -0.34$) and larger inflammatory infiltrates ($r = -0.34$). Severely distorted crypts were strongly associated with ruptured blood vessels, hemorrhage, and the presence of larger infiltrates ($r = 0.74$). Finally, the occurrence of ruptured blood vessels with hemorrhage was confirmed to be moderately associated with tissue inflammation ($r = 0.59$).

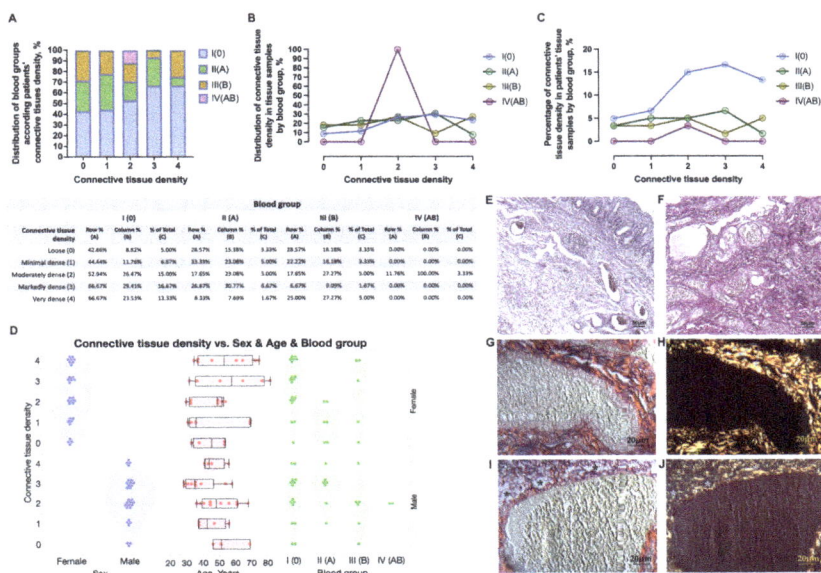

Figure 8. The histochemical assessment of connective tissue collagen fibers in HD males and females presented with different blood groups (**A–D**). Loosely (**E**) or more densely (**F**) structured submucosa houses thick and thin-walled congested blood vessels, Van Gieson's staining (**E,F**). Scale bars: 50 µm. Perivascular collagen is assessed in thick (**G,H**) and thin-walled (**I,J**) vessels using a differential interference (**G,I**) and a polarized light mode (**H,J**). When observed under polarized light, type I and type III collagen fibers are stained in yellow-red and green, respectively. Picro Sirius red staining (**H,J**). Scale bars: 20 µm.

Finally, a comparative analysis of the proportion of main categorical variables explored in this study for HD patients of blood type 0 and other blood types was performed (Figure 13). There were proportionally more surgeries performed below the dentate line for HD individuals of blood type 0 compared to other blood type patients (24% vs. 11%). Furthermore, the 0 blood type individuals presented more often with normally appearing mucosal glands compared to other blood type patients (24% vs. 11%). Proportions for minimally and markedly densely arranged connective tissue collagen fibers were differently presented in HD individuals of blood type 0 compared to other blood type patients, as it appears in a pie chart. Notably, dilated submucosal veins were two times more common (38% vs. 16%) in the samples of HD individuals with blood type 0 when compared to other blood types. Simultaneously, anorectal tissues obtained from the 0 blood type individuals were less inflamed (29% vs. 15%) when compared to other blood types. Finally, Longo surgery was equally applied in all HD patients.

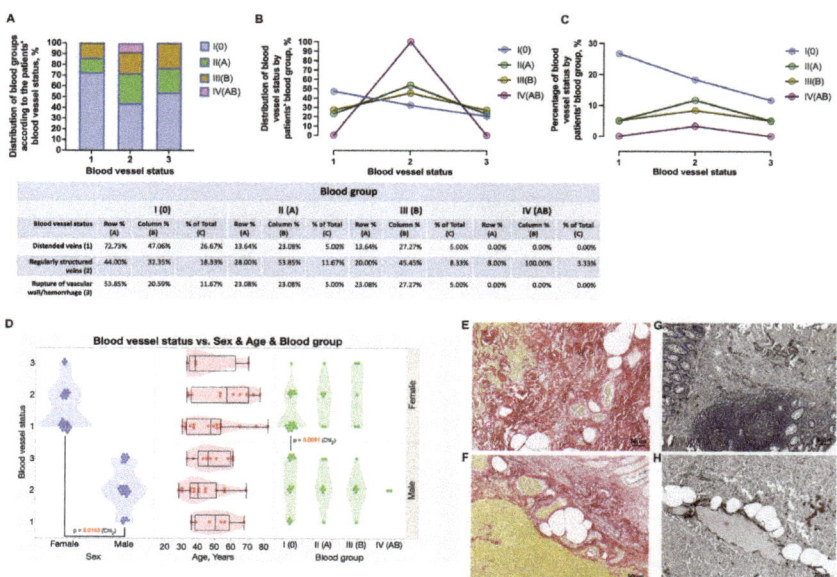

Figure 9. This figure illustrates the architectural peculiarities of collagen and its contribution to the maintenance of vascular integrity. Distribution of blood groups according to the patients blood vessel status (**A**). Distribution of blood vessels status by patients blood group (**B**). Distribution of blood vessel status by patients blood group in percentage (**C**). Blood vessel status vs. sex and age and blood group (**D**). Small arterioles are embedded in a collagenous matrix that reveals a haphazard orientation of fibers partly inserted into the hemorrhage area (**E**). Congested and markedly enlarged submucosal vessels (**F**). Inflamed mucosa with crypt distortion and thickened muscular mucosa; small mucosal and submucosal vessels are labeled with the anti-collagen type V antibody (**G**). Small dilated submucosal vessels labeled with the anti-collagen type V antibody are surrounded by a large hemorrhage (**H**). Picro Sirius red staining (**E**,**F**). Collagen type V immunohistochemistry (**G**,**H**). Scale bars: 50 µm (**E**–**G**), 20 µm (**H**).

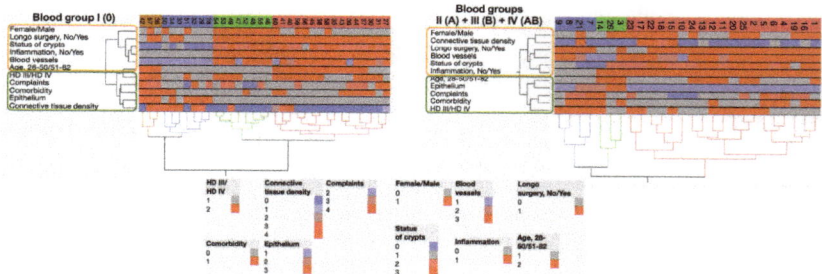

Figure 10. Hierarchical clustering shows the similarities of data points related to the studied system. The clades and leaves of a tree included data on the histopathological evaluations of a variety of anorectal tissue parameters in 60 subjects with grade III and IV HD submitted to surgical treatment, information about a patient's age and sex, complaints, and comorbidities.

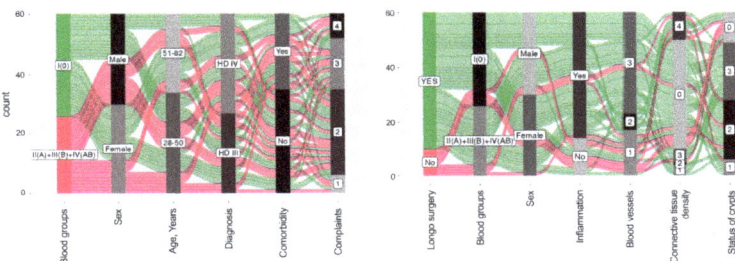

Figure 11. Alluvial diagrams represent flows among nodes. In these diagrams, individual observations are presented as rows, while characteristics are presented as columns. The width of each line and the flow path that stems from it are determined by the proportional fraction of the category total. The left panel illustrates how many patients of 0 blood type/patients of A, B, and AB blood types were males/females aged below or over 50 years, presented with HD grade III/IV, had comorbidities, and reported one or more complaints. The right panel shows how a high proportion of HD females and males have undergone Longo surgery or other types of surgical treatments, had 0 or A, B, and AB blood types, and presented with inflammation, damaged blood vessels and mucosal glands, and a certain density of connective tissue in their samples.

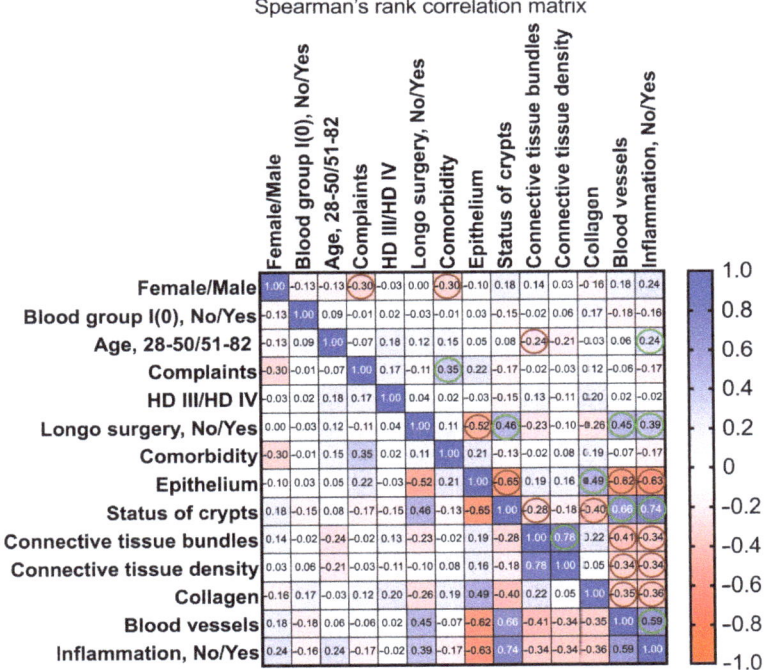

Figure 12. A correlogram of the studied variables. In this graph, correlation coefficients are colored according to the value. Positive correlations are displayed in blue, whereas negative correlations are shown in red. Color intensity is proportional to the correlation coefficients. Colored circles indicate associations with a significance level of $p < 0.05$.

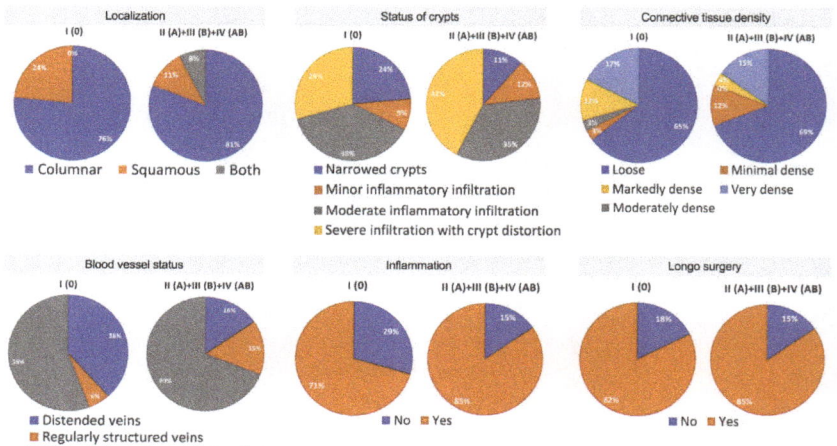

Figure 13. Comparison of the proportion of categorical variables studied for HD individuals of 0 blood type and other blood types.

4. Discussion

In this study, HD clinical manifestations, surgeries carried out, and the status of prolapsed anorectal tissues by exploring the associations with patients' ABO blood groups were analyzed. Younger and older male and female HD patients were investigated to target the possible differences between the aforementioned groups of subjects. To reach the goal, various histopathological methods, microscopies, and extensive bioinformatics tools were used. The given study also has some features of novelty. Firstly, the novelty of this study lies in exploring clinical manifestations and reported complaints among HD patients, particularly concerning their ABO blood types, which adds a novel perspective to understanding the disease's clinical presentation. Secondly, the association between ABO blood groups and the status of prolapsed anorectal tissues in HD patients has been investigated, thus contributing to a comprehensive understanding of the disease and its potential underlying mechanisms. Thirdly, the novelty lies in investigating the potential gender-specific differences in the presence of inflamed rectal mucosa among HD patients and the predisposition to tissue hemorrhage in HD patients, particularly in relation to blood type 0. Finally, the assessment of the integrity and density of collagen, a bulk of anorectal tissue, and its loosening, contributing to the development of HD, provides a better understanding of the disease's pathophysiology.

Hemorrhoids are vascular submucosal cushions that prevent stool leakage from the rectum [2,3,13,14,20]. They are classified based on their position relative to the dentate line: internal hemorrhoids above the line, covered by simple columnar epithelium, and external hemorrhoids below the line, covered by stratified squamous epithelium [1,2,21]. Studies have linked various factors, such as aging, genetics, intestinal issues, and dysbiosis, to the development of hemorrhoids [25,28,50]. Among other HD development promoting factors, abnormal connective tissue morphology and dysregulated blood flow in the affected anal cushions have been mentioned [1,2,7,15,18,37]. However, the complex analysis of tissue stratified by the location of the lesion and associated HD surgery has not yet been fully performed. Additionally, no prior research has explored potential connections between clinical symptoms, surgical treatments, and different ABO blood types in individuals with hemorrhoids, making this study novel.

Various surgical methods for hemorrhoid therapy have distinct benefits, indications, contraindications, and complications. However, no gold standard exists. Conventional excisional hemorrhoidectomy is commonly used for grade III and grade IV

HD treatment, with energy devices helping to reduce postoperative pain and bleeding [51]. The MM technique involves leaving wounds open for 3–5 weeks for healing. On the other hand, the Longo technique is considered safe and effective for grade II and III HD [2,4,11,13,14,26,27,32], showing excellent short-term results [2,8,16,18,19]. However, its efficacy for larger and more complicated HD treatments, as well as long-term follow-up, remains debated [8,13,19]. Other authors have found that conventional hemorrhoidectomy had more complications and a higher recurrence rate compared to stapled hemorrhoidopexy (Longo) within one year [1,4,32]. Long-term results of the Longo procedure with a 12-year follow-up were also evaluated [1,4,32]. Several systematic reviews suggested that stapled hemorrhoidopexy was less effective than conventional hemorrhoidectomy [1]. In Europe, particularly in France, Italy, and the United Kingdom, the MM-modified technique is widely used [51]. Modified techniques utilizing LigaSure tissue-sealing devices allow for faster operations with reduced bleeding and tissue damage, especially with increasing surgical experience [52]. In our study, stapled hemorrhoidopexy appeared as a surgical technique used most often and with fewer postoperative complications.

Numerous postoperative complications have been reported, including bleeding, relapses, surgical site hematoma, thrombosis, urine retention, incontinence, stenosis, and recto-vaginal fistula in female patients [42,53–56]. However, the frequency of complications has decreased since 2015 [36]. Postoperative pain after stapled hemorrhoidopexy is associated with various factors such as incorrect technique, anal wounds, inflammation in the stapled ring, age, or pelvic floor nerve stimulation [38,44,54,56–58]. Pain after the MM application is linked to bleeding and inflammation, often leading to acute reoperations to stop postoperative bleeding [6]. Delayed post-hemorrhoidectomy bleeding (DPHB) is an important complication that can occur between the fourth and eighteenth days after the procedure [26]. Risk factors for DPHB include the use of the LigaSure device by the surgeon and constipation, with an incidence of 0.9–49% [6]. On the contrary, other studies reported the early period hemorrhage—within three days [25]. In our study, DPHB was established on days 4, 5, 7, and 8 postoperatively when applying the Longo technique, and only once bleeding was demonstrated after LigaSure hemorrhoidectomy. Rates of postoperative bleeding have been reported as 2.4% and 5.7% in patients who underwent stapled procedures and hemorrhoidectomy, respectively [59]. Secondary bleeding after hemorrhoid surgery occurs in 0.6–2.4% of cases, with the highest probability on the sixth to ninth postoperative day [34]. Severe postoperative bleeding is recognized in 0.7% of patients only [60].

Previously, a reduction in the amount of connective tissue collagen was shown in HD. Other authors have reported a decrease in the ratio of type I to III collagen leading to the impaired mechanical stability of the perivascular tissue in HD patients [30,31,49,61]. However, approval of whether changes in collagen formation in HD are caused by external factors and metabolic changes or are influenced by genetic factors remains unsolved. Recently, connective tissue dysfunction was proven in HD-predisposed individuals conducting genome-wide analysis [23]. In the aforementioned study, prioritized genes encoding macromolecules, including collagens highly expressed in hemorrhoidal tissue, were identified. Furthermore, COL5A2, which encodes for type V collagen, was found to be implicated in the development of HD. Type V collagen is widely recognized as an essential molecule for major collagen types I and III fibril formation. The results of the collagen assessment obtained in the given study are in line with these observations. In this study, a decrease in the density of connective tissue was accompanied by gradual dilation of submucosal veins and hemorrhage. Furthermore, loosening and weakening of collagenous components of the rectal wall combined with vascular dilation and hemorrhage was found to differ in 0 blood type HD individuals compared to other types. HD males were demonstrated to develop the ruptures of vascular beds significantly more often when compared to HD females, and 0 blood type HD males were significantly more often presented with tissue hemorrhage compared to females. Other authors suggested that venous dilation and ruptures are the sources of bleeding. Furthermore, vascular malformations may become susceptible to injuries during defecation, and hemostatic failure may gradually develop in HD [47]. The exploration of the vascular supply and blood flow to the hemorrhoidal tissues is of value when developing advanced HD treatment techniques, including hemorrhoidal de-arterialization procedures [46,48,62]. Stapled hemorrhoidopexy lifts the hemorrhoidal cushions back up into their normal anatomical position and interrupts the mucosal and submucosal internal hemorrhoidal vascular pedicles, thus reducing the arterial flow.

HD is characterized by severe vasodilatation, which causes inflammation of the surrounding tissues and leads to extravasation in the interstitial space, increased permeability of blood vessels, fragility, and migration of inflammatory cells [24,63,64]. An increase in vascular permeability in chronically injured and inflamed tissue was shown to occur along with the elevation of the expression of CD34 and other adhesion molecules on the surface of vascular endothelial and immune cells [65].

In this study, we investigated the mucosa coat vascularity and the presence and distribution of immune cells contributing to crypt distortion using CD34 immunohistochemistry. Even rather small mucosal blood vessels were positively stained with the anti-CD34 antibody and easily tracked. The immunocompetent cells infiltrating mucosa were scored, and the contribution of larger inflammatory infiltrates to crypt distortion was estimated. HD males were found to present with significantly more often inflamed rectal mucosa. Elderly patients with HD were reported to develop inflammation more likely than younger patients in connection with the duration of the pathology, ischemia, vasculitis, toxins, medications, chronic tissue injury, diet (citrus, coffee, cola, beer, garlic, spices, and sauces), and smoking [64]. The presence of inflammation in the anorectal passage before the operation can be considered reliable when using preparations containing flavonoids, which are anti-inflammatory, antibacterial, vasoconstrictive, bleeding-reducing, and wound-healing [24,50,63]. Notably, some flavonoids were shown to inhibit gene expression and some pro-inflammatory cytokines [57].

The associations between ABO blood type and disease have been studied since the early 1900s when researchers determined that blood plasma antibodies and antigens on the surface of red blood cells are inherited [30,42,51,66]. The ABO blood group system consists of three main alleles and is controlled by a single gene located on the terminal portion of the long arm of chromosome 9 (9q34. 2) [32,42,43,52]. The link between the ABO blood type and thromboembolic diseases and bleeding risk is intervened by the glycosyltransferase activity and plasma levels, and the biologic activity of Von Willebrand factor, a carrier protein for coagulation factor VII which is low in the blood group 0 [24,27,47,52–54]. Previously, an ABO blood group 0 was demonstrated to have an important role in upper gastrointestinal bleeding [30]. The blood group 0 was shown to be associated with an increased risk of developing more severe hemorrhages and lower hemostatic potency [29,42,44,52,55]. Furthermore, blood group 0 was shown to be prevalent in patients with bleeding for unknown reasons compared to the normal population and to be associated with increased bleeding severity similar to bleeding from esophageal, gastric, and duodenal ulcers [29,44,66]. However, the difference was not confirmed when studying the associations between postpartum hemorrhage and blood type [23,53]. Simultaneously, the subjects other than the blood group 0 were reported to have an increased risk of developing coronary heart disease and venous thrombosis compared with 0 blood group individuals [12,44,52]. Therefore, the presence of non-0 blood type somehow may be assumed to be predisposing for thromboses [32,54,56]. Simultaneously, patients with blood group AB were shown to have a significantly higher 90-day survival compared with other blood groups [29,55]. In turn, this investigation proved that individuals with 0 blood type who have hemorrhoids (HD) show differences in the rectal wall's collagenous components, vascular dilation, and hemorrhage compared to individuals with other blood types. Additionally, HD males with 0 blood type are more prone to developing ruptures of vascular beds and experiencing tissue hemorrhage compared to HD females with 0 blood type.

The results of this study must be viewed in light of some limitations. The relatively small sample size is one of the limitations of the given study. It was performed on a small-sized HD patient cohort. This limitation may affect the generalizability of the findings to a larger population. The authors acknowledge that certain characteristics were assessed mainly through categorical variables. This might limit the depth of analysis and understanding of complex relationships between variables. The study aimed at the anorectal tissue assessment, and the resected tissues were obtained from advanced HD grade III and IV patients. Therefore, the authors did not explore the plausible tissue changes to occur earlier in HD grade I-II patients. Next, due to the retrospective character of the study, some clinical data remained not specified and analyzed in the present study, which might bring some new results and interpretations. Finally, realizing that the 0 blood group individuals constitute the majority worldwide, we created a non-0 group representatives' group by combining A, B, and AB blood group patients. This grouping might not account for potential differences between individual blood groups. However, a combined group of patients with blood groups A, B, and AB and a group of the 0 blood group individuals contrasting them were equalized, and the proportions of characteristics were assessed.

5. Conclusions

This retrospective study provides valuable insights into a spectrum of clinical manifestations and surgical treatments applied to treat prolapsing HD, as well as the assessment of anorectal tissue changes associated with the disease. The observed mucosal inflammation, connective tissue loosening, and vascular wall ruptures leading to hemorrhage are symptoms of prolapsing HD across all blood types—additionally, the presence of multiple complaints increases in patients with comorbidities. The study demonstrates the effectiveness of the most commonly used surgical therapy for curing HD and offers important information on the origin of patients' complaints, the applied therapy, and the localization of tissue lesions subjected to further resection. There was a higher level of tissue inflammation observed in men. However, further investigation is needed to understand its potential impact on the presentation of local symptoms in the context of edema. Notably, anorectal tissues obtained from HD individuals with blood type 0 showed relatively lower levels of inflammation compared to other blood types, while congested and markedly dilated submucosal veins were more frequently found in HD individuals with blood type 0. Given the relatively small cohort size, future studies should aim for a larger sample to enhance the generalizability of the findings and improve the statistical power for detecting significant associations. To gain a comprehensive understanding of the disease progression, future studies, when possible, should include patients with HD grades I and II, allowing for a comparison of tissue changes at different disease stages. Future studies should carefully account for confounding variables, such as age, gender, and comorbidities, to obtain more robust and reliable findings. Finally, collaborating with multiple medical centers can increase the diversity of the patient population and improve the external validity of the findings.

Author Contributions: Conceptualization, I.F. and V.G.; methodology, I.F., V.G. and Š.S.; formal analysis, I.F. and V.G.; investigation, I.F., V.G. and E.S.; data curation, I.F. and Š.S.; writing—original draft preparation, I.F. and V.G.; writing—review and editing, I.F. and V.G.; visualization, I.F., V.G. and Š.S.; bioinformatics—Š.S.; supervision, V.G. and A.G. All authors have read and agreed to the published version of the manuscript.

Funding: This research received funding (Nr. 6-DN-20/2/2023) from Riga Stradiņš University Department of Doctoral Studies for the purchase of reagents and coverage of the article processing charge.

Institutional Review Board Statement: This study was conducted in accordance with the Declaration of Helsinki and was approved by the Institutional Ethics Committee of Riga Stradiņš University (decision No. 22-2/264/2021).

Informed Consent Statement: Patient consent was waived due to the analysis of retrospective anonymous patient data.

Data Availability Statement: A publicly available bibliographic database, PubMed.gov, was used in this study (accessed from May 2020 till July 2023). The complete search query is specified in Section 2 of the article. The full bibliographic reference list is available upon request from the corresponding author.

Acknowledgments: The authors would like to acknowledge the Riga Stradiņš University Department of Doctoral Studies for support in acquiring the reagents. We would also like to thank Elza Rate for additional support during the collection of some tumor specimens.

Conflicts of Interest: The authors declare no conflict of interest.

References

1. Migaly, J.; Sun, Z. Review of Hemorrhoid Disease: Presentation and Management. *Clin. Colon Rectal Surg.* **2016**, *29*, 22–29. [CrossRef]
2. Lohsiriwat, V. Treatment of hemorrhoids: A coloproctologist's view. *World J. Gastroenterol.* **2015**, *21*, 9245–9252. [CrossRef]
3. Kibret, A.A.; Oumer, M.; Moges, A.M. Prevalence and associated factors of hemorrhoids among adult patients visiting the surgical outpatient department in the University of Gondar Comprehensive Specialized Hospital, Northwest Ethiopia. *PLoS ONE* **2021**, *16*, e0249736. [CrossRef] [PubMed]
4. Mott, T.; Latimer, K.; Edwards, C. Hemorrhoids: Diagnosis and Treatment Options. *Am. Fam. Physician* **2018**, *97*, 172–179. Available online: http://www.ncbi.nlm.nih.gov/pubmed/29431977 (accessed on 3 January 2021). [PubMed]
5. Rubbini, M.; Ascanelli, S. Classification and guidelines of hemorrhoidal disease: Present and future. *World J. Gastrointest. Surg.* **2019**, *11*, 117–121. [CrossRef]
6. Gallo, G.; Martellucci, J.; Sturiale, A.; Clerico, G.; Milito, G.; Marino, F.; Cocorullo, G.; Giordano, P.; Mistrangelo, M.; Trompetto, M. Consensus statement of the Italian society of colorectal surgery (SICCR): Management and treatment of hemorrhoidal disease. *Tech. Coloproctol.* **2020**, *24*, 145–164. [CrossRef] [PubMed]
7. De Marco, S.; Tiso, D. Lifestyle and Risk Factors in Hemorrhoidal Disease. *Front. Surg.* **2021**, *8*, 729166. [CrossRef]
8. Pata, F.; Gallo, G.; Pellino, G.; Vigorita, V.; Podda, M.; Di Saverio, S.; D'Ambrosio, G.; Sammarco, G. Evolution of Surgical Management of Hemorrhoidal Disease: An Historical Overview. *Front. Surg.* **2021**, *8*, 727059. [CrossRef]
9. Jayaswal, M.K.; Maurya, O.K. Retrospective Assessment of the Outcome of the Stapled Haemor-rhoidopexy for Haemorrhoids against Conventional Open Technique. *Int. J. Pharm. Clin. Res. Orig. Res. Artic.* **2022**, *14*, 705–711. Available online: www.ijpcr.com (accessed on 3 January 2021).
10. Hong, Y.S.; Jung, K.U.; Rampal, S.; Zhao, D.; Guallar, E.; Ryu, S.; Chang, Y.; Kim, H.O.; Kim, H.; Chun, H.-K.; et al. Risk factors for hemorrhoidal disease among healthy young and middle-aged Korean adults. *Sci. Rep.* **2022**, *12*, 129. [CrossRef]
11. Mir Mohammad, P.; Sadeghi, P.M.M.; Rabiee, M.; Darestani, N.G.; Alesaheb, F.; Zeinalkhani, F. Short term results of stapled versus conventional hemorrhoidectomy within 1 year follow-up. *Int. J. Burn. Trauma* **2021**, *11*, 69–74.
12. Sahin, M.; Emektar, E.; Kılıç, N.A.; Ozturk, D.; Bulus, H. The role of platelet parameters in thrombosed hemorrhoids. *J. Coloproctol.* **2020**, *40*, 362–367. [CrossRef]
13. Percalli, L.; Passalia, L.; Pricolo, R.; Riccò, M. Pre-operative assessment of internal mucosal rectal prolapse in internal hemorrhoids: Technical details and results from a single institution. *Acta Bio Medica Atenei Parm.* **2019**, *90*, 308–315. [CrossRef]
14. Salgueiro, P.; Caetano, A.C.; Oliveira, A.M.; Rosa, B.; Mascarenhas-Saraiva, M.; Ministro, P.; Amaro, P.; Godinho, R.; Coelho, R.; Gaio, R.; et al. Portuguese Society of Gastroenterology Consensus on the Diagnosis and Management of Hemorrhoidal Disease. *GE-Port. J. Gastroenterol.* **2020**, *27*, 90–102. [CrossRef] [PubMed]
15. Aigner, F.; Gruber, H.; Conrad, F.; Eder, J.; Wedel, T.; Zelger, B.; Engelhardt, V.; Lametschwandtner, A.; Wienert, V.; Böhler, U.; et al. Revised morphology and hemodynamics of the anorectal vascular plexus: Impact on the course of hemorrhoidal disease. *Int. J. Color. Dis.* **2009**, *24*, 105–113. [CrossRef]
16. Watson, A.J.; Cook, J.; Hudson, J.; Kilonzo, M.; Wood, J.; Bruhn, H.; Brown, S.; Buckley, B.; Curran, F.; Jayne, D.; et al. A pragmatic multicentre randomised controlled trial comparing stapled haemorrhoidopexy with traditional excisional surgery for haemorrhoidal disease: The eTHoS study. *Health Technol. Assess.* **2017**, *21*, 1–223. [CrossRef]
17. Roervik, H.D.; Styr, K.; Ilum, L.; McKinstry, G.L.; Dragesund, T.; Campos, A.H.; Brandstrup, B.; Olaison, G. Hemorrhoidal Disease Symptom Score and Short Health ScaleHD: New Tools to Evaluate Symptoms and Health-Related Quality of Life in Hemorrhoidal Disease. *Dis. Colon Rectum* **2019**, *62*, 333–342. [CrossRef]
18. Davis, B.R.; Lee-Kong, S.A.; Migaly, J.; Feingold, D.L.; Steele, S.R. The American Society of Colon and Rectal Surgeons Clinical Practice Guidelines for the Management of Hemorrhoids. *Dis. Colon Rectum* **2018**, *61*, 284–292. [CrossRef]
19. Maternini, M.; Guttadauro, A.; Chiarelli, M.; Bianco, G.L.; Pecora, N.; Gabrielli, F. Pervenuto in Redazione Dicembre 2018. *Ann. Ital. Chir.* **2018**, *89*, 101–106, pii:S0003469X1802818X.
20. Alonso-Burgos, A. Interventional Radiology Should be Competitive—If Haemorrhoids are Arteriovenous Connections, It is Now the Time for Liquids? Commentary on "Superior Rectal Artery Embolisation for Haemorrhoids: What do We Know so Far?". *Cardiovasc. Interv. Radiol.* **2021**, *44*, 686–688. [CrossRef]

21. Serra, R.; Gallelli, L.; Grande, R.; Amato, B.; De Caridi, G.; Sammarco, G.; Ferrari, F.; Butrico, L.; Gallo, G.; Rizzuto, A.; et al. Hemorrhoids and matrix metalloproteinases: A multicenter study on the predictive role of biomarkers. *Surgery* **2015**, *159*, 487–494. [CrossRef] [PubMed]
22. Labidi, A.; Maamouri, F.; Letaief-Ksontini, F.; Maghrebi, H.; Serghini, M.; Boubaker, J. Dietary habits asso-ciated with internal hemorrhoidal disease: A case-control study. *Tunis Med.* **2019**, *97*, 572–578. [PubMed]
23. Zheng, T.; Ellinghaus, D.; Juzenas, S.; Cossais, F.; Burmeister, G.; Mayr, G.; Jørgensen, I.F.; Teder-Laving, M.; Skogholt, A.H.; Chen, S.; et al. Genome-wide analysis of 944 133 individuals provides insights into the etiology of haemorrhoidal disease. *Gut* **2021**, *70*, 1538–1549. [CrossRef] [PubMed]
24. Said, O.; Khamaysi, I.; Kmail, A.; Sadiq, O.; Saied, B.; Fulder, S.; Abofarekh, B.; Masalha, M.; Amin, R.; Saad, B. Anti-Inflammatory, Antimicrobial, and Vasoconstriction Activities of an Anti-Hemorrhoidal Mixture of *Alchemilla vulgaris*, *Conyza bonariensis*, and *Nigella sativa*: In Vitro and Clinical Evaluations. *Immuno* **2022**, *2*, 132–150. [CrossRef]
25. Lee, K.-C.; Liu, C.-C.; Hu, W.-H.; Lu, C.-C.; Lin, S.-E.; Chen, H.-H. Risk of delayed bleeding after hemorrhoidectomy. *Int. J. Color. Dis.* **2019**, *34*, 247–253. [CrossRef]
26. Ng, K.-S.; Holzgang, M.; Young, C. Still a Case of "No Pain, No Gain"? An Updated and Critical Review of the Pathogenesis, Diagnosis, and Management Options for Hemorrhoids in 2020. *Ann. Coloproctol.* **2020**, *36*, 133–147. [CrossRef]
27. Willis, S.; Junge, K.; Ebrahimi, R.; Prescher, A.; Schumpelick, V. Haemorrhoids—A collagen disease? *Color. Dis.* **2010**, *12*, 1249–1253. [CrossRef] [PubMed]
28. Palumbo, V.D.; Tutino, R.; Messina, M.; Santarelli, M.; Nigro, C.; Lo Secco, G.; Piceni, C.; Montanari, E.; Barletta, G.; Venturelli, P.; et al. Altered Gut Microbic Flora and Haemorrhoids: Could They Have a Possible Relationship? *J. Clin. Med.* **2023**, *12*, 2198. [CrossRef]
29. Mehic, D.; Hofer, S.; Jungbauer, C.; Kaider, A.; Haslacher, H.; Eigenbauer, E.; Rejtő, J.; Schwartz, D.; Jilma, B.; Ay, C.; et al. Association of ABO blood group with bleeding severity in patients with bleeding of unknown cause. *Blood Adv.* **2020**, *4*, 5157–5164. [CrossRef]
30. Bayan, K.; Tüzün, Y.; Yılmaz, Ş.; Dursun, M.; Canoruc, F. Clarifying the Relationship Between ABO/Rhesus Blood Group Antigens and Upper Gastrointestinal Bleeding. *Dig. Dis. Sci.* **2009**, *54*, 1029–1034. [CrossRef]
31. Lin, W.-Y.; Hong, M.-Y.; Lin, C.-H.; Chang, P.-P.; Chu, S.-C.; Kao, C.-L. Association of ABO Blood Type with Bleeding Severity in Patients with Acute Gastroesophageal Variceal Bleeding. *Medicina* **2021**, *57*, 1323. [CrossRef]
32. Ewald, D.R.; Sumner, S.C. Blood type biochemistry and human disease. *Wiley Interdiscip. Rev. Syst. Biol. Med.* **2016**, *8*, 517–535. [CrossRef]
33. Langenbach, M.R.; Lisovets, R.; Varga-Szabo, D.; Bonicke, L. Decreased collagen ratio type I/III in association with hemorrhoidal disease. *J. Transl. Sci.* **2018**, *5*, 1–4. [CrossRef]
34. Sturiale, A.; Dowais, R.; Fabiani, B.; Menconi, C.; Porzio, F.C.; Coli, V.; Naldini, G. Long-term Outcomes of High-Volume Stapled Hemorroidopexy to Treat Symptomatic Hemorrhoidal Disease. *Ann. Coloproctol.* **2021**, *39*, 11–16. [CrossRef]
35. Kim, J.S. Partial Stapled Hemorrhoidopexy Versus Circular Stapled Hemorrhoidopexy. *Ann. Coloproctol.* **2017**, *33*, 7–8. [CrossRef]
36. Maemoto, R.; Tsujinaka, S.; Miyakura, Y.; Machida, E.; Fukui, T.; Kakizawa, N.; Tamaki, S.; Ishikawa, H.; Rikiyama, T. Effect of Antithrombotic Therapy on Secondary Bleeding After Proctological Surgery. *Cureus* **2021**, *13*. [CrossRef]
37. Kraemer, M.; Paulus, W.; Kara, D.; Mankewitz, S.; Rozsnoki, S. Rectal prolapse traumatizes rectal neuromuscular microstructure explaining persistent rectal dysfunction. *Int. J. Color. Dis.* **2016**, *31*, 1855–1861. [CrossRef] [PubMed]
38. Porrett, L.J.; Porrett, J.K.; Ho, Y.-H. Documented Complications of Staple Hemorroidopexy: A Systematic Review. *Int. Surg.* **2015**, *100*, 44–57. [CrossRef] [PubMed]
39. Plocek, M.D.; Kondylis, L.A.; Duhan-Floyd, N.; Reilly, J.C.; Geisler, D.P.; Kondylis, P.D. Hemorrhoidopexy Staple Line Height Predicts Return to Work. *Dis. Colon Rectum* **2006**, *49*, 1905–1909. [CrossRef] [PubMed]
40. Hong, Y.K.; Choi, Y.J.; Kang, J.G. Correlation of Histopathology with Anorectal Manometry Following Stapled Hemorrhoidopexy. *Ann. Coloproctol.* **2013**, *29*, 198–204. [CrossRef] [PubMed]
41. Eberspacher, C.; Magliocca, F.M.; Pontone, S.; Mascagni, P.; Fralleone, L.; Gallo, G.; Mascagni, D. Stapled Hemorroidopexy: "Mucosectomy or Not Only Mucosectomy, This Is the Problem". *Front. Surg.* **2021**, *8*, 655257. [CrossRef] [PubMed]
42. Abegaz, S.B. Human ABO Blood Groups and Their Associations with Different Diseases. *BioMed Res. Int.* **2021**, *2021*, 6629060. [CrossRef] [PubMed]
43. Groot, H.E.; Sierra, L.E.V.; Said, M.A.; Lipsic, E.; Karper, J.C.; van der Harst, P. Genetically Determined ABO Blood Group and its Associations with Health and Disease. *Arter. Thromb. Vasc. Biol.* **2020**, *40*, 830–838. [CrossRef] [PubMed]
44. Dahlén, T.; Clements, M.; Zhao, J.; Olsson, M.L.; Edgren, G. An agnostic study of associations between ABO and RhD blood group and phenome-wide disease risk. *Elife* **2021**, *10*, e65658. [CrossRef]
45. Yu, H.; Xu, N.; Li, Z.-K.; Xia, H.; Ren, H.-T.; Li, N.; Wei, J.-B.; Bao, H.-Z. Association of ABO Blood Groups and Risk of Gastric Cancer. *Scand. J. Surg.* **2019**, *109*, 309–313. [CrossRef]
46. Sardinas, C.; Díaz, D.; Oropeza, M.E.; Parrella, M.; Merheb, M. Rectal Prolapse due to Adenomatous Polyp: Case Report. *J. Hepatol. Gastrointest. Disord.* **2016**, *2*, 2. [CrossRef]
47. Deng, Y.-J.; Li, S.-L.; Jing, F.-Y.; Ma, L.-L.; Guo, L.-L.; Na, F.; An, S.-L.; Ye, Y.; Yang, J.-M.; Bao, M.; et al. Myofibrotic malformation vessels: Unique angiodysplasia toward the progression of hemorrhoidal disease. *Drug Des. Dev. Ther.* **2015**, *9*, 4649–4656. [CrossRef]

48. Symeonidis, D.; Spyridakis, M.; Zacharoulis, D.; Tzovaras, G.; Samara, A.A.; Valaroutsos, A.; Diamantis, A.; Tepetes, K. Milligan–Morgan hemorrhoidectomy vs. hemorrhoid artery ligation and recto-anal repair: A comparative study. *BMC Surg.* **2022**, *22*, 416. [CrossRef]
49. Matkovic, Z.; Zildzic, M. Colonoscopic Evaluation of Lower Gastrointestinal Bleeding (LGIB): Practical Approach. *Med Arch.* **2021**, *75*, 274–279. [CrossRef]
50. Cafaro, D.D.; Sturiale, D.A.; Sinicropi, D.M.S.; Onofrio, D.L.; Catalano, A.; Naldini, G. Topical Treatment with Bergamot Flavonoid-Based Gel in Post-Surgical Wounds after Hemorrhoidectomy: Preliminary Results. *Int. J. Innov. Res. Med. Sci.* **2022**, *7*, 33–36. [CrossRef]
51. Takahashi, Y.; Hayakawa, A.; Sano, R.; Fukuda, H.; Harada, M.; Kubo, R.; Okawa, T.; Kominato, Y. Histone deacetylase inhibitors suppress ACE2 and ABO simultaneously, suggesting a preventive potential against COVID-19. *Sci. Rep.* **2021**, *11*, 3379. [CrossRef]
52. Marano, G.; Vaglio, S.; Catalano, L.; Pupella, S.; Liumbruno, G.M.; Franchini, M. The Role of ABO Blood Type in Thrombosis Scoring Systems. *Semin. Thromb. Hemost.* **2017**, *43*, 525–529. [CrossRef] [PubMed]
53. Bade, N.A.; Kazma, J.M.; Amdur, R.L.; Ellis-Kahana, J.; Ahmadzia, H.K. Blood type association with bleeding outcomes at delivery in a large multi-center study. *J. Thromb. Thrombolysis* **2020**, *50*, 439–445. [CrossRef] [PubMed]
54. Albánez, S.; Ogiwara, K.; Michels, A.; Hopman, W.; Grabell, J.; James, P.; Lillicrap, D. Aging and ABO blood type influence von Willebrand factor and factor VIII levels through interrelated mechanisms. *J. Thromb. Haemost.* **2016**, *14*, 953–963. [CrossRef] [PubMed]
55. Slade, R.; Alikhan, R.; Wise, M.P.; Germain, L.; Stanworth, S.; Morgan, M. Impact of blood group on survival following critical illness: A single-centre retrospective observational study. *BMJ Open Respir. Res.* **2019**, *6*, e000426. [CrossRef] [PubMed]
56. Scheiner, B.; Northup, P.G.; Gruber, A.B.; Semmler, G.; Leitner, G.; Quehenberger, P.; Thaler, J.; Ay, C.; Trauner, M.; Reiberger, T.; et al. The impact of ABO blood type on the prevalence of portal vein thrombosis in patients with advanced chronic liver disease. *Liver Int.* **2020**, *40*, 1415–1426. [CrossRef] [PubMed]
57. Danilo, C.; Felipe, C.; Alessandro, S.; Stefania, S.M. Innovative results in the treatment of inespecific anusitis-proctitis with the use of bergamot gel (Benebeo gel)®. *Insights Clin. Cell. Immunol.* **2019**, *3*, 020–024. [CrossRef]
58. de Freitas, M.O.S.; Santos, J.A.D.; Figueiredo, M.F.S.; and Sampaio, C.A. Analysis of the main surgical techniques for hemorrhoids. *J. Coloproctol.* **2016**, *36*, 104–114. [CrossRef]
59. Naldini, G.; Caminati, F.; Sturiale, A.; Fabiani, B.; Cafaro, D.; Menconi, C.; Mascagni, D.; Celedon Porzio, F. Improvement in Hemorrhoidal Disease Surgery Outcomes Using a New Anatomical/Clinical–Therapeutic Classification (A/CTC). *Surg. J.* **2020**, *6*, e145–e152. [CrossRef]
60. Taieb, S.; Atienza, P.; Zeitoun, J.D.; Taouk, M.; Bourguignon, J.; Thomas, C.; Rabahi, N.; Dahlouk, S.; Lesage, A.C.; Lobo, D.; et al. Frequency and risk factors of severe postoperative bleeding after proctological surgery: A retrospective case-control study. *Ann. Coloproctol.* **2022**, *38*, 370–375. [CrossRef]
61. Yoo, B.E.; Kang, W.H.; Ko, Y.T.; Lee, Y.C.; Lim, C.H. The importance of compression time in stapled hemorrhoidopexy: Is patience a virtue? *Ann. Coloproctol.* **2022**, *20*, 1–6. [CrossRef]
62. Ratto, C.; de Parades, V. Doppler-guided ligation of hemorrhoidal arteries with mucopexy: A technique for the future. *J. Visc. Surg.* **2015**, *152*, S15–S21. [CrossRef]
63. Varut, P.S.; Shelygin, L.Y. Micronized Purified Flavonoid Fraction in Hemorrhoid Disease: A Systematic Review and Meta-Analysis. *Adv. Ther.* **2020**, *37*, 2792–2812. [CrossRef]
64. Loste, M.A.; de la Peña, J.; Terán, A. Patología inflamatoria de recto y ano. *Med.-Programa Form. Médica Contin. Acreditado* **2012**, *11*, 413–419. [CrossRef]
65. Li, Z.; Dong, S.; Huang, S.; Sun, Y.; Sun, Y.; Zhao, B.; Qi, Q.; Xiong, L.; Hong, F.; Jiang, Y. Role of CD34 in inflammatory bowel disease. *Front. Physiol.* **2023**, *14*, 1144980. [CrossRef] [PubMed]
66. Bahardoust, M.; Naghshin, R.; Mokhtare, M.; Hejrati, A.; Namdar, P.; Talebi, A.; Tavakoli, T.; Amiri, H.; Kiapey, S.H. Association between ABO Blood Group and Clinical Outcomes in Patients with Gastrointestinal Bleeding. *J. Clin. Cell. Immunol.* **2018**, *8*. [CrossRef]

Disclaimer/Publisher's Note: The statements, opinions and data contained in all publications are solely those of the individual author(s) and contributor(s) and not of MDPI and/or the editor(s). MDPI and/or the editor(s) disclaim responsibility for any injury to people or property resulting from any ideas, methods, instructions or products referred to in the content.

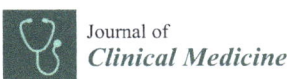

Article

Tunneling of Mesh during Ventral Rectopexy: Technical Aspects and Long-Term Functional Results

Paola Campennì [1], Angelo Alessandro Marra [1], Veronica De Simone [1], Francesco Litta [1], Angelo Parello [1] and Carlo Ratto [1,2,*]

[1] Proctology Unit, Fondazione Policlinico Universitario "Agostino Gemelli" IRCCS, 00168 Rome, Italy
[2] Department of Medicine and Translational Surgery, Università Cattolica del Sacro Cuore, 00168 Rome, Italy
* Correspondence: carloratto@tiscali.it; Tel.: +39-3356886968

Abstract: Avoiding the extensive damage of pelvic structures during ventral rectopexy could minimize secondary disfunctions. The objective of our observational study is to assess the safety and functional efficacy of a modified ventral rectopexy. In the modified ventral rectopexy, a retroperitoneal tunnel was created along the right side of rectum, connecting two peritoneal mini-incisions at the Douglas pouch and sacral promontory. The proximal edge of a polypropylene mesh, sutured over the ventral rectum, was pulled up through the retroperitoneal tunnel and fixed to the sacral promontory. In all patients, radiopaque clips were placed on the mesh, making it radiographically "visible". Before surgery and at follow up visits, Altomare, Longo, CCSS, PAC-SYM, and CCFI scores were collected. From March 2010 to September 2021, 117 patients underwent VR. Modified ventral rectopexy was performed in 65 patients, while the standard ventral rectopexy was performed in 52 patients. The open approach was used in 97 cases (55 and 42 patients in modified and standard VR, respectively), while MI surgery was used in 20 cases (10 and 10 patients in modified and standard VR, respectively). A slightly shorter operative time and hospital stay were observed following modified ventral rectopexy (though this was not statistically significant). Similar overall complication rates were registered in the modified vs. standard ventral rectopexies (4.6% vs. 5.8%, $p = 0.779$). At follow-up, the Longo score (14.0 ± 8.6 vs. 11.0 ± 8.2, $p = 0.042$) and "delta" values of Altomare (9.2 ± 6.1 vs. 5.9 ± 6.3, $p = 0.008$) and CCSS (8.4 ± 6.3 vs. 6.1 ± 6.1, $p = 0.037$) scores were significantly improved in the modified ventral rectopexy group. A similar occurrence of symptoms recurrence was diagnosed in the two groups. Radiopaque clips helped to accurately diagnose mesh detachment/dislocation. The proposed modified VR seems to be feasible and safe. Marking the mesh intraoperatively seems useful.

Keywords: ventral rectopexy; rectal prolapse; obstructed defecation syndrome; fecal incontinence; pelvic disorders

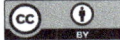

1. Introduction

Ventral rectopexy (VR) is an effective surgical option for the treatment of obstructed defecation syndrome (ODS) due to internal rectal prolapse (IRP), enterocele and rectocele, or external rectal prolapse (ERP). D'Hoore et al. [1] first described the VR procedure in patients with ERP, with VR progressively emerging as the procedure of choice for ERP [2–4]. To reduce the rectal-prolapse recurrence, several modifications of "standard" VR have been proposed, mainly concerning the mesh placement [5–8]. However, no superiority has been demonstrated. Since 2014, our group has modified the standard VR by introducing retroperitoneal tunneling of the mesh (preserving both lateral and utero-sacral ligaments) and marking the mesh with radiopaque clips (although radiopaque meshes are already provided), making it "radiologically visible" when mesh detachment or prolapse recurrence should be investigated. The aim of this study was to assess the feasibility and safety of the modified VR and to evaluate its long-term functional outcomes. The results observed in modified VR patients were compared with data from a control group of patients treated with standard VR.

2. Materials and Methods

2.1. Study Design

The study is reported according to the Strengthening the Reporting of Observational Studies in Epidemiology (STROBE) statement [9]. All patients gave their written, informed consent for data analysis. The study was approved by the ethical committee of the Institution Fondazione Policlinico Universitario Agostino Gemelli IRCCS, Rome, Italy (ID 2574).

Surgery was performed after a complete work-up that included the patient's history, validated questionnaires administration, a physical examination, and a radiological evaluation (dynamic evacuation proctography or MRI defecography) of the pelvic floor. All patients were discussed by a multidisciplinary pelvic team including proctologists, urogynecologists, and radiologists. All operations were performed by the same expert colorectal surgeon (C.R.).

Demographic data, operation time, hospital stay, and perioperative complications were collected retrospectively and gathered into a database. The recurrence of prolapse, rectocele and/or enterocele, and the functional results were assessed prospectively during the patients' follow-up visits at 1, 6, and 12 months and then annually.

2.2. Patients' Assessment

Patients' histories were accurately collected, specifically regarding defecation and urinary disorders, sexual activity impairments, and anatomic abnormalities of pelvic organs. Physical examinations were meticulously performed.

The severity of ODS was assessed by the following validated scoring systems, administered in a face-to-face interview: Altomare score (range: 0–32; no symptoms = 0) [10]; Longo score (range: 0–40; no symptoms = 0) [11]; Cleveland Clinic Constipation Scoring System or CCSS (range: 0–30; no symptoms = 0) [12]; Patient Assessment of Constipation-Symptoms questionnaire or PAC-SYM (including the assessment of twelve items assigned to three subscales, i.e., abdominal, stool, and rectal symptoms; scoring range for each item: 0–4; no symptoms = 0) [13]; and Fecal incontinence (FI) was assessed by the Cleveland Clinic Fecal Incontinence or CCFI score (range: 0–36, perfect continence = 0) [14].

Following the first visit, all patients underwent either a dynamic evacuation proctography or MRI defecography (using intra-rectal, intravaginal, and small bowel contrast, allowing their classification according to the Oxford rectal prolapse grading system) [15], an endoanal ultrasound and anorectal manometry. Colorectal screening was conducted in all cases with a colonoscopy. Indications for surgery were discussed by the multidisciplinary team.

2.3. Surgical Technique

Before 2014 (when the proposed new approach with the tunnelling of the mesh was introduced), the traditional technique using the inverted-J-shaped peritoneal incision was used; thereafter, the tunnelling of mesh was used in all patients. Similarly, when the MI approach was introduced in our experience (September 2018), the traditional technique of VR was used along the first period, and then the tunnelling of mesh was performed in all patients.

Preoperatively, bowel preparation (two enemas) and a single dose of broad-spectrum antibiotic were administrated.

Despite using either an open (LT, Pfannenstiel or umbilico-pubic incision) or minimally invasive (MI, robotic, or laparoscopic) approach to the pelvis, the bowel was retracted to the middle-upper abdomen to expose both the pouch of Douglas and the sacral promontory with the patient in the Trendelenburg position.

2.4. Modified VR: The Study Group

The modified VR approach provided a 5 cm peritoneal incision at the pouch of Douglas. Rectovaginal space was dissected up to the pelvic floor. The ventral rectum was fully exposed; in case of rectocele, particular attention was paid to the rectovaginal dissection to safely reach the perineum. A combined anorectal–vaginal digital examination confirmed the complete dissection. Any redundant pouch of Douglas was excised so that a longer tract of anterior rectum was available for mesh placement. A strip of polypropylene (Ethicon, Johnson & Johnson, Brussels, Belgium), trimmed to 10–14 cm, was introduced into the abdominal cavity; two radiopaque clips were previously placed on its distal edge. The mesh was sutured over the ventral rectum with a total of six 3-0 PDS sutures arranged. The two most proximal sutures were preserved for further fixation at the proximal vagina. The other two radiopaque clips were placed on mesh sides at the level of its proximal fixation over the rectum.

Thereafter, a small (2–3 cm) peritoneal incision was performed at the level of sacral promontory and the periosteum was freed, avoiding damages to the autonomic nerve fibers (Figure 1). A retroperitoneal tunnel from the promontory incision to the pelvic incision was accurately performed, avoiding damages to lateral and utero-sacral ligaments (Figure 2). The proximal mesh was then pulled up, reaching the sacral promontory. Under a gentle tension (in order to prevent future rectal intussusception and the persistence of rectocele), the mesh was fixed at the sacral promontory with two stitches of 2-0 PDS. Two clips were placed on the mesh and another one was placed on the sacral periosteum to allow for a further radiographic check of the mesh position at follow-up (Figure 3). The redundant mesh was trimmed. To prevent further enterocele, the posterior proximal vagina was approximated to the mesh using the two most proximal sutures left in place before. A full thickness passage with the needle through the posterior vaginal wall should be avoided. The peritoneal incisions were closed with V-loc sutures or absorbable running sutures. A video vignette of the modified VR using robotic approach is available. [16]

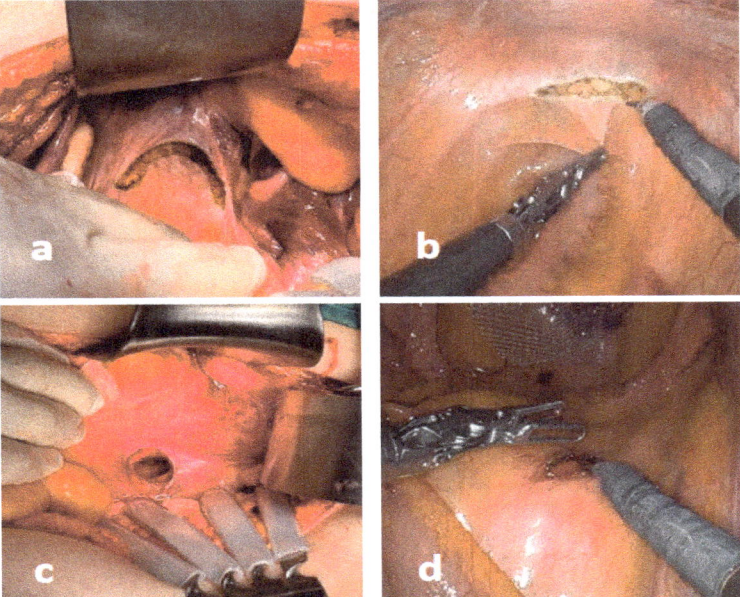

Figure 1. Peritoneal incisions were performed at the pouch of Douglas (**a**,**b**) and sacral promontory (**c**,**d**) in open and robotic surgery.

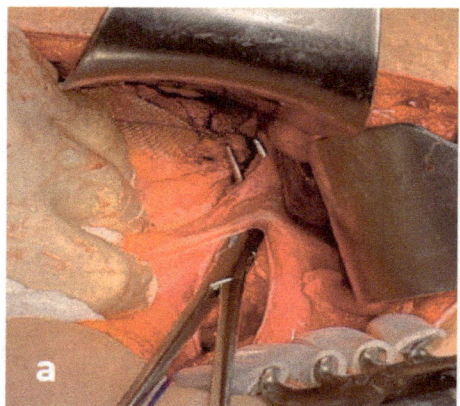
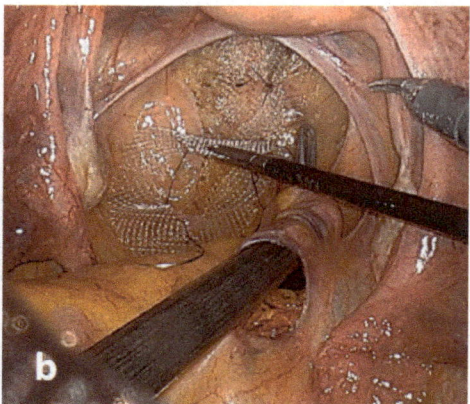

Figure 2. A retroperitoneal tunnel was created in open (**a**) and robotic (**b**) surgery.

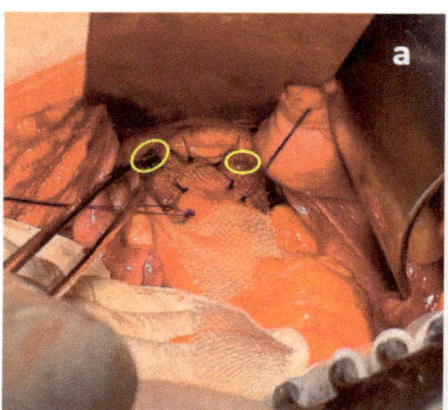
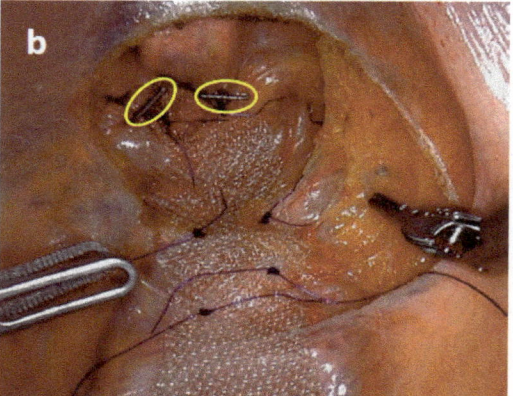

Figure 3. The mesh was sutured over the ventral rectum with three couples of 3-0 PDS stitches in open (**a**) and robotic (**b**) surgery. Two radiopaque clips were positioned at the distal edge of the mesh (circles).

2.5. Standard VR: The Control Group

A group of patients was treated with the "standard VR," provided an inverted-J-shaped incision of the pelvic peritoneum [1] and served as the control group. The recto-vaginal dissection, mesh conformation, placement, and fixation at the sacral promontory were all executed similarly to the modified VR.

2.6. Postoperative Management

Postoperatively, analgesics drugs were administered. A fiber-enriched diet was generally prescribed and resumed on the second postoperative day. Straining efforts were discouraged.

2.7. Data Collection

The mean duration of surgical procedure, intraoperative and postoperative complications (classified with Clavien–Dindo grade system) [17] and their management, conversion rate, postoperative hospital stay, and early reoperations (within 7 days) were analyzed. Follow-ups were scheduled at 1, 6, 12 months, and once a year thereafter. Postoperative symptoms were recorded, as in our daily clinical practice. Altomare, Longo, CCSS, PAC-SYM, and CCFI scores were completed under the supervision of a surgeon at each visit. Functional scores have usually been used in our clinical practice to evaluate and standardize the clinical approach to obstructed defecation syndrome. It is very useful during the first visit, when discussing the clinical case in the multidisciplinary team meeting and to evaluate the results after the treatment. In case of persistent constipation symptoms, patients were deeply investigated using a bowel transit study with radiopaque markers and dynamic evacuation proctography or MRI defecography. If a mesh detachment was suspected, a pelvic X-ray assessment (with antero-posterior, latero-lateral and oblique projections) was performed in order to check the position of the radiopaque clips placed at the operation.

2.8. Statistical Analysis

Continuous data were described as means with standard deviations and analyzed by the Wilcoxon and Mann–Whitney tests for paired and unpaired data, respectively. Categorical data were reported as frequencies and percentages and analyzed with a chi-squared test. Clinical scores in modified VR and standard VR patients were compared calculating the differences between preoperative and follow up values (delta-Δ). A p-value < 0.05 was considered to be significant. Data were analyzed using IBM SPSS Statistics for Windows, Version 25.0 (IBM Corp, Armonk, NY, USA).

3. Results

3.1. Demographic Data

From March 2010 to September 2021, 117 patients (116 females) underwent a VR, 38 (32.5%) and 79 (67.5%) for ERP and IRP, respectively. The mean age at the time of operation was 60.8 ± 12.8 years (range: 16 to 94 years). The modified VR was performed in 65 patients (19 patients with ERP, 46 patients with IRP) and the standard VR was performed in 52 patients (19 patients with ERP, 33 patients with IRP).

Further details concerning the clinico-pathological features of patients are reported in Table 1. Concerning patients' history, 85 patients (73.3%) had at least one vaginal delivery, 66 of them (56.9%) received an episiotomy and 26 (22.4%) reported an obstetric anal sphincter injury; 37 patients (31.9%) were submitted to a hysterectomy. Twenty-three patients (19.7%) were previously submitted to surgery for pelvic floor dysfunctions (Standard VR: 1 Orr-Loygue, 5 STARR, 3 Delorme, 1 Altemeier; Modified VR: 1 Orr-Loygue, 8 STARR, 4 Delorme), with poor outcomes. No difference was detected comparing the two groups.

Regarding clinical features (Table 1), 109 patients (93.2%) had significant impairment of physiologic defecation (including prolonged straining, unsuccessful attempts to defecate, self-digitation for defecation, incomplete evacuation or sensation of anorectal obstruction/blockage, and stool frequency >3 times/week); 72 patients (61.5%) referred symptoms of FI; and 64 patients (54.7%) suffered from both conditions. No statistically significant differences in preoperative clinical scores were reported between the two groups. Urinary incontinence was reported by 69 patients (59.0%), similarly across the two groups.

Patients' distribution according to the Oxford criteria provided: 11 (9.4%) high recto-rectal intussusceptions (grade 1); 17 (14.5%) low recto-rectal intussusceptions (grade 2); 31 (26.5%) recto-anal intussusceptions onto the anal canal (grade 3), 20 (17.1%) recto-anal intussusceptions into the anal canal (grade 4); and 38 (32.5%) ERPs (grade 5). If stratified in the two groups, this distribution revealed no statistical difference. Interestingly, FI was more frequent in patients with higher Oxford grades (65.2% in grades 4 and 5) in both the modified and standard VR groups (62.2% and 68.6%, respectively; p = 0.582).

Table 1. Baseline characteristics of patients who underwent modified and standard ventral rectopexy.

	Modified VR—n° (%)	Standard VR—n° (%)	p
Patients	65	52	
Female	65 (100.0)	51 (98.1)	0.262
Age (years) *	60.9 ± 12.0	60.7 ± 13.9	0.251
Previous abdominal surgery	39 (60.0)	32 (61.5)	0.866
Previous hysterectomy	19 (29.2)	18 (35.3)	0.487
Previous abdominal surgery for RP	1 (1.5)	1 (1.9)	0.873
Previous perineal surgery	26 (40.0)	21 (40.4)	0.966
Previous perineal surgery for RP	12 (18.5)	9 (17.3)	0.645
Vaginal delivery	45 (69.2)	40 (78.4)	0.266
Episiotomy	35 (53.8)	31 (60.8)	0.454
Obstetric anal sphincter injury	9 (13.8)	17 (33.3)	0.188
Forceps/vacuum	1 (1.5)	6 (11.8)	0.402
Caesarean delivery	13 (20.0)	10 (19.6)	0.958
Preoperative ODS	61 (93.8)	48 (92.3)	0.743
Preoperative FI	37 (56.9)	35 (67.3)	0.251
Preoperative ODS + FI	33 (50.8)	31 (59.6)	0.339
Preoperative UI	39 (60.0)	30 (57.7)	0.801
Oxford classification for RP			
Grade I	7 (10.8)	4 (7.7)	
Grade II	12 (18.5)	5 (9.6)	
Grade III	18 (27.7)	13 (25.0)	
Grade IV	9 (13.8)	11 (21.2)	
Grade V	19 (29.2)	19 (36.5)	
Rectocele	51 (78.5)	30 (57.7)	0.174
Enterocele	35 (53.8)	35 (67.3)	0.677

* Data are shown as mean ± standard deviation. VR = ventral rectopexy; RP = rectal prolapse; ODS = obstructed defecation syndrome; FI = fecal incontinence; UI = urinary incontinence.

3.2. Operation Data

The modified procedure was introduced in 2014 and it was performed in all patients who gave their written, informed consent. A standard rectopexy was performed in the first period of the study and when the patients denied the consent to the modified procedure.

The open approach was used in 97 cases (55 and 42 patients in modified and standard VR, respectively) while MI surgery was used in 20 cases (10 and 10 patients in modified and standard VR, respectively).

In the modified VR group, six patients (9.2%) needed a conversion to a conventional, inverted-J-shape peritoneal incision; among them, in four LT patients the decision was due to fibrotic tissue secondary to a previous pelvic surgery that made the retroperitoneal tunnelling technically difficult and at risk of damages to the right lateral ligament of the rectum; in two MI cases the conversion was due to bleeding from pelvic varicocele (safely managed intraoperatively) and pelvic adhesions, respectively (Supplementary Material, Table S1). During the modified VR, four patients (6.2%) underwent additional surgical procedures: two hemorrhoidectomies, one cystopexy, and one pelvic biopsy. In standard VRs, give patients (9.6%) were submitted to additional procedures: three hemorrhoidectomies, one colposacropexy and one pelvic biopsy.

Although shorter, no differences in the operative time (92.3 ± 26.8 vs. 94.7 ± 28.9 min, $p = 0.572$, and 133.5 ± 30.7 vs. 145.3 ± 27.2 min, $p = 0.657$, in patients who underwent LT and MI surgery, respectively) and hospital stay (3.1 ± 0.9 vs. 3.3 ± 1.0 days, $p = 0.114$) were observed between the modified and standard VR. An intraoperative complication (bleeding from a pelvic varicocele, controlled by bipolar forceps) was registered in one modified VR patient (0.9%). Five patients (4.3%) experienced postoperative complications: three hematomas, one seroma, one urinary infection (Clavien–Dindo grade ≤ 3). No mesh erosion was recorded. Comparing two groups, the overall complication rates were 4.6% (three patients) in the modified VR group and 5.8% (three patients) in the standard VR group ($p = 0.779$). There were neither re-operations during the primary admission nor perioperative mortalities. No chronic pelvic pain or major morbidities were reported in both VR groups.

3.3. Clinical Outcomes

The mean overall follow-up was 40.6 ± 33.1 months (24.3 ± 14.8 and 61.0 ± 38.2 in modified and standard VR, respectively). Following both modified and standard VR, all scores showed a significant reduction compared to baseline (Figure 4).

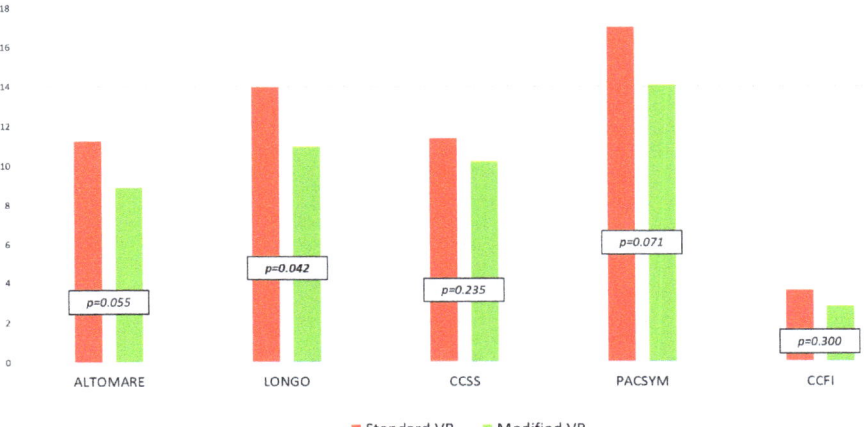

Figure 4. Comparison between postoperative values of clinical scores in patients who underwent standard vs. modified ventral rectopexy (Mann–Whitney U test). Altomare = Altomare score; Longo = Longo score; CCSS = Cleveland Clinic Constipation Scoring System; PACSYM = Patient Assessment of Constipation-Symptoms questionnaire; CCFI = Cleveland Clinic Fecal Incontinence score.

When comparing the long-term functional scores, the Longo score results were significantly improved after modified VR (p = 0.042). The decrease of the mean score from the preoperative to follow-up values (Δ) was always higher in the modified VR than in standard VR patients (Δ-Altomare score: 9.2 ± 6.1 vs. 5.9 ± 6.3, p = 0.008; Δ-Longo score: 11.5 ± 8.6 vs. 9.3 ± 9.0, p = 0.127; Δ-CCSS: 8.4 ± 6.3 vs. 6.1 ± 6.1, p = 0.037; Δ-PAC-SYM: 9.0 ± 9.4 vs. 6.7 ± 7.5, p = 0.059; Δ-CCFI score: 2.0 ± 3.6 vs. 1.7 ± 4.2, p = 0.900).

The comparison between pre- and postoperative values of clinical scores in patients with external rectal prolapse and internal rectal prolapse who underwent standard vs. modified ventral rectopexy is shown in Tables 2 and 3.

At the last follow up, 20 patients (17.1%) referred persistent constipation symptoms (12 modified VR patients, 18.5%; 8 standard VR patients, 15.4%; p = 0.660). All were re-evaluated by clinical and radiological examinations. In 13 cases (11.1%), slow-transit constipation was detected with a satisfying correction of preoperative pelvic organs prolapse; in 5 patients (4.3%), rectocele results were not completely corrected (2 modified VRs and 3 standard VRs). After evaluating the position of radiopaque clips placed intraoperatively with radiological imaging of the pelvis, a mesh detachment from the sacral promontory was diagnosed in 2 patients (1.7%, all standard VRs), probably due to severe and prolonged straining after surgery. These patients underwent surgical mesh re-fixation. Finally, 4 patients (3.4%) had new onset of FI. Preoperative urinary incontinence was reported in 69 patients (59.0%); 39 patients underwent modified VR and 30 patients underwent standard VR (p = 0.801). At the last follow-up, postoperative urinary incontinence was observed in 63 patients, 5 of which were cases de novo; 35 in the modified VR group and 28 in the standard VR group (p = 1.000).

Table 2. Comparison between pre- and postoperative values of clinical scores in patients with only internal rectal prolapse who underwent standard vs. modified ventral rectopexy (Mann–Whitney U test).

	Standard VR	SD	Modified VR	SD	p
Altomare pre	17.8	5.6	17.8	5.8	0.952
Longo pre	23.7	7.5	22.0	8.8	0.489
CCSS pre	18.2	4.9	18.7	5.4	0.383
PAC-SYM pre	23.9	5.5	23.2	5.6	0.643
CCFI pre	4.5	5.0	3.2	4.7	0.176
Altomare post	10.8	5.9	8.7	6.5	0.116
Longo post	13.5	7.8	10.5	8.4	0.050
CCSS post	11.4	5.4	10.0	6.3	0.289
PAC-SYM post	16.0	7.7	13.8	10.0	0.155
CCFI post	3.0	4.3	2.2	3.7	0.211

VR = ventral rectopexy; SD = standard deviation; Pre = preoperative; Post = postoperative; Altomare = Altomare score; Longo = Longo score; CCSS = Cleveland Clinic Constipation Scoring System; PAC-SYM = Patient Assessment of Constipation-Symptoms questionnaire; CCFI = Cleveland Clinic Fecal Incontinence score.

Table 3. Comparison between pre- and postoperative values of clinical scores in patients with only external rectal prolapse who underwent standard vs. modified ventral rectopexy (Mann–Whitney U test).

	Standard VR	SD	Modified VR	SD	p
Altomare pre	15.9	6.6	18.6	6.6	0.242
Longo pre	22.1	7.7	24.4	7.7	0.368
CCSS pre	16.3	6.2	19.0	4.6	0.106
PAC-SYM pre	23.8	7.4	23.7	5.8	0.927
CCFI pre	6.8	6.8	8.6	5.5	0.278
Altomare post	11.9	7.2	9.4	6.3	0.361
Longo post	14.9	10.2	12.2	7.6	0.447
CCSS post	11.2	6.4	10.5	5.8	0.703
PAC-SYM post	18.9	9.8	14.8	9.3	0.207
CCFI post	4.8	5.7	4.3	4.6	0.951

VR = ventral rectopexy; SD = standard deviation; Pre = preoperative; Post = postoperative; Altomare = Altomare score; Longo = Longo score; CCSS = Cleveland Clinic Constipation Scoring System; PAC-SYM = Patient Assessment of Constipation-Symptoms questionnaire; CCFI = Cleveland Clinic Fecal Incontinence score.

4. Discussion

VR is increasingly favored in the treatment of ERP and has been strongly proposed also for the IRP [18]. Although the literature is not conclusive, the evidence suggests that it is significantly better than posterior rectal prolapse repairs [19]. Its efficacy in regaining the anatomical position of pelvic organs has been largely documented. Moreover, when compared with the procedures using a posterior approach, the VR presents several opportunities: effective management of ERP or IRP; rectocele (even very large), and enterocele (by approximation of posterior vaginal wall to the mesh and ventral rectal wall); and availability for an integrated management of a central or anterior pelvic prolapse (i.e., with colposacropexy).

Although the primary purpose of rectal prolapse surgery would be the correction of the anatomical alterations of the rectum and surrounding structures, the improvement of anatomy does not systematically correspond to improving function due to several factors, some of them occult. The anatomical integrity of fundamental pelvic structures should be preserved, including the entire rectal wall, vascular and nerve supplies (passing through the lateral ligament of the rectum), and pelvic supportive structures, in particular the uterosacral ligaments. Standard VR (providing a long, inverted-J-shaped peritoneal incision) could be at risk of damage to the right lateral rectal and utero-sacral ligament.

The importance of lateral ligament preservation has been strongly highlighted: they contain autonomic nerves and are fundamental for the rectal motility. Their section/injury could lead to postoperative constipation and dyschezia following surgery (for neoplastic and non-neoplastic rectal diseases), including posterior and postero-lateral rectopexy procedures [20].

Recently, Petros has highlighted the role of utero-sacral ligaments in the biomechanics of pelvic floor organs prolapse [21]. Their pathologic progressive elongation may cause severe uterine prolapse. Moreover, they would progressively splay laterally, causing an enterocele and carrying the lateral rectal wall with them. The wider and weaker anterior rectal wall, due to its lateral stretching [22–24], would favor the rectal intussusception. Consequently, the anatomical distortion of the rectum would severely impact its biomechanical properties with significant functional impairments. All these etiopathogenetic events should strongly induce to spare the fundamental pelvic structures during surgery. However, in our opinion, the solution proposed by Petros (i.e., a posterior intravaginal slingplasty operation) would not seem to fit the purpose of an effective management of ERP and IRP. On the other hand, VR has demonstrated to be effective in regaining a correct anatomical organ configuration in the posterior-middle pelvic compartments, leading to significant functional improvements. Unfortunately, the heterogeneity in patient selections and pre- or postoperative assessments makes it impossible to compare the clinical results reported in literature. Among numerous studies published, only one randomized clinical trial compared laparoscopic VR and suture posterior rectopexy for ERP: the former approach gave a lower recurrence rate (8.8% vs. 23.3%) but was not statistically significant ($p = 0.111$), probably due to the small number of studied patients [25]. In a review of 26 studies on laparoscopic VR for ERP and IRP, the improvement of obstructed defecation ranged between 52% and 93%, and that of FI between 48% and 93%. On the contrary, persistent obstructed defecation symptoms may range from 2.6 to 20% [26]. A systematic review and meta-analysis of fourteen studies on laparoscopic VR for IRP reported a weighted complication rate of 13.6% and a mean recurrence of 6.5%. The main causes of recurrence were the incomplete dissection of anterior rectal wall and inadequate mesh fixation and/or position [27]. Later, another systematic review and meta-analysis by Emile et al. [28] on seventeen studies of 1242 patients submitted to a laparoscopic VR for ERP reported a weighted mean improvement of constipation in 71.0% and fecal continence in 79.3% of patients.

The reasons for symptom recurrence are not fully understood, and its predictors are still being investigated [28]. These might include multifactorial pathogenesis of constipation (drugs, depression, anxiety, obesity, etc.), coexistence of a slow-transit bowel constipation, and some technical aspects of surgery regarding the deepness of pelvic dissection, and the mesh chosen and its placement modality, tension, and fixation.

We have perfected the open technique and, more recently, we have also applied it to minimally invasive surgery. Our proposal seeks to improve such good data obtained with standard VR.

Reducing the length of peritoneal incision (splitting the single long peritoneal incision into two small incisions) would decrease the risk of possible iatrogenic damages to both the lateral rectal and utero-sacral ligaments. Although neither prospectively nor randomly performed (significant limitation for this study), the patients' selection to the operation was homogenous: preoperative patients' characteristics were similar in both standard and modified VRs in terms of clinico-pathological features and distribution, according to Oxford criteria. The two groups were also similar concerning the preoperative rectal prolapse type (ERP vs. IRP) and the surgical approach chosen (LT vs. MI).

Although other limitations (including the discrepancy of follow-up—which was longer for standard than for modified VRs—and the later adoption of the new technique of mesh tunnelling both in LT and MI groups), the adoption of modified VR was safe, with a low morbidity rate and limited recourse to conversion toward standard "inversed-J" peritoneal incision. The proposed modified VR obtained a slight reduction (not statistically significant) in operative time and postoperative hospital stay. A larger experience could further improve such results.

Concerning both ODS and FI, both the standard and modified VRs showed significant improvements in the severity of patients' symptoms. The modified VR produced a significantly lower Longo score ($p = 0.042$), and higher "Δ" of Altomare and CCSS scores ($p = 0.008$ and $p = 0.037$, respectively) between baseline and follow-up values, confirming a good trend of modified VR. When comparing the functional results for the two proposed rectopexy techniques, both techniques seem to be effective. This does not allow us to demonstrate a certain advantage of the modified approach, but certainly it seems to be a surgical option to be considered and studied further.

Interestingly, the adoption of marking the mesh with a few radiopaque clips during the operation allowed for its identification in follow-up. When a mesh detachment/dislocation was suspected, a simple pelvic X-ray series addressed the repair when confirmed, or to avoid a useless surgery when denied.

5. Conclusions

The retroperitoneal tunneling of mesh during the proposed, modified VR appears to be feasible and safe. Its long-term clinical results seem to be promising but without a great functional improvement. Further large and multicentric randomized trials will verify and clarify its role in managing ERP and IRP. Suspicious mesh detachment/dislocation can be settled simply and easily radiographically checking the position of intraoperatively placed radiopaque clips.

Supplementary Materials: The following supporting information can be downloaded at: https://www.mdpi.com/article/10.3390/jcm12010294/s1, Table S1: Patients' distribution between standard and modified ventral rectopexy in open and minimally invasive surgery.

Author Contributions: Conceptualization, P.C. and C.R.; data curation, V.D.S., A.A.M., F.L. and A.P.; formal analysis, A.A.M. and A.P.; investigation, P.C. and V.D.S.; methodology, P.C., A.A.M., A.P., F.L., V.D.S. and C.R.; project administration, P.C. and C.R.; validation, P.C. and C.R.; writing—original draft, P.C. and C.R.; writing—review & editing, P.C. All authors have read and agreed to the published version of the manuscript.

Funding: This research received no external funding.

Institutional Review Board Statement: This study was approved by the ethical committee of the Fondazione Policlinico Universitario "Agostino Gemelli" IRCCS, Rome, Italy; code: 2574.

Informed Consent Statement: The study protocol was approved by our local Ethics Committee and an informed written consent form was signed by patients.

Data Availability Statement: The data presented in this study are available on request from the corresponding author.

Acknowledgments: We thank Kelly Baron for English-language editing of this manuscript.

Conflicts of Interest: The authors declare no conflict of interest.

References

1. D'Hoore, A.; Cadoni, R.; Penninckx, F. Long-term outcome of laparoscopic ventral rectopexy for total rectal prolapse. *Br. J. Surg.* **2004**, *91*, 1500–1505. [CrossRef] [PubMed]
2. Wijffels, N.; Cunningham, C.; Dixon, A.; Greenslade, G.; Lindsey, I. Laparoscopic ventral rectopexy for external rectal prolapse is safe and effective in the elderly. Does this make perineal procedures obsolete? *Color. Dis. Off. J. Assoc. Coloproctol. Great Br. Irel.* **2011**, *13*, 561–566. [CrossRef] [PubMed]
3. Gouvas, N.; Georgiou, P.A.; Agalianos, C.; Tan, E.; Tekkis, P.; Dervenis, C.; Xynos, E. Ventral colporectopexy for overt rectal prolapse and obstructed defaecation syndrome: A systematic review. *Color. Dis.* **2015**, *17*, O34–O46. [CrossRef] [PubMed]
4. Mercer-Jones, M.A.; Brown, S.R.; Knowles, C.H.; Williams, A.B. Position statement by the Pelvic Floor Society on behalf of the Association of Coloproctology of Great Britain and Ireland on the use of mesh in ventral mesh rectopexy. *Color. Dis.* **2020**, *22*, 1429–1435. [CrossRef]
5. Auguste, T.; Dubreuil, A.; Bost, R.; Bonaz, B.; Faucheron, J.L. Technical and functional results after laparoscopic rectopexy to the promontory for complete rectal prolapse. Prospective study in 54 consecutive patients. *Gastroenterol. Clin. Biol.* **2006**, *30*, 659–663. [CrossRef]

6. Sileri, P.; Capuano, I.; Franceschilli, L.; Giorgi, F.; Gaspari, A.L. Modified laparoscopic ventral mesh rectopexy. *Techol. Coloproctol.* **2014**, *18*, 591–594. [CrossRef]
7. Mäkelä-Kaikkonen, J.; Rautio, T.; Klintrup, K.; Takala, H.; Vierimaa, M.; Ohtonen, P.; Mäkelä, J. Robotic-assisted and laparoscopic ventral rectopexy in the treatment of rectal prolapse: A matched-pairs study of operative details and complications. *Techol. Coloproctol.* **2014**, *18*, 151–155. [CrossRef]
8. Mantoo, S.; Podevin, J.; Regenet, N.; Rigaud, J.; Lehur, P.A.; Meurette, G. Is robotic-assisted ventral mesh rectopexy superior to laparoscopic ventral mesh rectopexy in the management of obstructed defaecation? *Color. Dis.* **2013**, *15*, e469–e475. [CrossRef]
9. von Elm, E.; Altman, D.G.; Egger, M.; Pocock, S.J.; Gøtzsche, P.C.; Vandenbroucke, J.P. STROBE Initiative The Strengthening the Reporting of Observational Studies in Epidemiology (STROBE) Statement: Guidelines for reporting observational studies. *Int. J. Surg.* **2014**, *12*, 1495–1499. [CrossRef]
10. Altomare, D.F.; Spazzafumo, L.; Rinaldi, M.; Dodi, G.; Ghiselli, R.; Piloni, V. Set-up and statistical validation of a new scoring system for obstructed defaecation syndrome. *Color. Dis.* **2008**, *10*, 84–88. [CrossRef]
11. Jayne, D.G.; Schwandner, O.; Stuto, A. Stapled transanal rectal resection for obstructed defecation syndrome: One-year results of the European STARR Registry. *Dis. Colon Rectum* **2009**, *52*, 1205–1214. [CrossRef] [PubMed]
12. Agachan, F.; Chen, T.; Pfeifer, J.; Reissman, P.; Wexner, S.D. A constipation scoring system to simplify evaluation and management of constipated patients. *Dis. Colon Rectum* **1996**, *39*, 681–685. [CrossRef]
13. Frank, L.; Kleinman, L.; Farup, C.; Taylor, L.; Miner, P., Jr. Psychometric validation of a constipation symptom assessment questionnaire. *Scand. J. Gastroenterol.* **1999**, *34*, 870–877. [CrossRef] [PubMed]
14. Jorge, J.M.; Wexner, S.D. Etiology and management of fecal incontinence. *Dis. Colon Rectum* **1993**, *36*, 77–97. [CrossRef] [PubMed]
15. Wijffels, N.A.; Collinson, R.; Cunningham, C.; Lindsey, I. What is the natural history of internal rectal prolapse? *Color. Dis.* **2010**, *12*, 822–830. [CrossRef] [PubMed]
16. Ratto, C.; Marra, A.A.; Campennì, P.; De Simone, V.; Litta, F.; Parello, A. Modified robotic ventral mesh rectopexy—A video vignette. *Color. Dis.* **2022**, *24*, 142. [CrossRef] [PubMed]
17. Dindo, D.; Demartines, N.; Clavien, P.A. Classification of surgical complications: A new proposal with evaluation in a cohort of 6336 patients and results of a survey. *Ann. Surg.* **2004**, *240*, 205–213. [CrossRef]
18. Picciariello, A.; O'Connell, P.R.; Hahnloser, D.; Gallo, G.; Munoz-Duyos, A.; Schwandner, O.; Sileri, P.; Milito, G.; Riss, S.; Boccasanta, P.A.; et al. Obstructed defaecation syndrome: European consensus guidelines on the surgical management. *Br. J. Surg.* **2021**, *108*, 1149–1153. [CrossRef]
19. Bordeianou, L.; Paquette, I.; Johnson, E.; Holubar, S.D.; Gaertner, W.; Feingold, D.L.; Steele, S.R. Clinical Practice Guidelines for the Treatment of Rectal Prolapse. *Dis. Colon Rectum* **2017**, *60*, 1121–1131. [CrossRef]
20. Bachoo, P.; Brazzelli, M.; Grant, A. Surgery for complete rectal prolapse in adults. *Cochrane Database Syst. Rev.* **2000**, *2*, CD001758. [CrossRef]
21. Petros, P. The biomechanics of uterine prolapse impact rectal intussusception, ODS and surgical restoration. *Techol. Coloproctol.* **2022**, *26*, 161–162. [CrossRef] [PubMed]
22. Brunenieks, I.; Pekarska, K.; Kasyanov, V.; Groma, V. Biomechanical and morphological peculiarities of the rectum in patients with obstructed defecation syndrome. *Rom. J. Morphol. Embryol. Rev. Roum. Morphol. Embryol.* **2017**, *58*, 1193–1200.
23. Ren, X.H.; Yaseen, S.M.; Cao, Y.L.; Liu, W.C.; Shrestha, S.; Ding, Z.; Wu, Y.H.; Zheng, K.Y.; Qian, Q.; Jiang, C.Q. A transanal procedure using TST STARR Plus for the treatment of Obstructed Defecation Syndrome: 'A mid-term study'. *Int. J. Surg.* **2016**, *32*, 58–64. [CrossRef] [PubMed]
24. Siri, S.; Zhao, Y.; Maier, F.; Pierce, D.M.; Feng, B. The Macro-and Micro-Mechanics of the Colon and Rectum I: Experimental Evidence. *Bioengineering* **2020**, *7*, 130. [CrossRef]
25. Hidaka, J.; Elfeki, H.; Duelund-Jakobsen, J.; Laurberg, S.; Lundby, L. Functional Outcome after Laparoscopic Posterior Sutured Rectopexy Versus Ventral Mesh Rectopexy for Rectal Prolapse: Six-year Follow-up of a Double-blind, Randomized Single-center Study. *EClinicalMedicine* **2019**, *16*, 18–22. [CrossRef]
26. van Iersel, J.J.; Paulides, T.J.; Verheijen, P.M.; Lumley, J.W.; Broeders, I.A.; Consten, E.C. Current status of laparoscopic and robotic ventral mesh rectopexy for external and internal rectal prolapse. *World J. Gastroenterol.* **2016**, *22*, 4977–4987. [CrossRef]
27. Emile, S.H.; Elfeki, H.A.; Youssef, M.; Farid, M.; Wexner, S.D. Abdominal rectopexy for the treatment of internal rectal prolapse: A systematic review and meta-analysis. *Color. Dis.* **2017**, *19*, O13–O24. [CrossRef]
28. Emile, S.H.; Elfeki, H.; Shalaby, M.; Sakr, A.; Sileri, P.; Wexner, S.D. Outcome of laparoscopic ventral mesh rectopexy for full-thickness external rectal prolapse: A systematic review, meta-analysis, and meta-regression analysis of the predictors for recurrence. *Surg. Endosc.* **2019**, *33*, 2444–2455. [CrossRef]

Disclaimer/Publisher's Note: The statements, opinions and data contained in all publications are solely those of the individual author(s) and contributor(s) and not of MDPI and/or the editor(s). MDPI and/or the editor(s) disclaim responsibility for any injury to people or property resulting from any ideas, methods, instructions or products referred to in the content.

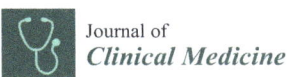

Article

The Emborrhoid Technique for Treatment of Bleeding Hemorrhoids in Patients with High Surgical Risk†

Paola Campennì [1], Roberto Iezzi [2,3], Angelo Alessandro Marra [1], Alessandro Posa [2], Angelo Parello [1], Francesco Litta [1], Veronica De Simone [1] and Carlo Ratto [1,3,*]

1. Proctology Unit, Fondazione Policlinico Universitario Agostino Gemelli—IRCCS, 00168 Rome, Italy
2. Dipartimento di Diagnostica per Immagini, Radioterapia Oncologica ed Ematologia, Istituto di Radiologia, Fondazione Policlinico Universitario Agostino Gemelli—IRCCS, 00168 Rome, Italy
3. Department of Medicine and Translational Surgery, Università Cattolica del Sacro Cuore, 00168 Rome, Italy
* Correspondence: carlo.ratto@policlinicogemelli.it; Tel.: +39-335-688-6968
† The abstract was a Plenary Presentation during the upcoming Annual Scientific Meeting of the American Society of Colon and Rectal Surgeons, in the "Abstract Session: Health Services Research", 30 April–4 May 2022, Tampa, FL, USA.

Abstract: The Emborrhoid is an innovative non-surgical technique for the treatment of severe hemorrhoidal bleeding. Patient selection and the impact on quality of life have not been fully investigated. This prospective observational study aims to evaluate the clinical outcomes after Emborrhoid in patients with high surgical risk. All patients with high surgical risk and anemia due to hemorrhoids were enrolled. Clinical data and previous blood transfusions were collected. The Hemorrhoidal Disease Symptom Score and Short Health Scala were completed before the procedure and during the follow-up visits at 1, 6 and 12 months. Transfusions and serum hemoglobin level variations were registered. Perioperative complications and the recurrence of bleeding were assessed. Trans-radial/femoral embolization of superior rectal artery, and/or middle rectal artery was performed with Interlock and Detachable Embolization Coils. From September 2020 to February 2022, 21 patients underwent a superselective embolization of all branches of the superior rectal artery. The transradial approach was most frequently performed compared to transfemoral access. After the procedure, no signs of ischemia were identified; three minor complications were observed. The mean follow-up was 18.5 ± 6.0 months. At the last follow-up, the mean increase of hemoglobin for patients was 1.2 ± 1.6 g/dL. Three patients needed transfusions during follow-up for recurrent hemorrhoidal bleeding. The Hemorrhoidal Disease Symptom Score and Short Health Scala decreased from 11.1 ± 4.2 to 4.7 ± 4.6 ($p < 0.0001$) and from 18.8 ± 4.8 to 10.2 ± 4.9 ($p < 0.0001$), respectively. Patients who had given up on their daily activities due to anemia have returned to their previous lifestyle. Emborrhoid seems to be a safe and effective option for the treatment of bleeding hemorrhoids in frail patients. The low complication rate and the significant reduction of post-defecation bleeding episodes are related to the improvement of the hemorrhoidal symptoms and patients' quality of life.

Keywords: Emborrhoid technique; arterial embolization; hemorrhoidal disease; hemorrhoidal bleeding

1. Background

Rectal bleeding is one of the main chronic symptoms of hemorrhoidal disease that severely affects patients' quality of life. It can cause severe anemia and drastically compromise the general state of health, especially in more frail patients. In order to reduce hemorrhoidal bleeding, phlebotonics and/or topical treatments (corticosteroids or anti-inflammatory agents) often represent the first therapeutic approaches, such us the office-based procedures (rubber band ligation, infrared photocoagulation, radiofrequency and sclerotherapy). These treatments are highly well tolerated, with a low complication rate, but often provide only short-term relief [1,2].

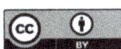

In all failures of the conservative management and severe anemia, surgery has to be considered. Several techniques have been proposed to treat symptomatic hemorrhoids, and the Doppler-guided hemorrhoidal artery ligation procedure (DG-HAL) is one of the most frequent minimally invasive approaches used [3,4]. The physiopathologic impact of DG-HAL on hemorrhoidal hyperflow is demonstrated by our recent study, which analyzed the hemodynamic effects after 12 months from the dearterialization. The study confirmed a significant decrease of the mean residual peak systolic velocity, pulsatility index and resistivity index with a drastic reduction of bleeding episodes [5].

Variable long-term results regarding the DG-HAL are reported in the literature, probably due to differences in the devices and stitches used, number and height of arterial ligations [6,7].

Based on the same principles, more recently, the Emborrhoid technique has proposed to perform a superselective endovascular occlusion of the terminal branches of the superior and middle rectal arteries. It is an innovative non-surgical technique for the treatment of severe hemorrhoidal bleeding [8].

Thus far, several studies have been published that include patients with heterogeneous baseline characteristics in terms of: hemorrhoidal disease degree, severity of bleeding and patient comorbidities. Clinical indication to perform Emborrhoid, patient selection, and its long-term impact have not been fully investigated [9].

The main objectives of our prospective study were to increase data regarding safety and efficacy of the Emborrhoid technique in frail patients with anemia and to assess the changes of hemorrhoidal disease symptoms and its impact on patients' quality of life.

2. Materials and Methods

2.1. Study Design and Study Population

The study is reported according to the Strengthening the Reporting of Observational Studies in Epidemiology (STROBE) statement for cohort studies [10]. It was approved by the ethical committee of the Fondazione Policlinico Universitario Agostino Gemelli IRCCS, Rome, Italy; code: 3705.

From September 2020 to February 2022, all consecutive patients with bleeding hemorrhoids and anemia were evaluated to be enrolled in this prospective observational single-center study. All patients gave their written informed consent.

Demographic data, patient's history, laboratory exams and previous blood transfusions were collected during the first visit. Therefore, a complete preoperative work-up (physical examination, endoscopy, and unenhanced and contrast-medium enhanced abdominal angio-CT) was performed in order to evaluate inclusion/exclusion criteria.

Therefore, all patients underwent a multidisciplinary pre-evaluation by the colorectal surgeons, the interventional radiologists, anesthesiologist and cardiologist to assess the risks and share the indication.

We included only patients older than 18 years of age and affected by symptomatic hemorrhoidal disease with anaemia and high surgical risk due to severe cardiovascular, respiratory and neurological disorders, cirrhosis/portal hypertension, antiplatelet and/or anticoagulant therapy and ASA ≥ 3. Patients ineligible for hemorrhoidal surgery with contraindication to general and/or spinal anaesthesia, or in the case of anal stenosis, were also considered for the protocol. If patients were on anticoagulants, they had to be able to stop medication temporarily prior to transarterial chemoembolization to obtain an INR < 1.5 at the time of the procedure.

On the other hand, we considered as exclusion criteria the following conditions:

Platelet count < 40,000/μL and/or international normalized ratio > 1.5, severe renal impairment, severe allergy or intolerance to any contrast media or chemotherapeutic drugs not controlled with medication, no available vascular access and/or absence of pulse in femoral or radial arteries, previous rectosigmoid resection, diagnosis of colorectal cancer, colonic angiodysplasia, inflammatory bowel disease, proctitis, or acute anorectal sepsis and family, psychological, social, or geographical circumstances preventing the patients from undergoing follow-up and from complying with protocol procedures.

2.2. Treatment

All treatments were performed by two experienced interventional radiologists (with more than 5 and 15 years of experience), using patient monitoring and anaesthesiologist assistance, in an angiographic suite with characteristics of an operating room. No antibiotic was administered before or after the procedure. Diagnostic angiography was performed under local anaesthesia (10 mL Lidocaine) using the Seldinger technique through the femoral or radial artery (based on operator preference for a single case) with a 5 Fr introducer sheath. Superselective catheterization of the superior rectal arteries was then performed using a coaxial technique, placing a 2.4 or 2.7 Fr Progreat microcatheter (Radifocus, Terumo, Rome, Italy). The coils used for the embolization were Interlock and IDC detachable embolization coils, to offer precision and control combined with thrombogenicity and flexibility, ranging between 4 and 7 mm in diameter, and 10–20 cm long (Boston Scientific, Marlborough, MA, USA). Also evaluated were all potential anastomoses with other feeder arteries (middle rectal or inferior rectal branches), advancing the 5 Fr Optitorque Multipurpose in the iliac internal artery and carrying out superselective injection into each branch using a coaxial technique with the same microcatheter. The anastomoses identified were embolized only in the cases in which they were among the main arteries feeding the hemorrhoidal plexus. All patients underwent haemostasis of the puncture site (radial or femoral). They were observed for 2 h (in the case of the transradial approach) or 6–8 h (in the case of the transfemoral approach) and discharged, if no complications arose, within 24 h (only in the case of the radial approach) or 48 h. Patients who had undergone the radial approach were managed in an outpatient setting, as reported in our previous pilot study [11].

Treatments needed to resolve any complications and recurrences were recorded.

Perioperative minor/major complications and death occurring within seven days from the treatment were evaluated and categorized according to the common terminology criteria for adverse event [12].

2.3. Endpoints and Definitions

The aim of our study is to report data on safety, efficacy and patients' quality of life after the Emborrhoid technique in patients unsuitable for surgery with severe anemia due to hemorrhoidal bleeding. Technical success was defined as the correct and complete coil deployment, with a complete lack of opacification of the terminal branches of the superior/middle rectal arteries.

Major complications were defined as events determining substantial morbidity and disability, increased level of care, or lengthened hospital stay; all other complications were considered minor.

Follow-up was scheduled at 1, 6 and 12 months, and once a year thereafter, including a physical examination and a pulse check at the vascular access site.

Transfusions and serum hemoglobin level variations were registered at 6 and 12 months. Patients who experienced new onset of anemia during the follow-up were regarded as a treatment failure.

The Hemorrhoidal Disease Symptom Score (HDSS) and Short Health Scale (SHS) [13] were completed before the procedure after 1 month, 6 months and 1 year during control visits or via telephone interviews. The HDSS is based on five different parameters characterizing the hemorrhoidal disease, with a grading from 0 (no symptoms) to 4 (daily presence) for each symptom. The total score of all five parameters was used to evaluate the patient's condition: 0 indicated the total absence of a symptom, while a score of 20 represented the worst clinical conditions. The SHS is a QoL-based score that includes information on symptoms severity, impact on daily activities, patients' concerns, and personal feeling of well-being ranging from 1 (optimal clinical conditions) to 28 (worst clinical scenario). They have been validated only in the English language and have been internally translated for clinical practice. As a mitigation, surgeons were present to guarantee adequate comprehension of the questions.

2.4. Statistical Analysis

Continuous variables were reported as mean and standard deviation. Categorical variables were described by count and percentage. Comparisons between groups were performed using the Wilcoxon test for continuous variables and the Fisher exact test for categorical data. Statistical significance was defined for $p < 0.05$.

Statistical analysis was performed with SPSS statistics for Windows version 23.0 software (IBM, Armonk, NY, USA).

3. Results

From September 2020 to February 2022, 24 patients were evaluated for embolization. After complete pre-treatment work-up, three patients were excluded from our protocol, in particular, two patients for severe heart failure and one patient due to right colon cancer.

3.1. Patients Characteristics

After multidisciplinary discussion, 21 patients with high surgical risk (16 male, 76.2%; mean age 72.2 ± 10.9 range 47–92 years) were candidates for Emborrhoid. As highlighted in Table 1, 18 patients were affected also by severe cardiovascular disease, six patients presented with obstructive pulmonary disease, two patients had hematologic or immunological disorders, five patients had mild chronic kidney failure, obesity plus metabolic syndrome in 17 patients, and one case of paraplegia. Nine patients were in anticoagulant therapy, six in antiplatelet therapy and one in anticoagulant plus antiplatelet therapy. Six patients (28.6%) had previously undergone a hemorrhoidectomy and presented with recurrence of bleeding. According to Goligher's classification, II degree was identified in eight patients, III degree in 10 and IV degree in three cases. Flavonoids and iron were already used by 95.2% of patients. Nineteen (90.5%) patients were referred for daily post-defecation bleeding. Pre-treatment blood transfusions were required for 52.4% of patients with severe anemia.

Table 1. Baseline patients' characteristics.

	n (%)
Patients	21
Ratio M:F	16:5
Age (years) *	72.2 (10.9)
Comorbidities	
Cardiovascular	18 (85.7)
Respiratory	6 (28.6)
Hematological/immunological	2 (9.5)
Mild chronic kidney failure	5 (23.8)
Obesity/dyslipidemia	17 (81.0)
Paraplegia	1 (4.8)
History of smoking/smoker	10 (47.6)
Antiplatelet therapy	6 (28.6)
Anticoagulant therapy	9 (42.9)
Antiplatelet + anticoagulant therapy	1 (4.8)
Previous hemorrhoidal surgery	6 (28.6)
Goligher's classification	
Grade II	8 (38.1)
Grade III	10 (47.6)
Grade IV	3 (14.3)
Flavonoids before embolization	17 (81.0)
Iron therapy before embolization	10 (47.6)
Blood transfusion before embolization	11 (52.4)

* Data are shown as mean ± standard deviation. M = male; F = female.

3.2. Operative and Perioperative Data

Superselective embolization of all branches of the superior rectal artery was performed in all patients, obtaining a technical success rate of 100%. Left radial access was successfully performed in 17 cases, and a switch from radial access to femoral access was reported in one case (cross rate 4.8%). Total examination times ranged from 40 to 50 min with low radiation doses and contrast volumes administered between 70 and 80 mL.

Distal embolization of the middle rectal branches was also required in three patients (bilateral in two patients and unilateral in one), using the same coils (Figure 1).

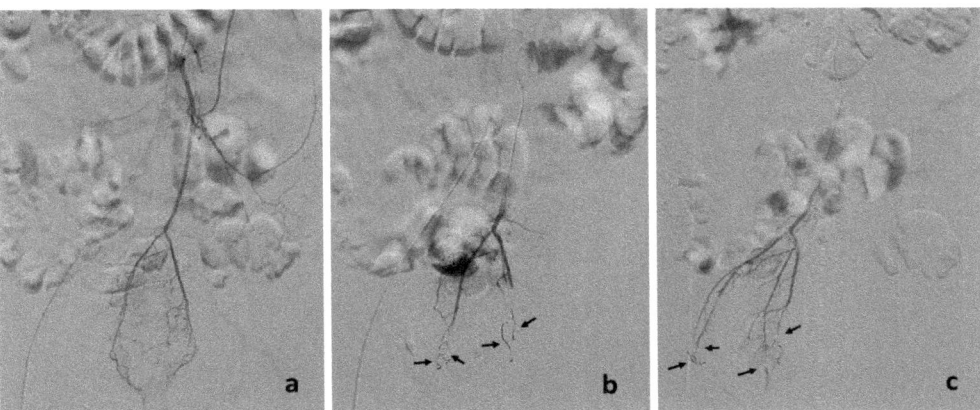

Figure 1. Diagnostic phase with hemorrhoidal arteries evaluation (**a**). Four Interlock and IDC coils (arrows) were positioned in the distal branches of the superior hemorrhoidal arteries ((**b**) = antero-posterior radiographic view; (**c**) = latero-lateral radiographic view).

Haemostasis was performed using a TR band radial compression device (Terumo medical corporation) in 13 patients who underwent transradial access, a 6 Fr Angio-seal vascular closure device (Terumo medical corporation) in four patients and manual compression of the femoral artery in four patients.

Stability of vital signs was registered in all patients, with adequate respiratory function. All patients had an adequate level of orientation and alertness, ability to tolerate a clear liquid diet, and absence of significant pain, with mild pain in one patient only, self-limited without requiring medical therapy.

Bowel movements were registered on the first and second days after the procedure, without severe bleeding.

All patients were discharged without complications, four patients after 48 h (all cases of femoral approach) and 17 patients who underwent transradial Emborrhoid, were managed in an outpatient setting, and discharged within 24 h of the procedure.

No signs of ischemia, radial or femoral pulse absence occurred. Three minor postoperative complications were observed (one ecchymosis, one arm pain, one pseudoaneurysm of radial artery), safely managed with conservative treatment. The overall complication rate was 14.3%.

Transient ischemic attacks, reversible ischemic neurologic deficits, and stroke, defined as a new, persistent neurologic disability lasting >24 h, were never registered.

All patients had reduction of hemorrhoidal congestion, no anal pain occurred after the procedure, tenesmus was referred by one patient.

No variations of anorectal sensitivity and of faecal continence were reported. Anal ulceration, ischemia and anorectal perforation were never diagnosed after the procedure and at the follow-up visits.

3.3. Middle- and Long-Term Follow-Up

Mean follow-up was 18.5 ± 6.0 months. One-year follow-up was assessed in 17 patients (81%).

Patients who daily experienced post-defecation bleeding episodes decreased from 19 to four. At the last follow-up, the mean increase of hemoglobin for a patient was 1.2 ± 1.6 g/dL. Three patients who experienced new onset of anemia during the follow-up were regarded as a treatment failure (overall recurrence rate was 14.3%). Two patients needed transfusions within one month and one patient within six months from the embolization. Consequently, one patient underwent surgical dearterialization, and two patients received sclerotherapy.

A case of death, for other causes (leukemia), was registered after five months from embolization.

At the 12-month follow-up visit, HDSS and SHS decreased from 11.1 ± 4.2 to 4.7 ± 4.6 ($p < 0.0001$) and from 18.8 ± 4.8 to 10.2 ± 4.9 ($p < 0.0001$), respectively, with a significant improvement of hemorrhoidal symptoms, except for itching. All patients referred the decrease of hemorrhoidal symptoms, especially for the bleeding severity ($p < 0.0001$), soiling ($p = 0.002$), frequency of postdefecatory hemorrhoidal prolapse ($p = 0.006$) and anal pain ($p = 0.001$); whereas, no significant difference was reported for the perianal itching ($p = 0.111$). The state of severity and anxiety/worry related to the hemorrhoidal disease referred by patients were greatly reduced ($p < 0.0001$ and $p = 0.002$) and associated with an improvement of general well-being ($p = 0.006$) (Figure 2).

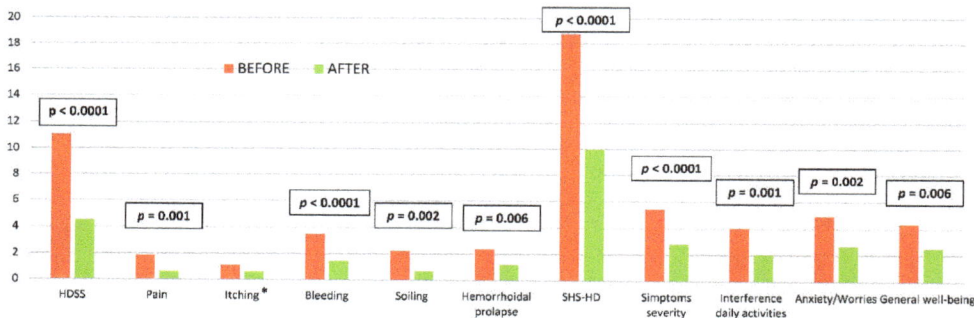

Figure 2. Comparison between HDSS and SHS-HD scores collected before Emborrhoid technique and at last follow-up visit (Wilcoxon test). * $p = 0.111$. HDSS = Hemorrhoidal Disease Symptoms Score; SHS-HD = Short Health Scale for Hemorrhoidal Disease.

Patients who had given up their daily activities due to hemorrhoidal disease have returned to their previous lifestyle. Moreover, the low complication rate and the significant reduction of post-defecation bleeding episodes are related to the improvement of the hemorrhoidal symptoms and patients' quality of life.

4. Discussion

Over the years, the therapeutic range available to treat the patient affected by hemorrhoidal disease has expanded, allowing a more individualized treatment [14]. Emborrhoid is a relatively new nonoperative treatment of hemorrhoidal bleeding, based on the same physiopathological principles of hemorrhoidal dearterialization. It consists in embolization with coils or microparticle of terminal branches of the superior and middle rectal arteries via the endovascular route. This approach was proposed by Vidal as a valid option for the treatment of chronic hemorrhoidal bleeding in patients with contraindications for surgery [8,15].

Although a recent case report described an event of sigmoid ischemia/stenosis after microparticles SRA embolization [16], several papers seem to demonstrate that this endovascular approach is safe and effective. Many authors supported the Emborrhoid technique either in the case of contraindication for surgery or as first line treatment in low grade of hemorrhoidal disease [17–20]. In these studies, the Emborrhoid technique has traditionally been performed on an inpatient basis, generally using the right femoral route, but the heterogeneity in patient selection (also in the same study) and pre- or postoperative assessment makes the results difficult to compare. Two reviews of literature underline the lack of homogeneous and comparable data, in particular, the evidence regarding appropriated indication, middle/long-term results, and cost-effectiveness remains insufficient [9,21].

Our prospective study aims to increase middle/long-term clinical results after embolization in selected patients with hemorrhoidal bleeding and to assess the impact of embolization on hemorrhoidal symptoms and patients' quality of life. Only patients with anemia and high surgical risk due to severe cardiovascular, pulmonary or absolute contraindication to anesthesia were enrolled. The technical success rate was 100%. Seventeen patients were treated via transradial access and four via transfemoral (including a case of a switch from radial to femoral access) without major intra- and perioperative complications. The overall recurrence rate was 14.3%.

Other studies investigating the impact of embolization in frail patients are available in the literature. In details, Moussa et al. reported a success rate of 72% in patients with contraindication for surgery (30 consecutive patients with hemostatic disorders, previous hemorrhoidectomy and affected by inflammatory bowel disease), after a single procedure or two procedures, with a significant improvement of the French bleeding score, of the general symptom score and of the patient's quality-of-life score, without complications (only a notable event of diarrhea self-limited) [22]. Similarly, in a case report of Venturini et al., two patients with heart disease and contraindication to suspension antiplatelet or anticoagulation therapy underwent coil embolization of SRA. No further blood transfusions and no complications were recorded at the one-month follow-up [23]. Two other case studies were published regarding the hemorrhoidal embolization in patients with portal hypertension. Both studies confirmed the safety and efficacy of the endovascular procedure in the short term, without major complications [24,25]. All these papers show encouraging perioperative results but lack long-term follow-up.

In our study, the mean follow-up was 18.5 ± 6 months. One-year follow-up was assessed in 17 patients (81%). Neither anorectal ischemia, ulceration nor perforation was recorded in short-term and one-year follow-ups. Three patients had new-onset anemia and received blood transfusions; of these, one patient underwent DG-HAL and in two cases sclerotherapy was performed. Considering the entire follow-up period, we recorded the relapse within the first six months.

Analyzing the HDSS and SHS scores showed a significant improvement of hemorrhoidal symptoms (expect for itching) and of the patient's quality of life. These positive results were obtained performing a standardized approach, using dedicated devices and based on an adequate screening process. Notably, the majority of our patients were treated in an outpatient setting and discharged within 24 h. No need for pre-procedural groin preparation, less post-procedural discomfort at the access route, and reduced limitations for the patient in performing basic activities are the main drivers for this relatively new approach. Therefore, in our opinion, any refinement in embolotherapy that reduces the impact on a patient's life, such as performing embolization during a single outpatient session, may bring benefits in terms of quality of cure and cost.

The limitations of our study are represented by the single-center study and by the small number of patients.

5. Conclusions

The Emborrhoid technique seems to have a promising role in the clinical practice for the treatment of patients with chronic hemorrhoidal bleeding and high surgical risk. Future multicenter prospective trials performed on larger populations will be necessary to more thoroughly evaluate the clinical efficacy of Emborrhoid techniques and to clarify the indication and clinical management.

Author Contributions: Conceptualization, P.C. and C.R.; data curation, R.I., A.A.M., A.P. (Alessandro Posa), F.L. and V.D.S.; formal analysis, A.A.M. and A.P. (Angelo Parello); investigation, R.I. and A.P. (Angelo Parello); methodology, P.C., R.I., A.A.M., A.P. (Alessandro Posa), F.L., V.D.S. and C.R.; project administration, C.R.; validation, A.P. (Alessandro Posa), A.P. (Angelo Parello), F.L., V.D.S. and C.R.; writing—original draft, R.I.; writing—review & editing, P.C. All authors have read and agreed to the published version of the manuscript.

Funding: This research received no external funding.

Institutional Review Board Statement: This study was approved by the ethical committee of the Fondazione Policlinico Universitario Agostino Gemelli—IRCCS, Rome, Italy; code: 3705.

Informed Consent Statement: The study protocol was approved by our local Ethics Committee and an informed written consent was signed by patients.

Data Availability Statement: The data presented in this study are available on request from the corresponding author.

Acknowledgments: We thank Kelly Baron for English language editing of this manuscript.

Conflicts of Interest: The authors declare no conflict of interest.

References

1. Perera, N.; Liolitsa, D.; Iype, S.; Croxford, A.; Yassin, M.; Lang, P.; Ukaegbu, O.; van Issum, C. Phlebotonics for haemorrhoids. *Cochrane Database Syst. Rev.* **2012**, *8*, CD004322. [CrossRef] [PubMed]
2. Cengiz, T.B.; Gorgun, E. Hemorrhoids: A range of treatments. *Clevel. Clin. J. Med.* **2019**, *86*, 612–620. [CrossRef] [PubMed]
3. Gallo, G.; Martellucci, J.; Sturiale, A.E.; Clerico, G.; Milito, G.; Marino, F.; Cocorullo, G.; Giordano, P.; Mistrangelo, M.; Trompetto, M. Consensus statement of the Italian society of colorectal surgery (SICCR): Management and treatment of hemorrhoidal disease. *Tech. Coloproctol.* **2020**, *24*, 145–164. [CrossRef] [PubMed]
4. Ratto, C.; Donisi, L.; Parello, A.; Litta, F.; Zaccone, G.; De Simone, V. 'Distal Doppler-guided dearterialization' is highly effective in treating haemorrhoids by transanal haemorrhoidal dearterialization. *Colorectal Dis.* **2012**, *14*, e786–e789. [CrossRef] [PubMed]
5. Parello, A.; Litta, F.; De Simone, V.; Campennì, P.; Orefice, R.; Marra, A.A.; Goglia, M.; Santoro, L.; Santoliquido, A.; Ratto, C. Haemorrhoidal haemodynamic changes in patients with haemorrhoids treated using Doppler-guided dearterialization. *BJS Open* **2021**, *5*, zrab012. [CrossRef]
6. Pucher, P.H.; Sodergren, M.H.; Lord, A.C.; Darzi, A.; Ziprin, P. Clinical outcome following Doppler-guided haemorrhoidal artery ligation: A systematic review. *Colorectal Dis.* **2013**, *15*, e284–e294. [CrossRef]
7. Ratto, C.; Campennì, P.; Papeo, F.; Donisi, L.; Litta, F.; Parello, A. Transanal hemorrhoidal dearterialization (THD) for hemorrhoidal disease: A single-center study on 1000 consecutive cases and a review of the literature. *Tech. Coloproctol.* **2017**, *21*, 953–962. [CrossRef]
8. Vidal, V.; Louis, G.; Bartoli, J.; Sielezneff, I. Embolization of the hemorrhoidal arteries (the emborrhoid technique): A new concept and challenge for interventional radiology. *Diagn. Interv. Imaging* **2014**, *95*, 307–315. [CrossRef]
9. Talaie, R.; Torkian, P.; Moghadam, A.D.; Tradi, F.; Vidal, V.; Sapoval, M.; Golzarian, J. Hemorrhoid embolization: A review of current evidences. *Diagn. Interv. Imaging.* **2022**, *103*, 3–11. [CrossRef]
10. Cuschieri, S. The STROBE guidelines. *Saudi J. Anaesth.* **2019**, *13*, S31–S34. [CrossRef]
11. Iezzi, R.; Campenni, P.; Posa, A.; Parello, A.; Rodolfino, E.; Marra, A.A.; Ratto, C.; Manfredi, R. Outpatient Transradial Emborrhoid Technique: A Pilot Study. *Cardiovasc. Interv. Radiol.* **2021**, *44*, 1300–1306. [CrossRef] [PubMed]
12. US Department of Health and Human Services; National Institutes of Health; National Cancer Institute. Common Terminology Criteria for Adverse Events (CTCAE) Version 5. 2017. Available online: https://ctep.cancer.gov/protocoldevelopment/electronic_applications/docs/CTCAE_v5_Quick_Reference_8.5x11.pdf (accessed on 16 March 2022).
13. Rørvik, H.D.; Styr, K.; Ilum, L.; McKinstry, G.L.; Dragesund, T.; Campos, A.H.; Brandstrup, B.; Olaison, G. Hemorrhoidal Disease Symptom Score and Short Health ScaleHD: New Tools to Evaluate Symptoms and Health-Related Quality of Life in Hemorrhoidal Disease. *Dis. Colon Rectum* **2019**, *62*, 333–342. [CrossRef] [PubMed]
14. Simillis, C.; Thoukididou, S.N.; Slesser, A.A.P.; Rasheed, S.; Tan, E.; Tekkis, P.P. Systematic review and network meta-analysis comparing clinical outcomes and effectiveness of surgical treatments for haemorrhoids. *J. Br. Surg.* **2015**, *102*, 1603–1618. [CrossRef] [PubMed]
15. Vidal, V.; Sapoval, M.; Sielezneff, Y.; De Parades, V.; Tradi, F.; Louis, G.; Bartoli, J.M.; Pellerin, O. Emborrhoid: A new concept for the treatment of hemorrhoids with arterial embolization: The first 14 cases. *Cardiovasc. Interv. Radiol.* **2015**, *38*, 72–78. [CrossRef] [PubMed]

16. Eberspacher, C.; Ficuccilli, F.; Tessieri, L.; D'Andrea, V.; Lauro, A.; Fralleone, L.; Mascagni, D. Annoyed with Haemorrhoids? Risks of the Emborrhoid Technique. *Am. J. Dig. Dis.* **2021**, *66*, 3725–3729. [CrossRef]
17. Zakharchenko, A.; Kaitoukov, Y.; Vinnik, Y.; Tradi, F.; Sapoval, M.; Sielezneff, I.; Galkin, E.; Vidal, V. Safety and efficacy of superior rectal artery embolization with particles and metallic coils for the treatment of hemorrhoids (Emborrhoid technique). *Diagn. Interv. Imaging* **2016**, *97*, 1079–1084. [CrossRef]
18. Sun, X.; Xu, J.; Zhang, J.; Jin, Y.; Chen, Q. Management of rectal bleeding due to internal haemorrhoids with arterial embolisation: A single-centre experience and protocol. *Clin. Radiol.* **2018**, *73*, 985.e1–985.e6. [CrossRef]
19. Moggia, E.; Talamo, G.; Gallo, G.; Bianco, A.; Barattini, M.; Salsano, G. Do We Have Another Option to Treat Bleeding Hemorrhoids? The Emborrhoid Technique: Experience in 16 Patients. *Rev. Recent Clin. Trials.* **2021**, *16*, 81–86.
20. Han, X.; Xia, F.; Chen, G.; Sheng, Y.; Wang, W.; Wang, Z.; Zhao, M.; Wang, X. Superior rectal artery embolization for bleeding internal hemorrhoids. *Tech. Coloproctol.* **2020**, *25*, 75–80. [CrossRef]
21. Tradi, F.; Mege, D.; Louis, G.; Bartoli, J.M.; Sielezneff, I.; Vidal, V. Emborrhoïd: Traitement des hémorroïdes par embolisation des artères rectales [Emborrhoid: Rectal arteries embolization for hemorrhoid treatment]. *Presse Med.* **2019**, *48*, 454–459. [CrossRef]
22. Moussa, N.; Sielezneff, I.; Sapoval, M.; Tradi, F.; Del Giudice, C.; Fathallah, N.; Pellerin, O.; Amouyal, G.; Pereira, H.; De Parades, V.; et al. Embolization of the superior rectal arteries for chronic bleeding due to haemorrhoidal disease. *Colorectal Dis.* **2017**, *19*, 194–199. [CrossRef] [PubMed]
23. Venturini, M.; De Nardi, P.; Marra, P.; Panzeri, M.; Brembilla, G.; Morelli, F. Embolization of superior rectal arteries for transfusion dependent haemorrhoidal bleeding in severely cardiopathic patients: A new field of application of the "emborrhoid" technique. *Tech. Coloproctol.* **2018**, *22*, 453–455. [CrossRef] [PubMed]
24. Giurazza, F.; Corvino, F.; Cavaglià, E.; Silvestre, M.; Cangiano, G.; Amodio, F. Emborrhoid in patients with portal hypertension and chronic hemorrhoidal bleeding: Preliminary results in five cases with a new coiling release fashion "Spaghetti technique". *Radiol. Med.* **2020**, *125*, 1008–1011. [CrossRef] [PubMed]
25. Alves e Sousa, F.; Lopes, P.M.; Mónica, I.B.; Carvalho, A.C.; Sousa, P. Emborrhoid technique performed on a patient with portal hypertension and chronic hemorrhoidal bleeding as a salvage therapy. *CVIR Endovasc.* **2022**, *5*, 1–4. [CrossRef]

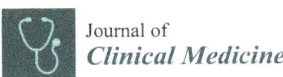 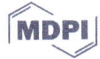

Article

Surgery for Ulcerative Colitis in the White British and South Asian Populations in Selected Trusts in England 2001–2020: An Absence of Disparate Care and a Need for Specialist Centres

Affifa Farrukh * and John Francis Mayberry

Nuffield Hospital, Leicester LE5 1HY, UK
* Correspondence: farrukh_affi@yahoo.com

Abstract: Over the last decade, there has been extensive evidence that patients with inflammatory bowel disease from minority communities in the UK receive less than optimal care. In none of the studies has the role of surgery in the management of acute and severe ulcerative colitis been considered in any detail. A freedom of information (FOI) request was sent to 14 NHS Trusts in England, which serve significant South Asian populations. Details of the type of surgery patients from the South Asian and White British communities received between 2001 and 2020 were requested. Detailed responses were obtained from eight Trusts. Four hundred and ten White British patients underwent surgery for ulcerative colitis over this period at these eight Trusts, together with 67 South Asian patients. There was no statistically significant difference in the distribution across the types of surgery undergone by the two communities overall ($\chi^2 = 1.3$, ns) and the proportions who underwent an ileo-anal anastomosis with pouch ($z = -1.2$, ns). However, within individual trusts, at the University Hospital Southampton NHS Foundation Trust, a significantly greater proportion of South Asian patients had an ileo-anal anastomosis with pouch compared to White British patients. At Cambridge University Hospitals NHS Foundation Trust, all 72 patients who underwent surgery for ulcerative colitis were White British. This study has shown that, in general, for patients with a severe flare of ulcerative colitis where medical treatment has failed and surgery is warranted, the nature of the procedures offered is the same in the White British and South Asian communities. However, of concern is the number of units with low volume procedures. For most Trusts reported in this study, the overall number of Ileo-anal pouch anastomosis or anastomosis of ileum to anus procedures performed over a number of years was substantially below that required for a single surgeon to achieve competence. These findings reinforce the argument that inflammatory bowel disease surgery should be performed in a limited number of high-volume centres rather than across a wide range of hospitals so as to ensure procedures are carried out by surgeons with sufficient and on-going experience.

Keywords: ulcerative colitis; surgery; ileostomy; ileo-anal anastomosis; ethnicity

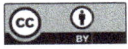

1. Introduction

Over the last decade, there has been extensive evidence that patients with inflammatory bowel disease from minority communities in the UK receive less than optimal care [1–5]. This has taken the form of less frequent consultations with senior clinicians, fewer investigations, more frequent discharge from follow-up clinics [3] and more limited access to expensive biologic therapies [1,2,4]. Such disparate care is not seen in all Trusts but is widespread and has been shown to effect patients who are from South Asian, Afro-Caribbean and Eastern European communities. In none of these studies has the role of surgery in the management of acute and severe ulcerative colitis been considered.

2. Method

A freedom of information (FOI) request was sent to the following 15 NHS Trusts in England which serve significant South Asian populations:

1. Barking, Havering and Redbridge University Hospitals NHS Trust
2. Barts Health NHS Trust
3. Bradford Teaching Hospitals NHS Foundation Trust
4. Cambridge University Hospitals NHS Foundation Trust
5. East Lancashire Hospitals NHS Trust
6. North West Anglia Foundation Trust
7. Northern Care Alliance NHS Foundation Trust
8. Sandwell and West Birmingham NHS Trust
9. The Hillingdon Hospitals NHS Foundation Trust
10. The Royal Wolverhampton NHS Trust
11. University Hospitals Coventry and Warwickshire NHS Trust
12. University Hospitals of Derby and Burton NHS Foundation Trust
13. University Hospitals of Leicester NHS Trust
14. University Hospital Southampton NHS Foundation Trust
15. Walsall Healthcare NHS Trust

The FOI request asked each hospital to provide information on the following types of surgery in the Trust between 1 January 2001 and 31 December 2020

1. Ileo-anal pouch anastomosis or anastomosis of ileum to anus (H042 and H043) (IPAA)
2. Total colectomy and anastomosis of ileum to rectum (H051)
3. Panproctocolectomy and ileostomy (HO41)

H041, H042, H043 and H051 are disease and procedure codes from ICD-10, which is the 10th revision of the International Statistical Classification of Diseases and Related Health Problems [6]. Data were not collected on the total number of patients with ulcerative colitis treated at each trust. Such data would have included outpatients who received medical treatment alone and these are not routinely collected by Trusts. Rather the purpose of the study was to consider whether patients from different ethnic groups who underwent surgery received similar operations or not. In addition, data on 30-day mortality rates, re-operation rates, leak and other complication rates were not requested. Such searches require more lengthy collection periods and often require access to data collected on local registers held by hospitals, surgical departments or individual surgeons. Within the Freedom of Information Act, such requests can be declined on the basis of cost and issues with lack of anonymity.

Trusts were asked to provide data for each quinquennium between 2001 and 2020 for two ethnic groups:

1. White British (National code A)
2. Asian (Pakistani, Indian, Bangladeshi origin) (National codes H, J and K)

A, H, J and K are ethnicity codes used by the NHS and defined in *The NHS Data Model and Dictionary* [7].

Data for each trust were summated for all the periods for which information was provided. A χ^2 test was performed to compare the forms of treatment received by the two groups of patients using the Social Science Statistics calculator [8]. In addition, a z test was used to compare the rates for ileo-anal anastomosis in the two populations for individual trusts and overall.

3. Results

Detailed responses were obtained from eight Trusts. However, three of these Trusts were only able to provide data for part of the period 2001–2020 (See Table 1). Seven of the Trusts, Barking, Havering and Redbridge (FOI 7981), Barts NHS Trust (FOI-0225-22), Coventry and Warwick (FOI 1732), Northern Care Alliance (FOI 11854), Wolverhampton

(FOI 100422) Hillingdon Hospitals (FOI 6782) and North West Anglia (FOI/2022/400), were unable to provide detailed breakdowns of their practice due to small numbers and concerns about patient anonymity.

Table 1. Types of Surgery for Ulcerative Colitis in the White British and South Asian Populations in Scheme 2001–2020.

Trust	Period	Ileoanal Anastomosis	Ileorectal Anastomosis	Ileostomy	Number	Significance
Southampton	2001–2020					
White		48	0	36	84	
Asian		7	0	0	7	$z = -2.23, p < 0.03$
Leicester	2001–2020					
White		59	6	86	151	
Asian		13	0	23	36	ns
Sandwell & West Birmingham	2001–2020					
White		3	0	8	11	
Asian		0	0	1	1	ns
Walsall	2014–2015					
White		1	0	1	2	
Asian		0	0	0	0	ns
Derby & Burton	2001–2020					
White		4	1	17	22	
Asian		1	0	1	2	ns
East Lancashire Hospitals	2006–2020					
White		7	0	16	23	
Asian		0	0	0	0	Ns
Bradford	2007–2020					
White		26	1	18	45	
Asian		13	0	8	21	Ns
Cambridge	2001–2020					
White		28	2	42	72	
Asian		0	0	0	0	
Total						
White		176	10	224	410	
Asian		34	0	33	67	ns

Four hundred and ten White British patients underwent surgery for ulcerative colitis over this period at the 8 Trusts, who provided a detailed response, together with 67 South Asian patients (Table 1). There was no statistically significant difference in the distribution across the types of surgery undergone by the two communities overall ($\chi^2 = 1.3$, ns) and the proportions who underwent an ileo-anal anastomosis with pouch ($z = -1.2$, ns). Although the value of statistical analysis within individual Trusts was limited by small numbers an analysis was performed to identify any Trusts which appeared to lie outside of the overall practice. Within individual trusts, at the University Hospital Southampton NHS Foundation Trust, a significantly greater proportion of South Asian patients had an ileo-anal anastomosis with pouch compared to White British patients (See Table 1). Indeed, all seven South Asian patients had a pouch procedure.

In order to assess the validity of the data obtained by Freedom of Information requests, the response from University Hospitals of Leicester NHS Trust was further scrutinised. The incidence of ulcerative colitis in the South Asian community is higher than in the White British community, and the disease is more aggressive in second generation migrants [9,10]. The population served by the Trust covers Leicester, Leicestershire and Rutland, with the South Asian community forming 17% of the population compared to 83% White British, excluding other communities [11]. If the disease is of comparable frequency and severity, then the expected number of patients in a group of 187, 32 would be South Asian. The group actually included 36 South Asian patients ($z = -0$–54, ns). Based on the data available from a study of surgical records of patients with ulcerative colitis in Leicester covering the period 1997 to 2007 [12], the expected number of South Asian patients would have been 37 ($z = -0.13$, ns). These latter data reflect differences in disease severity and yield an even closer match.

However, the results do raise various areas of concern. At Cambridge University Hospitals NHS Foundation Trust, all 72 patients who underwent surgery for ulcerative colitis were White British and none were South Asian. The very low overall number of patients reported by Barking, Havering and Redbridge, Coventry and Warwick, Northern Care Alliance, Wolverhampton, Hillingdon Hospitals and North West Anglia raises questions as to whether such surgery should occur at these centres or patients should be referred to a more experienced centre.

4. Discussion

This study has shown that, in general, for patients with a severe flare of ulcerative colitis where medical treatment has failed and surgery is warranted, the nature of the procedures offered is the same in the White British and South Asian communities. The choice includes a traditional ileostomy and proctectomy, with an associated significant impact on body image and the need to use stoma appliances. Both have been shown to have a significant impact for South Asian patients [13]. However, the surgery is relatively straightforward. Colectomy with an ileo-rectal anastomosis is, perhaps, the simplest procedure with a good continence outcome, but the patient remains at risk of colorectal cancer. It is for this reason that the procedure has never gained popularity in the UK, and in this study, only 10 of 477 patients underwent this procedure. An ileo-anal anastomosis is associated with an acceptable body image, but patients have a high frequency of defaecation and may develop pouchitis. It is a more complex procedure and ideally should be performed in centres with a large case load. The check on the data from an FOI in Leicester would indicate that the findings are robust with slightly more patients undergoing surgery, consistent with the greater frequency of the disease and its being more severe in South Asians. FOI data have previously been shown to be robust when considering data collected about the management of inflammatory bowel disease [2], and this study is consistent with such findings.

A recent study of Hospital Episode statistics has shown that Asian patients with ulcerative colitis are likely to experience a delay in colectomy surgery when admitted as an emergency [14]. In 1992, a study of Asian ostomists reported that only half of them had been able to discuss their management with a doctor or nurse who spoke the same language, whereas stoma care nurses thought that the service at that time was adequate [14]. In a later study of 107 patients with ulcerative colitis or familial adenomatous polyposis from Leicester, in 2009, complication rates and long-term outcome were comparable for White British and South Asian patients following a restorative proctocolectomy, with the exception of pouchitis, which was commoner in the latter group [12]. However, a separate study showed that language issues were clearly linked to a poorer quality of life and consistent with the views expressed by the ostomists [15]. Clearly, the fact that South Asian and White British patients experience the same types of surgery does not remove the need to explain their nature and consequences, such that these issues are understood by patients.

Of concern in this study is the number of units with low volume procedures. A study from the Cleveland Clinic, USA has shown that trainee staff undertaking stapled IPAA surgery only showed an improvement in the pouch failure rate following an initial training period of 23 cases versus 40 cases for senior staff [16]. The learning curve for hand-sewn IPAA surgery was quantified only for senior staff, who attained adequate results following an initial period of 31 procedures. This formed the basis for the recommendation in the 2019 British Society of Gastroenterology Guidelines that:

> "**Statement 22.** We suggest that pouch surgery should be performed in specialist high-volume referral centres (GRADE: weak recommendation, low-quality evidence. Agreement 97.4%) [17]."

In most Trusts reported in this study, the overall number of IPAA procedures performed over a number of years was substantially below that required for a single surgeon to achieve competence. These findings reinforce the argument that inflammatory bowel disease surgery should be performed in a limited number of high-volume centres rather than across a wide range of hospitals in order to ensure that procedures are carried out by surgeons with sufficient and on-going experience.

Reports from two trusts are worthy of comment. In Southampton, all 7 patients underwent an IPAA procedure, and in Cambridge, no South Asian patients underwent surgery for acute colitis compared to 72 White British patients over a 20-year period. FOI searches do not allow an explanation for these outliers, but such findings should prompt consideration by the relevant Trusts as to their approach to minority community patients.

In conclusion, although severely ill patients with ulcerative colitis receive the same range of surgical options regardless of whether they are of South Asian or White British origin there are trusts whose practice is outlying and the reasons are not known. In addition, this study has demonstrated the limited experience of such procedures in some trusts, all trusts were selected because they served significant South Asian communities and such a finding may not be more general. However, there is serious need to consider concentrating surgical expertise in high-volume centres.

Author Contributions: Conceptualization, A.F. and J.F.M.; formal analysis, A.F. and J.F.M.; investigation, J.F.M.; validation, A.F.; writing—original draft, A.F. and J.F.M. All authors have read and agreed to the published version of the manuscript.

Funding: This research received no external funding.

Institutional Review Board Statement: This study was conducted with publicly available data and did not require ethical approval or institutional review.

Informed Consent Statement: This study used anonymised publicly available data.

Data Availability Statement: These links are listed in the FOI Request References.

Conflicts of Interest: The authors declare no conflict of interest.

Ethical Approval

Ethical approval is not required for studies based on Freedom of Information requests. The data are publicly available and once requested responses to the original data can be accessed by any member of the public, who quotes the reference number. The nature of information that can be released is defined by the Freedom of Information Act (2000) and is anonymised. Where the number of patients is less than 5, many Trusts will not release specific figures but simply quote them as less than 5 (<5) so as to further protect anonymity.

FOI Request References

- Cambridge University Hospitals NHS Foundation Trust, 8053
- University Hospitals of Leicester NHS Trust, 45337
- Sandwell and West Birmingham NHS Trust, 22/022
- Walsall Healthcare NHS Trust, 637.21

- University Hospitals of Derby and Burton NHS Foundation Trust, 22.238
- East Lancashire Hospitals NHS Trust, 2022.017
- Bradford Teaching Hospitals NHS Foundation Trust, 22016
- Cambridge University Hospitals NHS Foundation Trust, 246.22

References

1. Farrukh, A.; Mayberry, J. Apparent discrimination in the provision of biologic therapy to patients with Crohn's Disease according to ethnicity. *Public Health* **2015**, *129*, 460–464. [CrossRef] [PubMed]
2. Farrukh, A.; Mayberry, J. Ethnic variations in the provision of biologic therapy for Crohn's Disease: A Freedom of Information Study. *Med. Leg. J.* **2015**, *83*, 104–108. [CrossRef] [PubMed]
3. Farrukh, A.; Mayberry, J.F. Patients with ulcerative colitis from diverse populations: The Leicester Experience. *Med. Leg. J.* **2016**, *84*, 31–35. [CrossRef] [PubMed]
4. Farrukh, A.; Mayberry, J.F. Apparent disparities in hospital admission and biologic use in the management of inflammatory bowel disease between 2014–2018 in some Black and Ethnic Minority (BEM) populations in England. *Gastrointest. Disord.* **2020**, *2*, 141–151. [CrossRef]
5. Farrukh, A.; Mayberry, J.F. Evidence of On-Going Disparate Levels of Care for South Asian Patients with Inflammatory Bowel Disease in the United Kingdom during the Quinquennium 2015–2019. *Gastrointest. Disord.* **2022**, *4*, 8–14. [CrossRef]
6. ICD-10 Version: 2010 International Statistical Classification of Diseases and Related Health Problems 10th Revision. Available online: https://icd.who.int/browse10/2010/en#/ (accessed on 5 June 2022).
7. The NHS Data Model and Dictionary. Available online: https://www.datadictionary.nhs.uk/data_elements/ethnic_category.html (accessed on 5 June 2022).
8. Social Science Statistics. Available online: https://www.socscistatistics.com/tests/ (accessed on 5 June 2022).
9. Probert, C.S.; Jayanthi, V.; Pinder, D.; Wicks, A.C.; Mayberry, J.F. Epidemiological study of ulcerative proctocolitis in Indian migrants and the indigenous population of Leicestershire. *Gut* **1992**, *33*, 687–693. [CrossRef]
10. Carr, I.; Mayberry, J.F. The effects of migration on ulcerative colitis: A three year prospective study among Europeans and first- and second-generation South Asians in Leicester (1991–1994). *Am. J. Gastroenterol.* **1999**, *94*, 2918–2922. [CrossRef]
11. Leicestershire Partnership NHS Trust. Demographic Profile of Leicester, Leicestershire and Rutland. Available online: https://www.leicspart.nhs.uk/wp-content/uploads/2019/11/2017-MYEs-and-2011-Census-demographic-profiles-LLR-LAs-UAs-DCs-v7.pdf (accessed on 7 June 2022).
12. Norwood, M.G.A.; Mann, C.D.; West, K.; Miller, A.S.; Hemingway, D. Restorative proctocolectomy. Does ethnicity affect outcome? *Colorectal Dis.* **2009**, *11*, 972–975. [CrossRef]
13. Bhakta, P.; Probert, C.S.J.; Jayanthi, V.; Mayberry, J.F. Stoma anxieties: A comparison of the attitudes of Asian migrants and the indigenous population in the United Kingdom towards abdominal surgery and the role of intestinal stomas. *Int. J. Colorectal Dis.* **1992**, *7*, 1–3. [CrossRef]
14. King, D.; Rees, J.; Mytton, J.; Harvey, P.; Thomas, T.; Cooney, R.; Patel, P.; Trudgill, N. The outcomes of emergency admissions with ulcerative colitis between 2007 and 2017 in England. *J. Crohn's Colitis* **2020**, *14*, 764–772. [CrossRef] [PubMed]
15. Soulsby, R.E.; Masterman, J.; Kelly, M.J.; Thomas, W.M. Stomas: Ethnicity and quality of life. *Colorectal Dis.* **2011**, *13*, 600–602. [CrossRef]
16. Tekkis, P.P.; Fazio, V.W.; Lavery, I.C.; Remzi, F.H.; Senagore, A.J.; Wu, J.S.; Strong, S.A.; Poloneicki, D.D.; Hull, T.L.; Church, J.M. Evaluation of the learning curve in ileal pouch-anal anastomosis surgery. *Ann. Surg.* **2005**, *241*, 262–268. [CrossRef] [PubMed]
17. Lamb, C.A.; Kennedy, N.A.; Raine, T.; Hendy, P.A.; Smith, P.J.; Limdi, J.K.; Hayee, B.H.; Lomer, M.C.E.; Parkes, C.C.; Selinger, C.; et al. British Society of Gastroenterology consensus guidelines on the management of inflammatory bowel disease in adults. *Gut* **2019**, *68*, s1–s106. [CrossRef] [PubMed]

MDPI
St. Alban-Anlage 66
4052 Basel
Switzerland
www.mdpi.com

Journal of Clinical Medicine Editorial Office
E-mail: jcm@mdpi.com
www.mdpi.com/journal/jcm

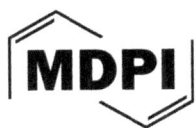

Disclaimer/Publisher's Note: The statements, opinions and data contained in all publications are solely those of the individual author(s) and contributor(s) and not of MDPI and/or the editor(s). MDPI and/or the editor(s) disclaim responsibility for any injury to people or property resulting from any ideas, methods, instructions or products referred to in the content.

www.ingramcontent.com/pod-product-compliance
Lightning Source LLC
LaVergne TN
LVHW070650100526
838202LV00013B/929